The Doctor in Literature

Volume 2
private life

Solomon Posen

Foreword by
Brian Hurwitz

D1372398

Radcliffe Publishing
Oxford • Seattle

Radcliffe Publishing Ltd
18 Marcham Road
Abingdon
Oxon OX14 1AA
United Kingdom

www.radcliffe-oxford.com
Electronic catalogue and worldwide online ordering facility.

British Library Cataloguing in Publication Data

A catalogue record for this book is available from the British Library.

ISBN-10   1 85775 779 3
ISBN-13   978 1 85775 779 8

Typeset by Anne Joshua & Associates, Oxford, UK
Printed and bound by TJ International Ltd, Padstow, Cornwall, UK

Contents

Foreword

'There was humanity there in the rough . . . and Philip felt a curious thrill when it occurred to him that he was in the position of the artist and the patients were like clay in his hands. . . . You saw in that room nature taken by surprise.'

W Somerset Maugham, *Of Human Bondage.*

In western societies, engagement with literature promotes the development and cultural orientation of children. For adults, reading novels, dramas and biographies can simultaneously be entertaining, escapist and intellectually and emotionally challenging. Reading brings individuals face-to-face with characters quite outside their present day experience – in literature, we become caught up in situations that transport us to times and places very different (even alien) from our own. Literature engenders new perspectives on life and work and inevitably provokes new thoughts, argument and emotions. Engaging with literature also helps develop narrative competences, the human abilities to 'acknowledge, absorb, interpret, and act on the stories and plights of others'[1] which healthcare practitioners should cherish.

Literary accounts of ill health and doctoring paint pictures that go far beyond the mere contours of disease descriptions found in medical textbooks. In *The Doctor in Literature* readers are introduced to accounts that allow them to enter into the lived experiences of the sick and the anxieties and perplexities of those who attempt to respond to them. The second of Solomon Posen's four volume *opus* deals with the lives, attitudes, work, family relationships and religious beliefs of physicians, as depicted in literature from the Egyptian era to the present day. Posen, a retired Professor of Endocrinology from Sydney who studied literature as a first degree, has created in this volume an anthology that threads quotations telling of the triumphs and failures of doctoring with those that weave a different story, concerning the more humdrum pattern of daily practice, of medical addiction, poor care, burnout, hypocrisy and 'patient pilfering'. The works he refers to illuminates the aberrant and anomalous, but in their barometric tracings of daily life they also tend to idealise the ordinary: 'The world with which literature deals', Aldous Huxley once wrote, ' is the world into which human beings are born and live and finally die; the world in which they love and hate, in which they experience triumph and humiliation, hope and despair; the world of sufferings and enjoyments, of madness and common sense, of silliness, cunning and wisdom; the world of social pressures and individual impulses, of reason against passion, of instincts and conventions of shared language and unshareable feeling and sensation; of innate difference and the rules, the roles, the solemn or absurd rituals imposed by the prevailing culture'.[2]

In offering some 1500 carefully chosen quotations from a wide range of major and minor literary works concerning doctoring, *The Doctor in Literature* reflects many of Huxley's themes. The result is a rich array of extracts – which are all well contextualised – on which the author builds interpretations. The volume contains excellent indices by title and subject, and can easily be read by anyone not familiar with the original texts, who may wish to learn how medical practice has been represented within the covers of a raft of literary works. In this second volume, Posen challenges us to repair to the original works to read and re-read them in their entirety (they are bibliographically well referenced here). Such renewed engagement will help us to step outside our 'presentist' intellectual and emotional frameworks, to appreciate these texts on their own terms. Do Posen's conclusions stand or are the quotations cited 'clay in his hands'? Read on and find out!

Brian Hurwitz MD FRCP FRCGP
Professor of Medicine and the Arts
King's College London
May 2006

References

1 Charon R (2001) Narrative medicine. *JAMA.* **286**: 1897–1902.
2 Huxley A (1963) *Literature and Science.* Chatto & Windus, London.

About the author

Solomon Posen majored in English before obtaining his medical degrees (MB BS, MD) at the University of Adelaide, Australia. He is a Fellow of the Royal Australasian College of Physicians, a Fellow of the Royal College of Physicians, London, and a past president of the Endocrine Society of Australia.

Professor Posen taught general medicine and endocrinology at Sydney University for almost 30 years. He served on the Editorial Boards of several medical journals, he is the author of some 130 scientific papers (mainly in the field of calcium metabolism) and he co-authored a book on alkaline phosphatase. He has published a number of papers on the subject of the doctor in literature, some of which form the basis of this series. The first volume ('Satisfaction or Resentment') was published by Radcliffe in 2005. A third volume, titled 'Career Choices', is planned for 2007.

Professor Posen is married with three adult children and seven grandchildren. He lives in Sydney, Australia.

Acknowledgements

My sincere thanks are due to Dr Carolyn Brimley Norris, who generously made available a full copy of her unpublished PhD dissertation (*The Image of the Physician in Modern American Literature*, University of Maryland, 1969) and who introduced me to the concept of 'earthy' physicians. In addition, Dr Norris corrected multiple stylistic and punctuation errors, made many valuable suggestions concerning the organization of the material and gave me constant encouragement. Professor John Last of Ottawa, Canada, offered many constructive comments and provided several important references.

Numerous authors, including Susan Cheever, Patricia Cornwell, Alan Lightman, the late Derek Lindsay (AE Ellis), Tony Miksanek, Neil Ravin, Larry Schneiderman and Richard Selzer, provided copies of their books, background information, encouragement and photographs (*see* pp. xiv–xv) in various combinations. I am grateful to all of them.

The staff of the Douglas Piper Library, Royal North Shore Hospital, Sydney, particularly Agnes Wroblewski, were most helpful in obtaining books from libraries all over Australia. Paula Moran of Radcliffe Publishing was a meticulous editor for both this and the previous volume, and the pleasing appearance of the first two volumes of *The Doctor in Literature* series is largely due to her efforts. The staff in the Permissions Departments of Random House (Carol Christiansen and Caryn Burtt in New York, and Catherine Trippett in the UK) gave considerable help in locating copyright holders, particularly in cases where the authors were dead and the publishers defunct.

Most importantly, I thank my wife, Jean Katie Posen, for her love, her patience and her forbearance.

Reprint permissions for copyrighted material

renewed 1967 by Esme Valerie Eliot. Reprinted by permission of Faber and Faber Ltd., London, and Harcourt Inc.

Arthur Hailey, *The Final Diagnosis*. Copyright © 1959 Arthur Hailey. Reprinted by permission of Doubleday, a division of Random House Inc., and Souvenir Press Ltd.

Arthur Hailey, *Strong Medicine*. Copyright © 1984 Arthur Hailey. Reprinted by permission of Doubleday, a division of Random House Inc., and Souvenir Press Ltd.

Jeffrey* Hudson, *A Case Of Need*. Copyright © 1968 Jeffrey Hudson. Reprinted by permission of Dutton Signet, a division of Penguin Group, USA, Inc., and Random House, UK.

Roger Martin du Gard, *Les Thibault*. Copyright © 1936–1940 Editions Gallimard, Paris. Reprinted by permission of Editions Gallimard. Translation Copyright © Stuart Gilbert. Reprinted by permission of the Harry Ransom Humanities Research Center, University of Texas, Austin.

Roger Martin du Gard, *Summer 1914*. Copyright © 1936–1940 Editions Gallimard, Paris. Reprinted by permission of Editions Gallimard. Translation Copyright © Stuart Gilbert. Reprinted by permission of the Harry Ransom Humanities Research Center, University of Texas, Austin.

W Somerset Maugham, *Of Human Bondage*. Copyright © 1915 Estate of W Somerset Maugham. Reprinted by permission of the Estate of W Somerset Maugham, AP Watt Ltd on behalf of the Royal Literary Fund and Random House Group Ltd.

W Somerset Maugham, *Rain*. Copyright © 1920 Estate of W Somerset Maugham. Reprinted by permission of the Estate of W Somerset Maugham, AP Watt Ltd on behalf of the Royal Literary Fund and Random House Group Ltd.

W Somerset Maugham, *The Razor's Edge*. Copyright © 1944 Estate of W Somerset Maugham. Reprinted by permission of the Estate of W Somerset Maugham, AP Watt Ltd on behalf of the Royal Literary Fund and Random House Group Ltd.

Francois Mauriac, *The Desert of Love*. Copyright © 1925 François Mauriac, Éditions Bernard Grasset. Reprinted by permission of Jean Mauriac and Éditions Bernard Grasset, Paris.

Francois Mauriac, *Therese*. Copyright © 1927 François Mauriac, Éditions Bernard Grasset. Reprinted by permission of Jean Mauriac and Éditions Bernard Grasset, Paris.

Alan Edward Nourse, *The Practice*. Copyright © 1978 Alan Edward Nourse. Reprinted by permission of Harper Collins Publishers and Brandt and Hochman, Literary Agents, Inc., agents for the Estate of Alan Edward Nourse.

Solomon Posen (1992) The portrayal of the physician in non-medical literature. 3. The physician and his family. *Journal of the Royal Society of Medicine*. 85: 314–17. Reprinted by permission of the Royal Society of Medicine, London.

Solomon Posen (1992) The portrayal of the physician in non-medical literature. 5. The physician and religion. *Journal of the Royal Society of Medicine*. 85: 659–92. Reprinted by permission of the Royal Society of Medicine, London.

Solomon Posen (1993) The portrayal of the physician in non-medical literature. 6. The physician who dislikes his trade. *Journal of the Royal Society of Medicine*. 86: 67–8. Reprinted by permission of the Royal Society of Medicine, London.

Solomon Posen (1993) The portrayal of the physician in non-medical literature. 8.

---

* Crichton's pseudonym is spelt 'Jeffrey Hudson' or 'Jeffery Hudson.' Both spellings are listed in the catalogue of the Library of Congress.

Photographs of four contemporary authors quoted in the first two volumes of *The Doctor in Literature*

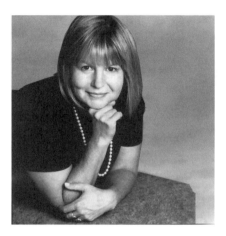

Susan Cheever, author of *Doctors and Women*, which illustrates the contrast between over- and under-involved physicians. Cheever also describes the reaction of doctors towards colleagues who develop an incurable illness. Ms Cheever, a professional writer, lives in New York City.
Photograph by Sigrid Estrada. Reproduced by courtesy of Simon and Schuster.

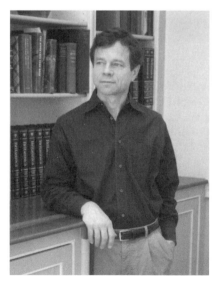

Alan Lightman, whose book *The Diagnosis* provides a graphic account of the frustrations of a patient whose illness remains undiagnosed to the end. Dr Lightman teaches humanities at the Massachusetts Institue of Technology, Cambridge.
Photograph by Jean Lightman.

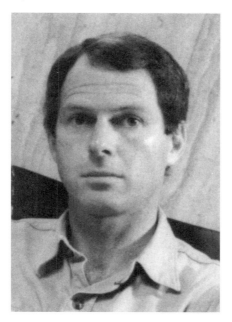

Neil Ravin, whose works (*MD, Seven North, Mere Mortals*) present the most detailed fictional descriptions of teaching hospitals at the end of the twentieth century. Dr Ravin is an endocrinologist practising in the Bethesda area.
Photograph by Claudia Reid Ravin.

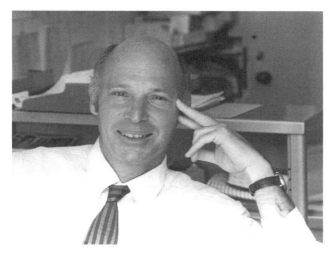

Lawrence Jerome Schneiderman, author of *Sea Nymphs by the Hour*, which satirizes various aspects of a twentieth-century Veterans' Hospital including the pretentious 'Teaching Round'. Dr Schneiderman is Professor of Family and Preventive Medicine at the University of California, San Diego.
Photograph by HD Teetzel.

Introduction

This book, the second volume in the series *The Doctor in Literature*, is intended, like the first,[1] to serve three purposes. First, it is an indexed anthology, bringing together a total of some 1500 extracts from approximately 600 works of fiction, describing medical doctors as major or minor characters. Second, it identifies and analyzes a number of themes that recur in the portrayal of physicians, some of them transcending time, place and cultural backgrounds. Third, it is hoped that medical and lay persons opening the book on any page will find some material of interest.

Because of the number of works involved, the citations have had to be kept brief. For readers in search of lengthy passages from well-known works of fiction, several conventional anthologies are available,[2-9] some of them containing excellent selections. The inclusion and exclusion criteria for this book are similar to those employed in the first volume.[1] Works that are not available in English are, with few exceptions, not included. Medical clowns and criminals, such as those portrayed in Elizabethan plays[10] or in contemporary clinical conspiracy novels, are omitted. Doctors whose medical qualifications are irrelevant to the story, such as Dr Jekyll,[11] are also excluded.

The witch doctor who 'treats' his patient's constipation without obtaining a relevant history and 'cures' her by extracting an evil spirit from her abdomen[12] is considered too far removed from genuine members of the profession to be included in a work of this nature. On the other hand, skilled advisers who practise recognizable medicine are included regardless of whether or not they are in possession of a licence issued by the relevant authorities. The arbitrary decisions that had to be made are explained in detail in the Introduction to the first volume.[13]

Apparently capricious choices also had to be made in the selection of particular editions and translations. Paperback editions, despite their disadvantages as reference sources, were frequently easier to obtain (and cheaper) than the relevant hardcover texts. In the case of books that are or were out of print, the decision to use a particular version was determined by its availability in accessible libraries. Once a selection had been made in favour of a particular edition, this version was used throughout the book, even when it appeared, in retrospect, that another text might have been more suitable. For instance, in the case of Scott Fitzgerald's *Tender is the Night*,[14,15] the edition describing the career of Dr Diver in chronological order[15] might have been more appropriate to an anthology concerned with the doctor in literature. However, the non-chronological text[14] had been used in the first volume so, for the sake of uniformity, no change was made for this book.

All biblical translations come from the Revised Standard Version. With few exceptions, the translations employed for classical works are those in Loeb's Classical Library. Of the various translations of *Madame Bovary*,[16] that of Francis Steegmuller seemed the most appealing, although some specialists may disagree with this choice. In the case of Céline's *Journey to the End of the Night*,[17,18] the copyright permission for Manheim's translation[17] was easier to obtain than that for the alternative.[18]

Unlike the first volume, which deals mainly with doctor–patient interactions, this book concerns itself with various aspects of the doctor's personal life as depicted in fictional literature. Acutely ill people seeking help from physicians do not, at the time, consider the private lives of their medical attendants. They may comment on their doctor's physical appearance, particularly his hands and eyes,[19] and on his behaviour during medical encounters,[20] but his family life (if any), his cultural attainments (if any), and his relationships with his sexual and practice partners (if any) are of little interest to the parents of a seriously ill child, to the woman with a fractured hip or to the man suffering from acute urinary retention.

When the medical emergency is over and the doctors are consulted in a more leisurely fashion or encountered on a social occasion, their private lives are subjected to intense scrutiny. The patients and their families want to know all about these powerful healers, their incomes and expenditures, their mode of transportation, their feasting and their fasting.[21] What are the doctor's views on political or religious topics? Does he ever become bored or frustrated with his trade? How does he react when ill health afflicts him? Most importantly, how does the doctor behave towards his own family members?

Fictional literature, from works by Nobel laureates to doctor–nurse romances, reflects this extraordinary interest in the doctor's private life. Multiple novels, short stories, plays and poems discuss doctors' families, their relationships with their colleagues, their attitudes towards religion and politics and their lack of attention to their own health. In general, the negative aspects predominate. Fictional doctors (mostly male) do not make good husbands, they relate poorly to their peers and they tend to be actively disinterested in intellectual pursuits such as art and classical music.

Six aspects of the male* doctor's personal life are portrayed in detail. The first concerns his family circumstances, which are generally far from agreeable. Doctors who are not single, widowed or divorced are trapped in dysfunctional marriages due to their inability to choose a suitable partner and their failure to communicate with their wives and children. Authors, especially twentieth-century authors, take an almost malicious delight in pointing out that supposedly wise and sophisticated healers are incapable of arranging a satisfactory home life for themselves. Incongruously, at the very moment when the doctor, at a patient's bedside, attempts to relieve suffering, his own bed is being polluted by his wife and her lover. Perceived reasons for the doctor's failure as a family man include his work habits and the 'temptations' associated with medical practice, especially hospital practice. Moreover, the doctor's priestly role characteristically turns him into a solitary figure. Wives, girlfriends and children have no place at 'The Altar of Asclepios'[22] (*see* p. 38). The perception of the doctor's unsatisfactory home life is so deeply ingrained that among the relatively few fictional physicians with happy families, several are portrayed as negative role models with the implied message 'He's great when it comes to playing with his kids, but he's not much of a doctor.'[23]

Chapter 2 describes doctor–doctor relationships as perceived in medical novels. Physicians are portrayed as socially segregated from the rest of the community but

---

* The fictional female doctor is discussed in detail in Volume 4 of this series.

unable to live and work in harmony with one another. Tensions, minor squabbles and vicious fights are described in great detail, while the genuine collegiate relationship that exists between doctors in real life is de-emphasized. Specialists look down on general practitioners. Academics despise 'merchant' physicians, who reciprocate by expressing their contempt for the inhabitants of the ivory towers.[24] Commercial rivalries lead to professional disagreements. The old fight the young. Self-appointed messiahs who want to reform the profession are universally unpopular.

This perceived lack of cooperation between the doctor and his peers may be due to selective reporting. War is more interesting to storytellers than peace, and acrimonious political disputes between colleagues make better reading than dull, harmonious case presentations. Furthermore, the doctor's training, with its emphasis on one-to-one interactions with patients, makes him almost the antithesis of a dedicated team player.

The doctor's perceived attitude towards organized religion is the main theme of Chapter 3. Even in the Middle Ages, when many doctors were in holy orders, members of the medical profession were usually regarded as lacking in piety. Nineteenth-century doctors were generally portrayed as practising Christian virtues but rejecting traditional religious practices or considering them unimportant. Presumably, the doctor's personal experiences with human suffering and unanswerable medical questions, have made him suspicious of pious platitudes. He is mistrustful of traditional religions as well as modern cults and mass movements, and he is particularly wary of individuals and groups who claim a monopoly on the truth. Religion is barely mentioned in recent medical or hospital novels, although the rare physician who displays signs of piety is likely to generate embarrassment among his colleagues.

Chapter 4 is concerned with the doctor's knowledge (or ignorance) of extra-medical subjects. Authors are divided in their perception of whether or not doctors devote (or should devote) all of their time to their chosen subject. While warnings against becoming too diffuse in their studies were issued to physicians in classical times, it is only in the last half century that the thoroughly proficient technocrat has become a standard figure. Aggressive, foul-mouthed and supremely competent in his own field, the contemporary doctor, especially the surgeon, is devoid of any general culture.

The frustrated and demotivated physician is described in Chapter 5. Minor annoyances, such as demanding patients or the latest asinine regulation promulgated by a Health Maintenance Organization (HMO), make doctors declare, with mock regret, that they wish they had chosen a different profession. In general, such grievances do not indicate that the doctor is contemplating a career change. However, when he becomes bored with his work and/or doubts his own capacity to be of any use to his patients, his practice is likely to disintegrate. Chekhov's doctors in particular repeatedly express their disillusionment with their profession. What their patients need is decent living conditions, not medicine.

Chapter 6, on 'The Impaired Doctor,' deals with physicians who are unable to 'heal themselves.' Their disabilities include a variety of acute, self-limiting illnesses which are likely to be treated with self-medication, while more chronic problems are ignored, denied, or concealed until such manoeuvres are no longer possible. Severe disfigurement leads to a loss of popularity among patients and colleagues. Despite their marginalization, severely ill and dying individuals retain features of their medical behaviour patterns. Old age is mentioned more frequently as a disability than extreme youth. The male physician-hero is expected to behave as if he were invulnerable and immortal. Under no circumstances must he become a patient with 'complaints.'

Three indices are provided. The bibliography, which is based on authors' names listed in alphabetical order, enables the reader to find what part of a particular work is quoted and where to find the relevant quotation in the original novel, play or short story, as well as in this book. For instance, the reader searching for works by John Irving will find that material from *Hotel New Hampshire* is quoted on p. 226 of this book, *Cider House Rules* on pages 7 and 122 and *The Fourth Hand* on pages 41, 84 and 107–8. The name index provides a list of fictional physicians, such as Dr Richard Diver, and fictional patients, such as Thérèse Desqueyroux, as well as the names of the novels where these characters are to be found. The name index also contains the titles of some secondary sources that have been cited, place names and names of institutions of higher learning. The subject index contains aphorisms, such as Henry James' 'once a doctor, always a doctor,' various diagnoses, such as diphtheria and bacterial endocarditis, as well as multiple other captions of potential interest to browsers.

References

1 Posen S (2005) *The Doctor in Literature. Satisfaction or resentment?* Radcliffe Publishing, Oxford.
2 Cole H (ed.) (1963) *Under the Doctor.* Heinemann, London.
3 Ceccio J (ed.) (1978) *Medicine in Literature.* Longmans, New York.
4 Cousins N (ed.) (1982) *The Physician in Literature.* Saunders, Philadelphia, PA.
5 Mukand J (ed.) (1990) *Vital Lines.* St Martin's Press, New York.
6 Reynolds R and Stone J (eds) (1991) *On Doctoring: stories, poems, essays.* Simon and Schuster, New York.
7 Gordon R (ed.) (1993) *The Literary Companion to Medicine.* St Martin's Press, New York, 1996.
8 Ballantyne J (ed.) (1995) *Bedside Manners.* Virgin, London.
9 Bamforth I (ed.) (2003) *The Body in the Library.* Verso, London.
10 Kolin PC (1975) The Elizabethan stage doctor as a dramatic convention. In: Hogg J (ed.) *Elizabethan and Renaissance Studies.* Institut für Englische Sprache und Literatur, Universität Salzburg, Salzburg, Austria.
11 Stevenson RL (1886) *The Strange Case of Dr Jekyll and Mr Hyde.* Heinemann, London, 1934.
12 Barker P (1995) *The Ghost Road.* Viking, London, pp. 50–1.
13 Posen S, op. cit., pp. 3–7.
14 Fitzgerald FS (1934) *Tender is the Night.* Penguin, London, 2000.
15 Fitzgerald FS (1934) *Tender is the Night.* Penguin, Harmondsworth, 1974.
16 Flaubert G (1857) *Madame Bovary* (translated by Steegmuller F). Modern Library, New York, 1982.
17 Céline LF (1932) *Journey to the End of the Night* (translated by Manheim R). New Directions, New York, 1983.
18 Céline LF (1932) *Journey to the End of the Night* (translated by Marks J). Chatto and Windus, London, 1934.
19 Norris CB (1969) *The Image of the Physician in Modern American Literature.* PhD Dissertation, University of Maryland, Baltimore, MD, pp. 37–43.
20 Posen S, op. cit., pp. 72–8.
21 Sams F (1987) Big Star Woman. In: *The Widow's Mite and Other Stories.* Penguin, New York, 1989, p. 161.
22 Bennett A (1923) *Riceyman Steps.* Cassell, London, 1947, pp. 178–80.
23 Lewis S (1924) *Arrowsmith.* Signet Books, New York, 1961, pp. 193–7.
24 Roe F (1989) *Doctors and Doctors' Wives.* Constable, London, p. 241.

CHAPTER 1

The doctor and his family

Physicians make good husbands.[1,2]

A girl is a fool to marry a doctor.[3]

The typical fictional doctor is not a happily married man who enjoys helping his children with their homework or taking the family on camping vacations. Even during the nineteenth century, and long before the current epidemic of marital failures, physicians were widely portrayed as single, widowed, unhappily married or divorced. A few medical marriages produced six or eight children,[4-6] but with rare exceptions[7,8] one hears little about these large families and, from the point of view of the medical plots, they are irrelevant. The theme of the unmarried or unhappily married physician recurs in so many works of fiction and across such varied cultural settings that the list of doctors without families or with dysfunctional families seems almost endless. The marriages of female physicians are discussed in Volume 4 of this series.

The unmarried doctor

In accordance with their priestly tradition, a great many physicians from a range of cultural backgrounds have never been married. Balzac's saintly Dr Benassis,[9] Bernard Shaw's precise Dr Colenso Ridgeon[10] and Söderberg's evil Dr Tyko Glas[11] are all single men, mothered and bullied by their housekeepers. Benassis' celibate lifestyle[9] is part of a penance. He has to atone for a sin committed many years previously, when he abandoned his mistress and their child. Ridgeon,[10] who has spent his life in the laboratory, talks unrealistically about marrying the widow of his star patient (who dies in curious circumstances), but the romance does not prosper and he remains a middle-aged bachelor.[10] Glas, with his strange views on morality in general (*see* p. 193) and sexual behaviour in particular[11] (*see* pp. 114–15), is impossible to envisage as a husband or a father.

Among Chekhov's wretched pre-revolutionary Russian district medical officers, the unmarried state seems almost the norm.[12-25] Dr Chebutykin, the ignorant, drunken stage clown in *Three Sisters*,[12] 'never got round to marrying.' Dr Michael Astrov in *Uncle Vanya*,[17] conservationist[18] and vegetarian,[19] is intellectually and emotionally isolated in his semi-rural surroundings. He has no friends,[19] and although not beyond a transient liaison with the wife of one of his patients,[20] he has evidently given up all thoughts of ever establishing a long-term attachment to any woman.[19] By the time the play ends, Astrov is well on the way to alcoholism.[21]

Another of Chekhov's physicians, Eugene Dorn in *The Seagull*,[22] is a relatively serious and 'successful' character. Dorn is not rich,[23] but he enjoys life, he is keen on his work in an emotionally detached way (*see* Volume 1, Chapter 7), and he shows no signs of having become bored, disillusioned or alcoholic. Nevertheless, his personal relationships are no more satisfactory than those of Chekhov's burnt-out medical types. A bachelor at 55 years of age,[24] Dorn has had a long-standing affair with Polina Shamrayev, whose brutish husband has made her life miserable, but her appeal to let her come and live with him is rejected out of hand on the grounds that 'it's too late for me to change my life.'[25] Polina's daughter, Masha Shamrayev, who may be Dorn's natural child,[26] does not fare much better. He feels sufficiently paternalistic towards the girl to take away her snuffbox, hurl it into the bushes and tell her 'that's disgusting,'[25] but when she comes to him for love and advice ('help me, or else I'll do something silly and make a mess of my life'[25]), Dorn refuses to become involved in her emotional problems. 'How can I help you?' he responds, 'What can I do, my child?'[25]

Dostoyevsky's Dr Herzenstube, from a different generation and a different background, retains his idealism and his faith (*see* p. 129) but, like his cynical Chekhovian colleagues, he remains 'a confirmed bachelor all his life.'[27]

The single status of these Russian doctors is presumably the consequence of their paltry earnings and their geographical isolation, but unmarried doctors also abound in Western countries, where isolation is not a major factor and medical poverty is neither as pervasive nor as prolonged as in Russia. Francis Brett Young's dedicated Dr Marshall,[28] whose tastes are 'simple and inexpensive,' and who sends out his accounts once every three years, is of course a bachelor. Another of Young's medical characters, Dr Jonathan Dakers,[29] despite his fine physique is awkward in his dealings with young women and fails miserably in his quest for a suitable female companion. His brief engagement to one of the operating-room nurses comes to an abrupt end, because

> he had suffered a sudden revulsion of feeling at [her] familiarity with anatomy. . . . She said she had been mistaken in Jonathan; he had a coarse mind. . . . Then there was a girl undergraduate . . . who had fallen in love with Jonathan's torso on the football field. Jonathan at her suggestion took her on the river and quoted poetry, which wasn't what she had expected of him. . . . She, too, was mistaken in Jonathan; his mind was not coarse enough.[29]

Next, Jonathan falls hopelessly in love with Edith Martyn who, instead of returning his affection, has an affair with his glamorous younger brother. When the brother is reported missing in action during the First World War, Edith, pregnant and unmarried, turns to Jonathan for help. Jonathan, by this time an old-fashioned, decent but somewhat pedestrian general practitioner, marries her for the sake of appearances, but the marriage is not consummated.[30] The dashing young brother, upon his return from a prisoner-of-war camp, finds this act of abstinence amusing and somewhat contemptible. In the meantime, 'dark', faithful Rachel Hammond grows old as she waits for Jonathan, who fails to appreciate genuine happiness until it is too late.[31]

Ravic, the hard-drinking, cynical and nomadic refugee doctor in Remarque's *Arch of Triumph*,[32] is portrayed as a skilful surgeon and amateur philosopher. He lacks a residency permit, a licence to practise and a proper name,[33] but he gives every indication that even if he were to acquire these accoutrements, he would be emotionally incapable of forming a stable relationship with any woman. 'Neat little apartment[s and] ant-like attempt[s]' to build up an orderly 'bourgeois' existence[33] no longer attract Dr Ravic, and it seems unlikely that he ever found a 'regular' lifestyle appealing. The idea of a stable marriage is quite alien to this inhabitant of cheap hotels and prisons, who holds the view that 'women should be adored or abandoned.'[34]

In the American literature the unmarried doctor is less common, but by no means unknown. Faulkner's Dr Jules Martino,[35] a retired cardiologist who never marries and who 'didn't have any family at all', forms a strange relationship with Louise King, a girl young enough to be his granddaughter. Martino teaches Louise to be rebellious, 'not to be afraid', and dies the day she marries a colourless, conventional 'Yale man' who belongs to the right clubs and owns Oklahoma oil wells.[35]

Dr Rintman, one of the chief medical characters in *The Hospital Makers*,[36] is a woman hater. He is 'so much aware of his deep concealed hostility to women' that he goes out of his way to be excessively polite to them. Dr Rintman leads a solitary existence. 'No wife or children had ever entered his lonely life – only disciples, all male.' The relationship between the idealistic Dr Adam Stanton and his almost perfect sister in *All The King's Men*[37] may or may not have been incestuous at some stage,[38] but during the course of the story Stanton displays no overt physical interest in any woman (including his sister). The hero in Irving's *Cider House Rules*, Dr Wilbur Larch, obstetrician and abortionist, has had 'one sexual experience in his life.'[39]

The childless widower

Another standard figure in nineteenth- and early twentieth-century literature is the physician who succumbs to the temptations of connubial bliss, but who then, after the death of his wife, reverts to his natural celibate existence. Dr Leslie, the idealized, asexual, nineteenth-century New England *Country Doctor*,[40] is a widower and 'a lonely man in spite of his many friends.' Like Dr Benassis,[9] Dr Ridgeon[10] and Dr Glas,[11] Dr Leslie has a housekeeper who treats him like a naughty schoolboy. Leslie reacts, as might be expected, with little symbolic rebellious acts.

> Marilla called eagerly from the kitchen window to ask where he was going . . . but the doctor only answered that he should be back at dinner-time and settled himself comfortably in his carriage, smiling at Marilla's displeasure.[41]

Somerset Maugham's elderly Dr South in *Of Human Bondage*[42] is another typical medical widower.

> His wife had died thirty years before and his daughter had married a farmer in Rhodesia. He had quarrelled with him . . . she had taken her husband's part . . . and her children he had never seen. . . . It was just as if he had never had a wife or child. He was very lonely.[42]

Other widower doctors are described by Don Marquis, whose romanticized Dr Stewart, a horse-and-buggy *Country Doctor*,[43] dies on the job, and by Grace Metalious, whose Dr Matthew Swain,[44] an earthy but dedicated small-town family physician, is a central character in *Peyton Place*. The wife of *Doctor*

Serocold[45] died in childbirth 40 years earlier when she was 22 and he a 'tongue-tied young fellow, straight from hospital and knowing as little about women as he did about his work.' Dr Serocold has only dim recollections of his marriage, which lasted for one year, but he remembers his wife's unexplained 'fits of crying', and he now wonders whether he 'should have made her happy.' Helen Ashton does not provide an answer to this question, but hints that this kindly but impatient old man, who never remarries, is not cut out to be a good husband or father. Dr Richard Gaunt, Dr Serocold's senior partner, was the master of a 'jolly house' in his younger days, with a 'sweet and gentle wife' and two boys. However, this happy family life was not to continue: 'She died and the boys grew up and went away.' One son becomes a drifter, the other joins the navy, and both die during the First World War. Dr Gaunt, having been reduced to the 'natural' solitary state of a doctor, goes on practising for another 15 years with the widow of one of his sons acting as his housekeeper.[46]

Professor Van Helsing, the idealized, versatile, priestly nineteenth-century physician and scholar, who solves the Dracula mystery almost single-handedly, might as well be a widower. Van Helsing is a 'faithful husband', but his demented wife is 'dead to me',[47] and his only child did not survive. Martin Arrowsmith,[48] a widower, briefly remarries after the death of his childless first wife.[49] The second marriage produces a son,[50] but Martin is not happy (*see* p. 21). He walks out on his second wife and goes off into the 'desert' (*see* p. 181) to serve science together with another single and single-minded seeker after the truth.[51]

The irrevocably divorced doctor

In the contemporary real world, medical divorces, mostly stages on the road to remarriage, are common although, with the exception of those involving psychiatrists, no more so than in the general population.[52] Several fictional doctors stand out against this pattern and go through divorces or separations that are perceived to constitute the end of any kind of married life. Tomas, the hero in *The Unbearable Lightness of Being*,[53] neurosurgeon, political dissident and womanizer, realizes, after his divorce, that 'he was not born to live side by side with any woman.'

Dr Oliver Selfridge, the successful surgeon in *All The Little Heroes*,[54] has no family at all. An only child, he is brought up from the age of four by a disfigured aunt, after his mother dies and his father, an eccentric vagabond, abandons him.[55] His brief marriage ends in divorce[56] and 'he has told himself he cannot ever marry again',[57] even though there are casual affairs. Selfridge's loveless upbringing,[58,59] his social isolation and his 'burnout' at the age of 32 (*see* Chapters 5 and 6) make him an atypical character, but conclusive medical divorces are by no means confined to such individuals.

The doctors' competence, their idealism and their compassion afford no protection against the fatal breakdown of their marriages. Grisham's Dr Walter Kord,[60] the successful and kind-hearted oncologist of the 1990s, who gives absolutely trustworthy evidence on behalf of one of his patients (*see* Volume 1, Chapter 11), fares no better than the incompetent and unsuccessful Dr Al Blauberman,[61] whose inept psychiatric endeavours are a disgrace to New York University, which awarded him his MD in 1939. Both are in family situations best described in one, apparently decisive, term – 'divorced.' Similarly, in Galgut's story[62] neither the cynical and lazy Dr Frank Eloff nor the starry-eyed and childlike Dr Lawrence Waters manage to salvage their relationships. Frank's divorce is due to his indolence,[63] while Lawrence's partner decamps because, to him, 'work is the only thing that matters.'[63]

Robin Cook's *Brain*[64] contains a description of an entire building, adjacent to a medical centre, and occupied largely by divorced MDs: 'There were almost no children except for weekends when it was Dad's turn with the kids.' One of the inhabitants is Dr Martin Philips, whose wife had left him around four years earlier when she realized, after six years of 'matrimonial suburban stalemate', that Martin was 'married to medicine' and that she was only the mistress.[64]

Miserable medical marriages

Dysfunctional marriages are not restricted to the medical profession. However, the fact that one or both partners have a degree in medicine seems to aggravate rather than alleviate the inevitable tensions between lifelong companions. While the usual marital arguments over money, children and infidelity occur, peculiarly 'medical' difficulties intrude. For instance, boredom, which is circumvented by a busy professional schedule, becomes a major problem when, with increasing prosperity and age, the doctor reduces his working hours. Rinehart's Dr Grant and his wife have stayed together but when, in his decline, Grant has to give up night work, 'the long hours alone with Janet got on his nerves.'[65]

Medical 'shop talk' at social gatherings is a constant source of irritation for the non-medical partners, who are unable to join in and at times cannot even follow the gist of the conversation. Nourse, the author of *Intern*,[66] describes a pleasant (for him) Thanksgiving Dinner attended by three young medical couples, all from the same hospital.

> After dinner we sat around talking until almost midnight, and it was medicine all the way . . . you could change the subject to the state of the world or some other scintillating topic time and again, but the conversation always drifted back to some patient's breast abscess in about five minutes. Sometimes I think the girls must get damned sick of it, but they're married to it, so what are they going to do?[66]

Robin Cook goes into greater detail. His medical couples, who are sharing a lakeside cottage for a weekend,[67] are older than Nourse's interns,[66] and the 'girls', who have been exposed to medical jargon for considerably longer, are openly resentful.[67] After dinner the conversation turns to medicine, and one of the established doctors asks Dr David Wilson, the newcomer, how he is coping with his practice. Wilson replies:

> 'I've got more oncology patients than I'd anticipated.' . . . 'What's oncology?', Nancy Yansen asked. Kevin [Yansen, the aggressive ophthalmologist] gave his wife an irritated look of disbelief. 'Cancer,' he said disdainfully. 'Jesus, Nance, you know that.' 'Sorry,' Nancy said with equal irritation.

The doctors then go on to discuss their various oncology patients, including one Donald Anderson, who has pancreatic carcinoma.

'I recognize that name,' Trent [Yarborough, the surgeon] said. 'That patient had a Whipple procedure.' 'Thanks for telling us,' Gayle [Yarborough] said sarcastically.[67]

William Carlos Williams' works contain an entire catalogue of medical men beset by matrimonial calamities. One of his doctors dies in a hotel room making love to a friend's wife.[68] A second, in *Old Doc Rivers*,[69] 'had shot himself in despair at the outcome of an affair with the wife of another physician.' A third, also in *Old Doc Rivers*, 'had divorced his wife and married once again – a younger woman.'[69] A fourth 'had left town hurriedly, possibly to escape jail, leaving a wife and child behind.'[69] Williams does not tell us whether these doctors were good or bad, old or young, dedicated or disillusioned. He simply reports, as a matter of fact, the fate of four medical marriages.

Most fictional doctors do not enjoy even a semblance of marital happiness. The 'blame' for their unsatisfactory home life may rest squarely with one or the other spouse – such as the despotic husband or the stupid wife. Mostly, however, both partners are at fault, with the doctor's occupation not only failing to rescue the relationship, but actively contributing to its breakdown. The theme transcends historical and geographical boundaries.

Three nineteenth-century novels

Three major nineteenth-century novels[70–72] have as their main theme the story of medical men whose marriages turn into crosses that they have to bear. One of them, Dr Charles Bovary, who stumbles and falls under his load, barely deserves the title 'Doctor.' He fails the examination for his inferior medical qualification at the first attempt,[73] and when he does manage to pass after much cramming, his knowledge of medicine is so weak that during the central emergency of the story[74] he is as useless as the local pharmacist. Moreover, Charles is diffident and shy, so that from the moment he enters the schoolroom on the first page of the book to the time of his death he remains a victim, a dupe and a loser. This poor pretence of a doctor is married twice, and neither marriage is happy.[70] Charles' first bride, a hideous, ill-tempered, middle-aged widow, is selected by his mother, who believes that the lady's 'fortune' (later found to be non-existent) will help to set him up in practice.[75] When this scarecrow suddenly dies at the age of 46, of what sounds like cardiac arrhythmia or a pulmonary embolus, her place is taken by the famous Madame Emma Bovary, whose fanciful ideas of love[76] are rapidly followed by bitter disappointment. Instead of providing '"bliss", "passion" and "rapture", words that had seemed so beautiful to her in books,' marriage turns out to consist of her husband's medical prattle, with sexual congress determined by fixed schedules. Soon Emma displays overt signs of boredom, engages in unrealistic fantasies and makes pathetic attempts to relieve the monotony of her life. She behaves histrionically, neglects her family, and after the principal medical disaster of the story, she comes to despise Charles, goes on to cuckold and bankrupt him,[70] and finally poisons herself.

If this empty-headed, self-centred, manipulative woman had presented as a patient, even an accomplished physician might have found it difficult to deal with her constantly changing complaints. Charles Bovary is not an accomplished physician. Moreover, he has to take care of Emma not as a patient, but as a permanent companion, who eats at his table and sleeps in his house, if not in his bed.[77] In the process, this decent, simple fool is totally destroyed. Not only is he unable to manage his wife, he even lacks the emotional resources to look after his little daughter, who suffers the ultimate degradation of having 'to work for her living in a cotton mill.'[78] Bovary is not a good doctor. As a husband and a father he is totally useless.

Robert Gibson, the doctor in Elizabeth Gaskell's *Wives and Daughters*,[71] fares better. More competent and more intelligent than Bovary, Gibson converses with 'the leaders of the scientific world' as an equal,[79] and even submits 'contributions of his own to the more scientific of the medical journals.' Despite his accomplishments, he cannot escape his share of matrimonial annoyances.

An overt misogynist, Gibson expresses views like 'the world would get on tolerably well if there were no women in it'[80] and 'I'm not sure that reading or writing is necessary [for women]',[81] whose principal function in life consists of 'running up milliners' bills.'[82] Despite these notions, he has enjoyed several 'love' affairs,[83] he has been married at least once and he is now a widower with a 16-year-old daughter who, he believes, requires 'feminine' guidance. Rather than sending her to a boarding school or hiring a governess, Dr Gibson decides to enter into a marriage of convenience with Clare Hyacinth Kirkpatrick, a widow with a cynical and flirtatious teenage daughter of her own. The fact that this '*ménage à quatre*' functions at all is largely due to Gibson's diplomatic skills, although considerable tensions develop. The doctor's 40-year-old[84] 'faded bride',[85] with her shallow intellect,[86,87] her pretence of gentility[88] and her clumsy intrigues,[89] soon begins to irritate him. He

> had made up his mind before his second marriage to yield in trifles, and be firm in greater things. But the differences of opinion about trifles arose every day, and were perhaps more annoying than if they had related to things of more consequence.[90]

One constant source of friction is the midday meal. When the doctor comes home at lunchtime between house calls, he wants a quick snack so that he can set out again without delay.[91] A serving of bread and cheese together with a glass of beer is entirely satisfactory as far as he is concerned, but the new wife objects to this menu on the grounds that it lacks refinement: 'I cannot allow cheese to come beyond the kitchen',[90] 'It's such a strong-smelling coarse kind of thing, fit only for labourers.'[91]

More substantial disagreements follow. Listening at the surgery door, Mrs Gibson discovers that the heir to the estate of the local squire suffers from a serious heart condition (possibly bacterial endocarditis), and promptly encourages her daughter to become engaged to the younger son of the family.[89] The doctor, incensed at this breach of confidence, now 'had to face and acknowledge the fact that the wife he had chosen had a very different standard of conduct to that which he had upheld all his life.'

At the end of the unfinished version of *Wives and Daughters*,[92] Dr and Mrs Gibson are still cohabiting, although her shallow mind has not improved. Gaskell's editor surmises that the final chapter would have seen the doctor hire an assistant, to enable him to visit his married daughter in London for a few days now and then, and 'to get a little rest from Mrs Gibson.'[92]

Dr Tertius Lydgate in *Middlemarch*[72] proposes marriage almost on the spur of the moment to a tearful young woman whom he has been trying to comfort.[93] Rosamond Lydgate, pretty, stubborn and stupid, resents her husband's medical activities, especially his attempts at research.[94] 'You always want to pore over your microscope,' she sulks, 'confess you like those things better than me.' She expresses the wish that he had not been a medical man.[95] '"Don't say that", said Lydgate, drawing her closer to him. "That's like saying you wish you had married another man."' Rosamond resembles Emma Bovary[96] in her inability to think logically, her 'dream-world'[97] and her 'languid' posturings,[98–100] and it is largely through her machinations that Lydgate abandons his research ambitions (he had even entertained the idea of establishing a medical school in Middlemarch) and becomes a wealthy rheumatologist instead. His colleagues consider him a 'success', but he regards himself as a failure and blames his wife for the atrophy of his brain.[101] 'He had chosen this fragile creature and had taken the burthen of her life upon his arms. He must walk as he could carrying that burthen pitifully.'[102]

The intellectually limited wife

The *Middlemarch*[72] theme of a medical eagle wedded to a goose recurs many times in fictional literature. Obviously, unions between intellectually mismatched individuals, which were described in classical times,[103] are not restricted to physicians and their wives. However, the doctor's supposed knowledge of human nature, far from shielding him against disastrous matrimonial decisions, seems to render him particularly vulnerable to catastrophic blunders when it comes to choosing a partner. Physicians may indeed be able to identify physical and psychological defects, but this aptitude abandons them at the most critical moment of their lives. They select a wife or a girlfriend from among the mad, the bad, the dim and the cantankerous, with predictable results. Authors appear to take an almost malicious delight in revealing the prospective bride's blemishes to the reader, while the doctor, with all his experience, is either oblivious to these imperfections or ignores them.

Dorothy Sayers' 'Lady Mainwaring'[104] endows male doctors with a specific shrewdness of judgement when it comes to the choice of a mate. She wants to match up 'Dr Julian Freke', a rich and distinguished surgeon, with her eldest daughter, although she anticipates some problems. Freke has so far proved impervious to the charms of multiple English maidens because, Lady Mainwaring suspects, of his perspicacity in detecting physical shortcomings. One can hardly expect a surgeon who has 'so many opportunities of judging . . . to be taken in by a figure that . . . [is] all padding.'

She is quite wrong. Dr Freke's unmarried state is due to his freakish and criminal tendencies rather than to his acumen in recognizing artificial contours.

Two medical classmates and research collaborators, both with allegorical surnames (Dr Sidney Feeder and Dr Jackson Lemon), appear in Henry James' *Lady Barberina*.[105] One of the doctors thrives, while the other has his research career terminated by a wife with a severely restricted intellect.[106] Feeder, who 'enjoyed the highest esteem at the medical congress',[105] has no time to investigate 'the facilities for getting married.' Lemon, on the other hand, is very rich, and decides to marry Barberina, a 'flower of the English aristocracy', principally, Norris suggests, in order to beget a race of well-bred and statuesque little Lemons.[107] Barberina, handsome, stubborn, stupid and depressive, cannot bear to live anywhere outside England, so Lemon is forced to lead a life of idleness in London.

> He's exceedingly restless and is constantly crossing over to the Continent.
> . . . Sidney Feeder feels very badly about him; it's months since Jackson
> has sent him any results.[106]

Some physicians, having once made the wrong choice, go on to repeat their
mistakes. Danby's renegade Jew, Dr Benjamin Phillips, a popular general practitioner when he first appears in *A Maida Vale Idyll*,[108] subsequently decides to
specialize in surgery and becomes 'one of the first surgeons in England.'[109] This
brilliant, devious man, 'with all his knowledge of the world, of men and of
women',[110] is married to a simple, sterile, pious and placid invalid whom he
despises, insults[111] and finally murders (without getting caught). He then proposes
to marry his scheming mistress, despite her lack of affection for him or their
illegitimate little girl,[112] who dies as a result of her mother's neglect.[113] After this
woman leaves him for a younger man, Phillips reverts to the 'natural' solitary state
of a doctor. In public, he is 'the brilliant, keen, intellectual Benjamin Phillips . . .
[whose] name is in all men's mouths.'[109] His private life is conducted at a 'bachelor
retreat' where he is waited upon by a parlour maid 'whose services have other
rewards besides her yearly wages.'[109]

Similarly, Mauriac's Dr Paul Courrèges,[114] a talented and successful Bordeaux
physician, not only has a dull wife but, in addition, proposes to replace her with an
equally boring mistress. The lack of marital success in the Courrèges family is
portrayed as a generational phenomenon. Paul's father, a prominent surgeon, is a
lifelong womanizer[115] (*see* p. 27). Paul himself goes through a mid-life crisis at the
age of 52. 'His continued presence no longer served to bring contentment to an
embittered partner. . . . He found the thought of living [with her] any longer
unutterably boring.'[116] His daughter, on whom he has lavished all his affection
('people think you're my wife') is married to 'a well-off [army] officer of good
ancestry' but of limited intelligence.[117] His 17-year-old son has become totally
inaccessible. 'All he had to do was to break with his wife as he had seen many of his
colleagues do with theirs.'[116] This experienced doctor is evidently unable to
recognize that Maria Cross, the patient with whom he intends to elope, is highly
unlikely to provide him with the physical or emotional satisfaction he believes he
craves. Maria, sexually frigid,[118] incurably lazy[119] and domestically incompetent,[119]
does not become the doctor's wife or his mistress, and the doctor–patient relationship remains superficially correct. If she had agreed to accompany him to Algiers or
Santiago, her indolence and her habit of spending 'all day in an old dressing gown
and slippers'[119] would have made him nostalgic for his first wife within a month.

Towards the end of the story, Dr Courrèges reappears as an old man, afflicted by
Parkinsonism[120] and deserted by his patients (*see* p. 229). The doctor realizes that he
is largely to blame for his unsatisfactory marriage and that his wife 'now takes her
revenge by being over-attentive'[120] and performing tedious and unpleasant domestic
tasks. He advises Raymond, his estranged, non-medical son, who has inherited his
grandfather's promiscuity but not his professional dedication, to get married,
despite his own experiences. Like other male chauvinists, he believes that the
function of women is to look after children when they are young and after invalid
husbands when they are old. He articulates this conviction in medical terms:

> The great thing in life is to make some sort of refuge for yourself. At the
> end of one's existence, as at the beginning, one's got to be borne by a
> woman.[120]

Another doctor trapped in a loveless marriage to a dull woman is Mary Rinehart's Chris Arden, the medical hero of *The Doctor*.[121] Chris's partner, Catherine, the daughter of his former landlady, is an immature and manipulative woman, slatternly in her habits, surly in her behaviour, and shallow in her emotions and interests. She does not even excite him sexually.[122] However, she turns up without warning on the day of his departure for postgraduate study in Vienna, declaring that unless she can accompany him on his trip, she will kill herself or 'go on the streets.'[122] Chris, notwithstanding his medical training, is unable to rid himself of this burden, and marries her 'an hour before the ship sailed' because of a perverted sense of honour. The wretched marriage lasts 14 years before Catherine decides to divorce Chris. She has spent most of his money and leaves him a physical and emotional cripple.[123] Fortunately, after he recovers from his brachial plexus injury and his depression, his first love, Beverley, reappears with a perforated peptic ulcer. The book ends with Chris operating on Beverley, confident that she 'would make a home for him and bear his children',[124] leaving the reader with the impression that Beverley, who grew up in a luxurious home, will succeed where Catherine, the daughter of impoverished and disorganized parents, failed.

Dr Alan Gray, the romantic hero in Ruth Blodgett's *Home Is The Sailor*,[125] is a giant in the field of cardiac surgery, but a dwarf when it comes to choosing a partner. Gray, who sews up the lacerated heart of the town drunkard in a hut on the beach, is also an innovator. Using a cat model, he invents an instrument for the relief of mitral stenosis, and he is invited by a New York surgeon to demonstrate the use of his new gadget in humans.[126] The fact that the first patient happens to be his mother-in-law, who dies of 'pneumonia' five days after a 'successful' operation, adds interest to the plot but does not detract from Alan's stature.

This towering mastermind behaves like an oafish high-school student in his dealings with 'Elaine', with whom he fancies himself in love. During one of his clumsy attempts at physical contact he informs her that 'I've never had much time to get to know girls. Or much chance either.'[125] Elaine, the shallow and flirtatious belle of a small Maine coastal town, is not particularly turned on by Alan's serious and intense attitude,[125] and she is aggressively disinterested in his research activities.[127] Almost incomprehensibly to a contemporary reader, Alan and Elaine decide to get married after a very mild (by current standards) petting session.[128] They marry in haste and repent in haste. She does not want to hear about heart valves and he is not interested in her small domestic accomplishments. Like the unhappy Ardens,[122] the Grays do not even enjoy sex.

> Some attitude of hers, a fastidiousness bordering on prudery, got in his way to bother him . . . making him feel to blame for wanting her in just that way . . . [leaving him with] a dissatisfying feeling of unfulfilment.[127]

The inevitable separation follows. Elaine goes back to Daddy, while Alan heads off to Europe for a year's research.[129] His loyal and determined nurse-assistant will study at Johns Hopkins Hospital* during his absence, so that she can help him with his experiments on unwanted cats, as well as with other aspects of his life, upon his return.[129] Alan's father, an old seafaring man, attributes his son's restlessness and inability to 'settle down' to his descent from generations of sailors. As the title of the book suggests, a sailor's return from the sea is followed

---

* *See* footnote on pp. 21–2.

by a brief sojourn on shore before he is off again to parts of the world where his wife cannot follow.[130]

Multiple other stories involve gifted doctors and their brainless wives. The talented psychiatrist *Parris Mitchell of King's Row*,[131] despite his clinical skills, marries a 'Daddy's Darling' who 'used her pretty little helplessness to dominate the old man' and subsequently attempts to employ the same technique with her psychiatrist husband.[131] Parris tires of his child-bride, who dies, but not before she discovers that he is in love with another woman.[132]. By contrast, Dr Paul Nolan, the loyal and sensible friend of Parris, remains happily married.

Lucas Marsh, the medical crusader in Thompson's *Not As A Stranger*,[133] marries Kristina, a competent and dependable operating-room nurse, not because of her intellectual accomplishments (which are limited) or her physical charms (which are non-existent), but because of her savings (which will support him through medical school). After graduation, he becomes ashamed and openly contemptuous of Kristina, the trusting, unsophisticated daughter of immigrant parents, who decides to become a nurse because she likes the uniform.[134] Lucas has an affair with an emotionally unstable artist,[135] but then returns to his pregnant wife, who has been patiently waiting for him.[136]

There is no reconciliation between Stuart Bergman, MD, and his wife. Bergman, the hero of Harlan Ellison's *Wanted in Surgery*,[137] rescues the medical profession from its subservience to robots, but is unable to rescue his own flawed marriage. Thelma's 'insensitivity' originally strikes this priest-like surgeon as 'humorous', but after many 'barren years of . . . marriage . . . it was now a millstone he wore silently.' Thelma reciprocates in kind. Her husband's emotional turmoil leaves her quite indifferent. 'There just is no understanding that man', she declares as she rushes off to play electro-mah jong with her 'girl-friends.'

George Sava's *No Man is Perfect*,[138] a fanciful medical romance, describes the decline and fall of Dr Anthony Sommers, a leading British neurosurgeon. Sommers' disintegration begins when he is 39 and about to be offered the Chair of Neurosurgery at Oxford University. At this stage he decides to marry 21-year-old Patricia, a brainless and badly brought up English aristocrat, whose only accomplishment is a talent for insulting repartee. Naturally Patricia finds Anthony's work and aspirations totally uninteresting, and she promptly cuckolds him with a worthless member of her own set, the future Lord Marlowhope. Sommers discovers this relationship and the paternity of Patricia's child through a series of coincidences, and embarks on a new career, characterized largely by alcoholism.

The wrong sister

Several medical stories use the biblical theme of a pair of eligible sisters, one of whom is enchanting and the other hard-working.[139,140] Dr Edward Hope in the nineteenth century[141] and Dr Alan Beresford in the twentieth[142] are both confronted by this dilemma, and both choose the less intelligent and more dependent of the two. In each case, the doctor and both sisters subsequently live together, the Hopes and the unmarried sister on a permanent basis, the Beresfords and 'Jo' while she is on leave from Nigeria. Both doctors lie awake at night thinking of the woman in the next room. Harriet Martineau resolves the problem, somewhat unrealistically, by bringing adversity on the Hope family. Mrs Hope redeems herself by displaying a strength of character that is not at all obvious at the beginning of the story.[141] The resolution of the potential conflict in the Beresford household is more credible. The glamorous Jo goes back to her World Health Organization post in Africa, leaving her small-minded and dependent sister in possession of the field.[142]

Faith Baldwin also tells a story of two sisters, both of them nurses, but only one of them worthy to share Dr Peter McDonald's bed. The doctor's office nurse, Lydia Owens, serious, sensible and loyal, has been secretly in love with her chief for years, but the doctor who 'was quick to diagnose the symptoms of others' is unable to recognize her devotion.[143] Lydia's younger sister Sophie, a shallow, selfish and flirtatious creature, has no difficulty in attracting the doctor's attention, and the two actually become engaged.[144] Fortunately, Sophie (not the doctor) has the sense to realize that the two are ill matched, the engagement is terminated and Lydia is set to take her sister's place.[145] Despite the banality of the story and the predictability of the plot, Baldwin provides yet another illustration of the doctor's lack of judgement with regard to his own personal relationships.

Doctor–nurse romances

Doctor–nurse romances, which remain popular with some members of the reading public, invariably finish on a 'they lived happily ever after' note. A fairly typical tale involving 'mature' characters is that of an operating room nurse who falls in love with the chief of orthopaedic surgery, an MD for nearly 20 years,[146] 'who had taken his time about marrying, a big man with broad shoulders, powerful arms and a strong face.'[146] The nurse lives in an apartment which she has made into a mantrap.

> There was a round oak table with rush-bottomed chairs pulled up to it, a bowl of fruit hospitably inviting. . . . In the next room, her bed was covered with a patchwork quilt. . . . Their eyes met, their hands, their lips.[147]

It is not surprising that the hero's medical behaviour is no more convincing than his love life. A similar romance involving somewhat younger participants has as its central character a 19-year-old student nurse who lusts after and, despite some mishaps, finally captures a rich 35-year-old surgeon who drives a gold-coloured Rover car.[148] However, even such stereotyped stories contain hints that all may not conclude well, that the blushing bride of today ('orange blossom and six brides-maids') may become a middle-aged bore who resents her husband's medical conversations and turns to alcohol or other men for comfort.[148]

Richard Dooling provides a partial explanation for the propensity of doctors to enter into disastrous relationships with dim-witted women. Dr Werner Ernst, the only serious ('earnest') character among a series of medical freaks in *Critical Care*,[149] is having a transient, sexually unsatisfying affair with a brainless model who is intensely preoccupied with her own body. Unbelievably, the thought occurs to Dr Ernst that he might enjoy setting up house with this bimbo.

> She was dull, simple and shallow, but who wanted drama, complexity and depth after sixteen hours in the ICU? It might be pleasant to come home to a lovely simpleton.[149]

The wayward wife

The theme of the talented husband and his adulterous wife goes back to the Old Testament.[150] It recurs several times in medical novels, where doctors enter into their matrimonial predicaments as a result of misjudging their future partners' sexual behaviour as well as their intellectual capacity. They become infatuated with women who are not only short on brains but also exceptionally well endowed with lust, which, unfortunately for the doctor, is not satisfied by their exertions in the conjugal bed. Some of this marital infidelity is due to a discrepancy in age. Medical qualifications do not protect old fools from using their status or their money to entice young women to become their partners.

One of Boccaccio's physicians, Mazzeo della Montagna,[151] is very much in demand both in Salerno and in the surrounding villages. We see him in action preparing an opiate for a patient who requires surgery for the removal of a bony sequestrum, and providing very credible explanations to the relatives. Despite his medical skills, this elderly character with his diminished libido and potency marries a young woman who, unlike some later examples of the species, is 'of considerable spirit and intelligence.' The vigorous bride promptly becomes bored with her elderly husband and finds herself a lover.[151]

The theme recurs many centuries later when Dr Robert Munro's wife, who keeps her middle-aged husband out of her bed, develops a violent passion for James Dyer, Munro's young partner. The gossips of Bath, England, are amused but not surprised.[152]

> 'What did Munro expect, a man of his years marrying a green, head-strong woman like Agnes Munro? And then to invite that creature Dyer into his house?'[152]

Marital infidelity is not specifically mentioned by Chellis in his 'Temperance Tale',[153] which relates the story of old Dr Foster, who is generally regarded as a confirmed bachelor until he marries a woman 25 years younger than himself. However, it is implied that there is something unnatural about this marriage, which produces a single child, a son, who develops into an alcoholic doctor (*see* p. 215).

Jinny O'Brien, wife of Dr James M'Murdo O'Brien, Professor of Physiology at the University of Melbourne, who 'preserved a girlish and even infantile expression of innocence', is evidently disenchanted with her husband's researches into 'Bile Pigments with Special Reference to Urobilin' and 'The Comparative Anatomy of the Vermiform Appendix', and leaves a note announcing her imminent elopement.[154] She subsequently marries another professor, but eventually goes back to O'Brien, who still dotes on her and admits 'I thought too much of my work and too little of my wife.'[154] Conan Doyle leaves it to the reader to imagine whether the professor and his wayward wife live together harmoniously after their re-unification.

Another unfaithful medical spouse is described by Chekhov in *The Butterfly*.[155] Dr Osip Dymov, hard working and idealistic, stands in sharp contrast to Chekhov's miserable and demotivated medical vagabonds, who end up in remote Russian villages where they drink themselves to death. These drifters are generally unencumbered by wives and children (*see* p. 5) or, if married, become separated from their families.[156] Unlike these inferior medical types, Dymov, a talented physician, can look forward to a bright academic future. Unfortunately, the accomplishments of this potential pioneer (whose career ends prematurely) do not help him to establish a satisfying relationship. He marries Olga, the 'butterfly', nine years his junior, whom he meets in the course of his professional activities. Olga, 'fiendishly in love with herself', flits from painting to music to acting but shows no particular dedication to or talent for any of these pursuits. She takes no interest whatever in her husband's academic career, and openly engages in adulterous liaisons.[155]

Some doctors manage to extricate themselves from such ruinous associations before it is too late. Dr Sydney Archer, the hero of Weir Mitchell's *Circumstance*,[157] avoids the snares of a sex kitten (Kitty Morrow) who would undoubtedly have turned into an unfaithful partner. Archer is briefly attracted to this mindless 'rosebud with . . . [her] pretty ways [and her] vivacity . . . [and he becomes] conscious of an attraction which he did not care to analyze.'[157] Fortunately, his medical training enables him to recognize that even Kitty's flirtatious behaviour is counterfeit. She is a teaser who 'likes the pursuit, the game, not the final object.' There is at hand Kitty's more meritorious cousin, who possesses less well-developed physical allurements but a greater intellect than Kitty, and the book ends with Archer's engagement to this worthy woman.[158]

While Archer triumphs over the 'temptation of the flesh' by his own will-power, Bernard Malamud's Dr Simon Morris[159] is rescued from his folly by the object of his desires. Morris, a lonely, retired physician, has discovered that Evelyn, a 29-year-old woman living in his apartment block, is being implored by her parents to stop sleeping around and to settle down with a husband who will respect her. Quite implausibly, the 66-year-old doctor decides to assume the role of Evelyn's companion and protector, and writes her a letter to that effect. Dressed like a lorikeet ('green suit, blue striped shirt, pink tie'[159]), he waits in the lobby for her reaction. Whether from callousness or common sense, Evelyn takes the letter out of her pigeonhole, reads it, tears it into small pieces and flings them in the direction of her admirer.

Arthur Schnitzler's *Dr Graesler*,[160] a medical drifter and a bachelor at 47 years of age, has had multiple affairs over the years ('many a narrow escape') but no major relationships. When a serious and intelligent woman offers this timid and suspicious doctor a marital partnership based on mutual respect and trust, he reacts with 'fright and flight.'[160] Instead, he has an affair with a young shop assistant,[161] and when this girl dies from scarlet fever (probably transmitted by the doctor) he lets himself be comforted by a widow with a 'doubtful reputation', and her seven-year-old daughter whose paternity is uncertain.[162] The widow becomes Frau Graesler, but we do not hear how she and her daughter treat the doctor in his declining years.

The most detailed account of a relationship between a 'virtuous' medical man and a 'depraved' woman is to be found in Somerset Maugham's *Of Human Bondage*.[163] Philip Carey, the central character of the novel, a deformed, sensitive, introspective medical student with a 'passion for art and literature',[164] is almost destroyed by his obsession with Mildred Rogers, a stupid, slovenly and bad-tempered shop assistant, who subsequently changes professions and becomes a street prostitute.[165] Philip leaves Norah Nesbit, the 'agreeable chatterbox' who wants to mother and protect him,[166] to set up house with the unreliable and unclean Mildred, whose mind is totally closed to anything outside her limited sphere of experience. Fortunately for Philip, Mildred prefers the life of a common whore to chaste cohabitation with a cripple, and abandons him to his studies and his disastrous share speculations.[167] After finally graduating, at the age of 30, Dr Carey is so afraid of loneliness that he offers to marry Sally, yet another 19-year-old shop assistant (albeit a good-natured one), whom he does not love and whose education has been neglected by her eccentric father.[168] The views of the future father-in-law on the relationship between men and women are quite blatant. Notions of intellectual equality and comradeship are rubbish. 'A man doesn't want to talk politics to his wife . . . a man wants a wife who can cook his dinner and look after his children.'[168] When Philip marries a teenager raised on these principles, he has to give up his travel plans and his appointment at 'St Luke's Hospital.' He will practise among poor people who 'would not sneer at the simple manners of his wife.'[164] His 'dreams of a rich and varied life' will have to be realized in his children. We do not see Carey after 25 years of marriage, but we hear him proposing: 'I wonder if you'll marry me?'. Sally responds laconically: 'If you like.'[164]

The theme of the doctor and his whore spouse also occurs in Warwick Deeping's *Sorrell and Son*.[169] While still at medical school, Maurice Pentreath secretly marries a shop assistant with a 'baby face' and 'innocent eyes', who infects him with a disease that renders him 'polluted in body and shamed in soul.'[170] Pentreath's second wife, a cold and judgemental canon's daughter,[171] 'economizes on small talk', bullies her husband and, although the subject is not discussed in these terms, almost certainly keeps him on a very meagre sex ration.

Surprisingly, Dr Christopher Sorrell, the main medical character in the same novel, also lacks judgement when it comes to finding the right partner. Sorrell is much more capable than Pentreath. While Maurice tries hard (not very successfully) to function as a general practitioner in a country town, Christopher is appointed to a prestigious surgical position on the staff of a major London hospital.[172] He treats Pentreath, his former classmate, for his unmentionable disease,[170] and later assists him in avoiding what threatens to become a medico-legal predicament[171] (*see* Volume 1, Chapter 10). This potential leader of men pursues Pentreath's young sister Molly, a talented writer, with an ardour worthy of a medieval troubadour. Molly, a convoluted character, declares that she is not interested in men and, being of a literary turn of mind, she expresses this sentiment in metaphorical terms: 'Man has no spoon in my porridge plate.'[173] She informs Christopher that she dislikes children,[174] that she gets bored easily[173] and that she would not make him a good wife. She is happy to sleep with him, but she will not entertain the idea of marriage.[174] Christopher, the immature 'boy-man',[175] is not satisfied with this modern proposal (the year is 1925). Unless he can have 'permanence', 'possession' and the sanctity of marriage, he wants nothing to do with the affair.[174] The impasse is resolved during Christopher's near-mortal illness,* when Molly agrees to an official marriage ceremony and he concedes that she can go on working, unencumbered by the 'servitude' of bearing children.[176] Christopher's father believes that the marriage will be happy ('the fruit will retain its flavour and its tang'[176]), but the reader is left to wonder whether, in ten years' time, an essentially simple soul like Sorrell will be happy in a childless marriage with a tempestuous, colourful artist for a wife.

Yet another medical man in love with a 'loose woman' is Dr Edwin Ingleby in *The Young Physician*[181] by Francis Brett Young. Edwin, who is besotted with a chorus

---

* Christopher's arm becomes infected due to an inadvertent 'needle-stick' during surgery.[176] Similarly, Bashford's neurosurgeon loses an arm[177] and Francis Brett Young's Dr Jonathan Dakers dies[178] as a consequence of infections acquired in the operating room or the mortuary. The 1931 President of the American College of Surgeons ridiculed the apparent obsession of fictional authors with such accidents,[179] but the theme was recently revived by Peter Goldsworthy.[180]

girl, discovers the night before his final examination results are announced, that the young lady is deceiving him. He bursts in on his inamorata, who is closeted with his old enemy Griffin, a womanizer and a syphilitic. There is a fight, Griffin dies (of cardiac arrhythmia), and Edwin is instantly cured of his infatuation. Dr John Hammond, another of Francis Brett Young's physicians,[182] is less fortunate. Hammond, an earthy character, has 'a strong taste for women', but his taste lacks discernment. Soon after setting up in practice in 'Wednesford' he proceeds to marry 'Hilda', a local girl who is so coarse and so devoid of formal education that 'the people [the doctor] mixed with couldn't stomach [her].' She has various sexual affairs both before and after her marriage, she drinks immoderately and eventually Hammond divorces her on the grounds of adultery.[182]

An American instance of the medical cuckold is Collier's Dr Rankin, 'a decent and straightforward guy', who at the age of 45 sets up in practice in a small town and proceeds to marry the local strumpet.[183] The girl is young, stupid and useless as a housekeeper, but her promiscuity is a byword among the locals: 'Everybody just watches and laughs.' The doctor's rough and simple fishing friends who provide him with detailed information about local real estate, cannot bring themselves to warn him about the reputation of his future wife, presumably because they believe (wrongly, as it turns out) that he is more knowledgeable about women than they are.[183]

Tennessee Williams' Dr John Buchanan, the complex principal character in *Summer and Smoke*,[184] appears to give some consideration to the selection of a steady partner, although at the end of the play the audience is left speculating as to whether he makes the right choice. John, an only child, comes from a blighted medical family. His mother dies when he is quite young, but he vividly recollects the painful deathbed scene.

> 'She didn't look like my mother. Her face was all ugly and yellow and – terrible – bad-smelling. . . . She caught hold of my hand and wouldn't let me go – and so I screamed and hit her. . . . They told me that I was a devil.'[184]

John is then raised by his elderly medical father,[185] who persuades the boy to attend college and the Johns Hopkins* Medical School, where he graduates *magna cum laude*.[186] He returns to his home town of 'Glorious Hill' with the vague intention of joining his father's practice, but there is a problem. In addition to his medical training, John has also acquired a taste for 'wild living', so that he scandalizes the small Gulf town by gambling, drinking and fornicating.[185] For a while he is not even certain that he wants to practise medicine. Everything changes when old Dr Buchanan dies as a result of John's riotous living. Young Dr John undergoes a Pauline conversion; he takes over his father's practice and becomes the local hero after 'stamping out' an epidemic in a nearby town.[187]

Three young women aspire to the distinction of becoming the consort of this 'Promethean' character with his demoniacal energy.[185] Alma Winemiller, the preacher's daughter from next door, is rejected because of her sexlessness.[188] Rosa Gonzales, a gangster's daughter, is sexy enough (she never makes love 'without scratching or biting'[189]) but in the end she draws too much blood – Papa Gonzales

---

* *See* footnote on pp. 21–2.

shoots the old doctor during an altercation. The successful candidate for the position of 'Mrs Dr Buchanan' is Nellie Ewell, the daughter of the town's lady of easy virtue. Nellie's chief qualifications appear to consist of her youth (she is still attending a finishing school), her good looks and her ability to enjoy herself without pondering unduly over problems of 'soul' or 'conscience.'[190] Nellie is last seen displaying her engagement ring, but Tennessee Williams does not foreshadow whether her inattention to matters of conscience will ultimately lead her in the direction of her mother's profession.

Jonathan Ferrier, the hero of *Testimony of Two Men*,[191] is yet another doctor married to an unfaithful woman with sexual problems. Despite his great medical skills and extremely critical attitude, which extends to his colleagues[191] (*see* pp. 80–1) as well as his patients,[192] he becomes infatuated with Mavis Eaton, a 'brainless and shallow [woman] except where it concerned her demands.'[193] Mavis is well endowed with physical charms but 'almost incapable of being aroused' and 'devoid of sensual passion.'[194] Ferrier's disillusionment with Mavis begins on their wedding night,[193] and soon turns into a murderous hatred, thoroughly reciprocated by the scheming, unfaithful Mavis. This disastrous marriage, which almost destroys the doctor's career,[191] is followed years later by matrimony with a rather withdrawn woman who suspects Jonathan of conspiring to murder her mother.[195] The fate of that marriage is not revealed.

The rich wife

Sinclair Lewis[196] presents a marital combination that is almost guaranteed to lead to disaster. A dedicated physician (Martin Arrowsmith) marries a fabulously wealthy woman (Joyce Lanyon). The driven, tireless doctor fascinates the pampered heiress who has never had to do a day's work, and who fancies that she would like to share his labours. The doctor, who comes from an impoverished background and has had to struggle all his life, is in turn attracted to the 'cool' creature who is used to giving orders and who seems to be totally in control. Martin, the widower, whose first marriage was almost ideal ('the real thing'; *see* p. 43), finds it impossible to live with Joyce, despite her generosity and despite their son (*see* p. 8). He can adjust to her prejudices and her lifestyle, but he rejects her plans to control his career. He walks out and goes to live in a rustic shack where he and a friend will be free to pursue 'pure research' unrestricted by political or family considerations. When Joyce, who is shallow but genuinely fond of Martin, proposes reconciliation, Martin refuses: 'You want a playmate and I want to work.'[197] The same theme is used by Cave in *The Doctor's Wife*,[198] where the rich woman soon tires of her medical husband's punishing work schedule, his refusal to talk platitudes to her circle of friends and his dedication, which she finds 'disgustingly noble.'

The 'mad' wife

One of the best-known fictional physicians, Scott Fitzgerald's Dr Richard Diver – Yale graduate, Rhodes scholar, alumnus of the Johns Hopkins* Medical School and

---

* In literature dating from the first half of the twentieth century, the Johns Hopkins Medical Establishment is mentioned by name more frequently than any other single hospital or medical school. An entire novel[199]

Vienna-trained psychiatrist[202] – finds it hilarious that the immensely rich Devereux Warren proposes to 'buy' himself a young doctor who will marry Nicole, his schizophrenic daughter, in order to care for her on a full-time basis.[203] The situation becomes less amusing when Richard himself takes on the position of Nicole's husband, physician and custodian and, in the process, destroys his career and himself. He has to participate in Nicole's recurrent delusions[204] rather than analyze them under the protection of a white coat (*see* Volume 1, Chapter 3) and from behind a physician's desk. By way of compensation, the Warren fortune sustains Richard as the spiritual head of the idle rich on the French Riviera, so long as he remains married to Nicole.[205] When he can no longer cope with his wife/patient and the marriage falls apart, Richard's attempts to resume clinical practice[206] are unsuccessful. His powers of analysis and detachment have become blunted, his encounters with patients are painful or confrontational,[206] and refuge in alcoholism is the inevitable outcome.[206] As his marriage to Nicole (and his association with the Warren millions) is nearing its end, Dick briefly reflects on how and why he has ruined his career and his life.

> He had made his choice, chosen Ophelia, chosen the sweet poison and drunk it. Wanting above all to be brave and kind he had wanted even more than that to be loved.[207]

Even medical classmates may enter into disastrous unions. Dr Katrina Silverstaff,[208] who goes through medical school with her future husband, Dr Otto Silverstaff, chooses a particularly bizarre method to injure him and herself. After ten years of marriage, Katrina can evidently no longer endure Otto with his 'dedicated round little body' and his punctuality. She takes leave of reality and speaks only in incomprehensible riddles. Not content to simply walk out or to act like a 'regular' psychotic, Katrina punishes her boring spouse by taking an unkempt itinerant pedlar into her bed the night before her death. It comes almost as a relief when, at the end of the story, Otto and the children are still alive, although the one-night lover is shattered by his experience and turns into a drunkard.

Mary Ann Herndon, a nurse who has 'landed' a doctor,[209] becomes morbidly possessive during her second pregnancy:

> and her jealousy expanded with the size of her stomach. And Mary Ann knew women too. They couldn't keep their hands off him. Wedding rings? Children? For a woman after a man they didn't exist.[209]

She becomes fat and depressed; 'dishes were piled in the sink, the bathroom smelled of unwashed diapers, dust rolls were everywhere.' After a trip to a psychiatric establishment, Mary Ann

> returned home cured. . . . She had both children in her complete charge, did the housework and laundry meticulously and renewed her own wardrobe. . . . She never complained, seemed very happy but would never discuss anything with him but the children, her plans for a garden,

---

forms a thinly disguised hagiography of the founders of this legendary institution. In the more recent literature, the 'place of honour' has been taken over by the Harvard Medical School and its associated hospitals, with Johns Hopkins being actively disparaged, as in 'What the hell do you expect of a Hopkins man?'[200] or '[What are] the two most overrated things in the world? Answer: sexual intercourse and Johns Hopkins University.'[201]

her bridge club. . . . She would hear nothing about his professional life which occupied eighty-five per cent of his time. . . . She was cured but he was living with a stranger.[209]

The story ends with the termination of an extramarital affair between the doctor and a patient, but there will no doubt be others.

It is difficult to assign Dr James Dyer, the central, semi-allegorical character in *Ingenious Pain*,[210] to any sort of medical category. Dyer, with his congenital insensitivity to pain, is an uncaring, highly efficient surgeon whose dramatic operations result in miraculous cures, a large and distinguished clientele, and an impressive bank balance. This emotionless surgical robot is magically transformed into a compassionate, vulnerable human fellow-sufferer, but in the process he loses not only his clinical skills, but even his elementary medical behavior pattern[211] (*see* pp. 211–12).

One feature spans the two phases of Dyer's life: His inability to establish satisfactory sexual relationships. He loses his virginity to a set of conjoined twins but a day later watches, quite unmoved, the murderous operation that separates the girls and leaves both of them dead on the operating table.[212] Neither the adulterous passion of his partner's wife[152] (*see* p. 17) nor the subsequent suicide of the husband[213] engage him emotionally. The woman's infatuation is aggravated by his indifference, but 'he understands what is required of him. She is there to be taken.' When, after her husband's death, she takes to her bed, Dyer does not even bother to visit her.

After his metamorphosis and his rapid progress in the 'school of suffering', he fantasizes about setting up in general practice, with Dorothy Flyer ('Dot'), a violent, alcoholic, epileptic fellow inmate of a lunatic asylum,[214] as his companion. He proposes to marry this woman, who is sufficiently sane to reject the offer. Dorothy dies the next day but she leaves James one legacy: a taste for alcohol.

'The doctor's wife is generally to blame'

Mary Rinehart, writing in the pre-feminist, pre-managed care, general practitioner days, blames failed practices (and failed marriages) almost entirely on the doctor's wife. She expresses this view through a 'saintly' old nurse[215] who

> had seen a good many medical men ruined by the women they married; common wives; jealous wives; over-ambitious wives. The ordinary man could leave his wife at home and go to his business. The average doctor could not.[215]

It was the duty of the doctor's wife to achieve 'the necessary compromise',[215] and it was her fault if the practice or the marriage (or both) failed. This one-sided view was laid to rest well before Rinehart's time, when writers such as Henry Handel Richardson[216] and Virginia Woolf[217] portrayed medical marriages that were destroyed by the doctor's behaviour.

The domineering husband

The theme of the overbearing husband who treats his wife like one of his children is not confined to medical novels. However, the doctor, who possesses specialized knowledge that his wife does not share, and is revered by patients who treasure his most trivial remarks, is particularly prone to become paternalistic towards his spouse.

Some medical wives are prepared to tolerate this state of affairs. Proust's 'good-natured' Léontine Cottard, who is anxious to please her prominent medical husband, 'and trembled lest she failed to do so',[218] shows no signs of resenting his contemptuous observations which are shouted across the room during a card party at a friend's home: 'Look at yourself in the mirror. You're as red as if you had ... acne. You look just like an old peasant.'[218] Maria Howe, wife of Dr Elijah Howe in *Miss Susan Slagle's*,[199] is completely under the domination of her husband, who even dictates what clothes their daughter is to wear at a dance. Mrs Howe and her daughters seem comfortable with their subordinate status, although Dr Howe's young son, Elijah, shows signs of rebelliousness. Rinehart's Dr David Mortimer and his wife form 'a great team' because she does not object to the doctor 'throwing his boots at her when he felt so inclined'[215] (*see also* 'Happy marriages: subservient but contented wives', p. 39).

Mary, the loyal wife of Dr Richard Mahony,[219] does not have to put up with this kind of indignity, but she does endure a great deal of verbal abuse. Mahony, a deeply flawed character, is selfish, capricious, impulsive and prone to outbursts of temper as well as bouts of morbid introspection, long before he develops organic dementia. When his wife becomes pregnant after many years of childlessness

> he no longer wished for children. One needed to be younger than he, still in the early years of married life, to accept their coming unconcernedly. (Nor was he enough of a self-lover to crave to see himself reduplicated.) [The children] dimly conscious of his perpetual uneasiness . . . never really warmed towards their father.[219]

Mary endures constant irrational reproaches, while Richard cannot tolerate even the slightest suggestion that he might be mistaken.[220] The two stay together – indeed, Mary nurses her demented, paraplegic husband during his final illness.[221] However, Richardson leaves the reader in little doubt that if Mahony had retained his health and his capacity for physical violence, Mary would have left him.

The Bradshaws' marriage in Virginia Woolf's *Mrs Dalloway*[222] remains officially intact. Lady Bradshaw's photographs 'in court dress and ostrich feathers' still adorn Sir William's office, but the lady herself has become totally crushed by her authoritarian psychiatrist husband, and no longer possesses a personality of her own. 'There had been no scene, no snap, only the slow sinking, water-logged, of her will into his.' She has become obese and she displays symptoms of vague ill health.[222]

Hemingway does not provide any background information about the couple in *The Doctor and the Doctor's Wife*,[223] but suggests that the wife copes with her aggressive husband and her own lot in life by lapsing into bouts of invalidism (possibly migraine). She calls out from 'the room where she was lying with the blinds drawn', and her illness (whatever its nature) obviously constitutes a major factor in the family dynamics.

François Mauriac, like Hemingway a Nobel laureate and son of a physician, describes two dysfunctional medical families in considerable detail. Dr Paul Courrèges and his wife in *The Desert of Love*[114] are discussed on p. 13. The other miserable marriage involves Dr Élisée Schwartz, a Jewish doctor, and Catherine, his aristocratic wife, who met during their undergraduate days when both of them supported 'left-wing' causes.[224] Unlike the stupid Madame Courrèges, whose husband ignores her, the intelligent Catherine has to endure constant verbal harassment and ridicule. Schwartz, now a prominent psychiatrist rather than a radical student, treats his wife

> especially when other people were present, with an extraordinary lack of consideration. His language when he addressed her was carefully designed to wound. After twenty years he had got so much into the habit of humiliating her on every possible occasion that he did so . . . quite automatically and without any deliberate intention.[225]

When, at ten o'clock one night, Catherine tells her husband's secretary to go home, assuming that the doctor will not be doing any more work, Schwartz promptly and offensively countermands his wife's instructions.

> No sooner had Élisée Schwartz heard Catherine's words through the wall, than he opened the door of his consulting room. Without so much as a glance at his wife he said to his secretary: 'I will call you in a moment. Please remember that in this house it is I who give orders.'[225]

Listening at the door while Dr Schwartz examines Thérèse, a woman who has tried to poison her husband and who still harbours murderous tendencies, Catherine

> could have sworn that it was another man he had in there with him, some good-natured friend whom she did not know. She realized why . . . his patients so often said: 'He's perfectly charming, so kind, so gentle' . . . The doctor . . . never used . . . [his] grave tone on her.

Later that evening Catherine tells her husband that she no longer loves him, causing the reader to speculate why it has taken her 20 years to discover that her husband is an aggressive tyrant and her marriage a total debacle.[225]

Dr Edward Loring, a minor character in Raymond Chandler's *The Long Good-bye*,[226] is pompous, self-righteous and morbidly jealous, and suffers from chronic fatigue punctuated by outbursts of belligerence. His wife, a multi-millionaire's daughter, who presumably married Loring for the magic letters after his name, can no longer tolerate his antics and his pathetic attempts to assert himself, and leaves him (with Daddy's approval).[227]

Fay Weldon, herself the daughter of an unsuccessful medical marriage, examines the frustrations of Margot, wife of Dr Philip Bailey, a general practitioner in a London suburb.[228] Philip is not by nature an aggressive bully. Indeed, set among the marital infidelities, the bastard children and the ghastly, lacerating family squabbles of *Remember Me*,[228] the Baileys' marriage seems relatively successful. However, over the years, Margot, a nurse, has turned herself into the doctor's slave, 'cleaning up, picking up, bending down and putting back. Philip's dirty socks and Philip's shoes; Philip's wallet, always lost; Philip's memos here and there; Philip's tissues, nail parings, hair clippings.'[229]

After 15 years of this kind of life, Margot's resentment begins to come to the surface: 'I am the doctor's wife,' she ruminates,

> 'mother of the doctor's children; I am used, put up with, ignored; I am . . . my husband's adjunct, neither smart nor beautiful nor successful.'[230]

Like Catherine Schwartz,[225] Margot Bailey adds a medical flavour to her complaints. She contrasts her husband's tolerance and compassion for his patients with his attitude towards herself.

> 'He sympathizes with, understands and heals the whole world and its populace with the single exception of . . . [myself].'[231]

The accomplishments of Dr Stephen Courtney-Briggs in *Shroud for a Nightingale*[232] do not extend to a harmonious family life. Courtney-Briggs, a successful, wealthy and egotistical surgeon, is ashamed of his late brother Peter, a homosexual actor and compulsive gambler who hanged himself. 'Peter had violated his brother's first principle, the necessity of being successful.'[232] Stephen speaks with obvious distaste of his brother's suicide, which he considers, like everything else,

> in relationship to himself. 'Not a very dignified or pleasant way to go, but the poor boy hadn't my resources. The day when they make my final diagnosis I shall have more appropriate measures available than doing myself to death on the end of a rope.'[233]

Muriel, Courtney-Briggs' wife, is independently wealthy[234] and able to deal with her overbearing husband in her own way. 'She goes around with a smart set and . . . doesn't . . . qualify for the League of Purity.' Dr Courtney-Briggs has a transient affair, with a nurse 20 years younger than himself, and bitterly resents this young woman 'who had the temerity to reject him before he had chosen to reject her.'[234]

Habitual or occasional philanderers

The inclination to seek multiple sexual partners, and the problems that stem from this propensity, are clearly not confined to members of the medical profession. However, there is a widespread perception that marital infidelity is an occupational hazard for doctors, and that the wife of a lecher with a medical degree has to cope with risk factors over and above those facing the wife of a lay Casanova.

Physicians working in large institutions are regarded as particularly prone to the lures of the flesh. 'These doctors and nurses', says the deputy sheriff in Faulkner's *Wild Palms*,[235]

> 'What a fellow hears about hospitals. I wonder if there's as much laying goes on in them as you hear about.' 'No,' Wilbourne said, 'there never is any place.' 'That's so. But you think of a place like a hospital, all full of beds every which way you turn. And all the other folks flat on their backs where they can't bother you. And after all doctors and nurses are men and women.'[236]

Slaughter expresses the same notion: 'Kay had worked enough in a big teaching hospital . . . to know what goes on in one of the most highly sexed atmospheres existing anywhere, except maybe a brothel.'[237]

Whether the promiscuous doctor is at his hospital, in his office or in the process of making house calls, his jealous partner continually has to worry about the latest temptation to which he might succumb. Moreover, the doctor has been trained to lie to his patients (*see* Volume 1, pp. 129–31), so the insecure wife suspects that the signals of affection emanating from her husband are as dishonest as the 'good' news he provides to sick and dying people. Cynthia Derry, the anorexic wife of Dr Kevin Derry,[238] admires and envies her calm and competent husband, who can change their little girl's nappies and handle their boy's tantrums as easily as he reassures his patients. After overhearing a telephone conversation between Kevin and one of his patients, Cynthia comments somewhat wistfully on his ability as a 'healer.' He responds, 'Why make people gloomy? Tell them the best. I lie a great deal in my work.' Cynthia is not happy with Kevin's mendacious talents. '[Lying] seems to come easily to you. Do you lie to me?' she asks.

An early example of the medical lecher is to be found in Hardy's *The Woodlanders*,[239] where Dr Edred Fitzpiers has an affair with a village girl while engaged to be married to Grace Melbury, and continues to be unfaithful to Grace within a few months of their wedding. The two ultimately become reconciled, but Grace's father expresses considerable doubts about his philandering son-in-law. He does not specifically mention Fitzpiers' profession, but it would be surprising if the temptations associated with the young doctor's women patients did not enter Melbury's mind.

> 'Well – he's her husband', Melbury said to himself, 'and let her take him back to her bed if she will. . . . But . . . it's a forlorn hope for her and God knows how it will end!'[239]

Rinehart's mayor[3] is more open about the snares that beset doctors:

> 'A girl is a fool to marry a doctor . . . out at all hours, sitting by other women's beds and holding their hands.'[3]

Dr Solomon Margolin's adulterous behaviour[240] is not the only reason for the dreariness of his marriage, but it is certainly a major factor. Dr Margolin's career has survived his migration from Europe to New York City, but his childless marriage to Gretl, a German nurse, has turned exceptionally dull. Gretl, a loyal creature, has tried for years to adapt to the doctor's Jewish ways and to atone, single-handedly, for the Holocaust by performing the most menial domestic chores. She suffers from dyspareunia and other menopausal symptoms, while he 'had always had a way with women . . . [and] still pursued them more than was good for him at his age.' Understandably, Gretl 'suspected him of carrying on with every female patient.' The two are separated by 'a strangeness that comes of great familiarity.'

In *A Wedding in Brownsville*,[240] Margolin meets a middle-aged woman who claims to be his teenage sweetheart and, for a brief moment, this medically trained man entertains the bizarre idea of running away from Gretl in order to recapture his lost youth with this complete stranger.[240]

The theme of the seasoned medical fornicator and his unsatisfactory family life reappears in several other works of fiction. Dr Courrèges Senior, a famous surgeon and lifelong lecher in Mauriac's *The Desert of Love*,[115] 'had never paid the slightest attention to his son, to whom he habitually referred as "the young 'un" as though he had forgotten his name' (*see* p. 13). Thomas's *Pictures at an Exhibition*[241] contains an account of a neurosurgeon who has retired from his professional but not his libidinous activities (*see* p. 37). In novels that describe unhappily married partners in group practices,[242,243] at least one couple is miserable because of the husband's habitual philandering.

Peter Straub's Dr Michael Poole,[244] a paediatrician and Vietnam veteran, is not a habitual philanderer. However, he has lost interest in his intelligent and attractive wife and is now prone to the temptations that beset medical doctors. Instead of finding himself a 'proper' girlfriend, he forms an unhealthy relationship with a teenage patient who suffers from a terminal malignancy.

Medical practice and family dynamics in late Edo Japan were both so different from their contemporary Western equivalents that any comparisons seem inappropriate. Yet even in this insular setting, one can find hints that the doctor's relationship with his wife may be complicated by his medical activities. When Sawako Ariyoshi's Doctor Hanaoka and his wife Kae finally consummate their marriage, the virgin bride

> who had no knowledge of bedroom intimacies . . . and . . . was quite uninformed about foreplay . . . concluded that [her husband's] actions were motivated by professional curiosity. . . . It appalled her to see him acting like a doctor in these circumstances.[245]

The doctor's work habits

Both in real life and in fiction, medical marriages are under constant strain because of the doctor's commitment to his work and his constant absences from home. The neglected wife reacts by taking a lover, drinking alcohol, or simply becoming bored and bad-tempered, driving the doctor even further towards the sirens awaiting him at the office or in hospital.

Nitzberg's *Hippocrates' Handmaidens* contains endless accounts of disgruntled and angry doctors' wives who no longer wish to be 'patient and understanding.'[246] Nitzberg, who writes from the point of view of a committed feminist and 'stress reduction therapist', gained her insight into unsatisfactory medical marriages during interviews with unhappy 'sisters' who felt left out of their husbands' professional lives[247] and dissatisfied with their own 'lack of power.'[248] One fairly typical wife describes herself as suffering from 'isolation, disconnection, not feeling important or understood.'[249] Most of the time she does not know where her husband is or what he is doing. The husband, 'a big lung specialist,' naturally won't go to counselling; he despises psychiatrists and their activities. He cannot see anything amiss and does not understand what is distressing his wife.

> 'I've provided a good life, I've worked like a dog. What's wrong with you? Why are you angry and upset?'[249]

Dr Marian Crowder, a fictional feminist, addressing a group of doctors' wives at a medical convention,[250] warns her middle-aged audience that in a year or two some of them will no longer be attending medical conferences. Their hard-working, successful husbands will still be there, accompanied by new partners: 'nurses, technicians and other women on the make with which the average hospital population virtually teems.'[250]

The concept of the totally dedicated doctor and his 'neglected' wife is not new. The eighteenth-century Dr Oloroso,[251] 'though a Spaniard and already well stricken in years', is too absorbed in his work to worry about his wife's fidelity or to develop any jealousy towards young Gil Blas, who serenades her in the evenings.

His profession engrossed him wholly and as he returned fatigued from his patients in the evening, he went to bed betimes without being alarmed at his wife's attention to our concerts.[251]

Paradoxically, the doctor's busy practice, which is the basic cause of his wife's waywardness, ultimately prevents the consummation of an adulterous act. The doctor's young wife smuggles Gil Blas into her house 'but just as Cupid . . . was about to crown the lovers' happiness' their 'conference' is interrupted by an emergency call.[251]

Conversations, if any, between medical husbands and their wives are restricted to the doctor's limited field of endeavour – clinical medicine. During the brief period when the Bovarys' marriage seemed happy,[76] Charles

> came home from his rounds late – ten o'clock, sometimes midnight. He was hungry at that hour and . . . Emma served him. . . . He would . . . tell her [about] . . . every person he had seen, . . . every prescription he had written; and he would complacently eat what was left of the stew. . . . Then he would go up to bed, fall asleep the minute he was stretched on his back and begin to snore.[76]

The negative effects of the doctor's working hours on his marriage are stressed repeatedly in Mary Rinehart's *The Doctor*.[121] The future father-in-law of Dr Chris Arden is not at all pleased when he learns that his daughter may be interested in marrying a young doctor. 'What kind of life will she have? At everybody's call, all hours of the night and day. And no future in it.'[215] One of Rinehart's interns, 'laying down the law after the fashion of all interns', echoes these sentiments:

> 'We doctors make rotten husbands. . . . A man who is really set on getting anywhere in medicine or surgery can only have one job. He can't strike a balance. Either he's a good husband or he's a good doctor. He can't be both.'[252]

Even Chris, the medical hero of the novel, agrees.

> All the women who married into the profession took the chance of . . . being only a part of [their husbands' lives]. . . . Their men lived vicariously a thousand lives but they lived only one; and it was only when night came and . . . a tired man turned to some woman for comfort, that their men were their own.[215,253]

Black Dr Benedict Copeland in *The Heart is a Lonely Hunter*,[254] a philanthropist and idealistic revolutionary, becomes estranged from his wife and children because of his radical views. A solitary figure, Copeland is disappointed in his children, who revert to traditional black forms of speech, modes of dress and behaviour patterns.[254] He compensates for his unsatisfactory family life with a grueling work schedule, which further aggravates the process of alienation.

Just before the outbreak of *The Plague*,[255] Dr Bernard Rieux, hero and chronicler of Camus' novel, is shown bidding farewell to his wife at the train station. Madame Rieux, who has tuberculosis, is leaving for a mountain sanatorium on one of the last trains out of Oran.

> Then hurriedly he begged her to forgive him. He felt he should have looked after her better; he'd been most remiss. When she shook her head

as if to make him stop, he added: 'Anyhow, once you're back, everything will be better. We'll make a fresh start, you and I, dear.'[255]

Rieux and his wife are not given the opportunity to make 'a fresh start.' She dies in the sanatorium, while Rieux is trapped in the plague-stricken city.[256]

Frank Slaughter[257,258] repeatedly uses the theme of physical exhaustion combined with sexual boredom to explain marital problems among physicians. Dr Jethro Forbes' childless marriage[258] is particularly stale.

> Twice-a-week sex had dwindled years ago to Saturday nights only, and lately they hadn't even bothered. General practice in Revere, Kansas was a twelve- to sixteen-hour day job with only a few hours off for golf on Sunday morning if you were lucky. And a man as tired as Jethro . . . could hardly get much pleasure out of panting over a woman whose only response was to ask 'Are you through?' and reach for the remote-control unit that activated the TV set.[258]

Forbes, a kind and sensible man as well as a skilled and compassionate doctor, makes up his mind to walk out on his wife and his general practice in Revere, Kansas, and to join an old classmate who runs an Albert Schweitzer-type of medical practice in Guatemala.[259] Incredibly, he has barely left home when he meets Alice Perrault, a classical 'convention strumpet' who, he decides, would make an ideal companion to take along with him to his jungle practice.[260] Alice, of course, would have found life in a Guatemalan village totally unbearable. The trip never takes place.

The relationship between Dr Greg Alexander, Chief of Surgery at a Baltimore Clinic, and his wife, Jeanne, although not as loathsome as that of Jethro and Sarah Forbes,[258] is nonetheless under considerable strain because of Greg's persistent absences from home.[257]

> Jeanne Alexander was in the living room of the apartment, nursing a highball glass morosely, when Greg let himself in. One look at her flushed face and glittering eyes told him it was not her first drink, and probably not her second. 'Hello, darling.' He leaned down to kiss her, but she turned her head and his lips touched only her hair. 'I'm sorry I was late.' 'It's nothing new', she said dully.[257]

(There is a subsequent reconciliation.)

In *Women in White*,[237] Slaughter offers the same explanation except that in the standard scenario of this work, the roles are reversed. The wife feels tired and the husband is getting bored.

> I've seen too many of these medical center marriages turn sour after the husband finishes a residency or a fellowship and goes out into practice . . . [The wives] exhaust themselves at the wheels of a station wagon, taking the kids to speech class and ballet school or working with the medical auxiliary because they think it will help their husband's practice. But when hubby comes home at night, what does he find? A tired wife who doesn't feel like taking a bath and dousing herself with perfume before putting on the sexiest lounging pajamas she can buy and making like Cleopatra giving Julius Caesar the hots.[237]

Quite the reverse, the hard-working wives and mothers in *Women in White*, who wear 'plaid skirts and loose sweaters', cannot compete with the younger and sexually more attractive nurses who wear tight-fitting nylon uniforms, and are quite shameless in their hunt for medical husbands.[237]

The workaholic doctor's marriage may survive, at least outwardly, if his wife finds an intellectually satisfying occupation. Claire Barrett (daughter of Dr Richard Barrett) and Dr Mark Harrison (who has just joined her father's clinic) are discussing one of the partners who has been recently divorced from his second wife.[261] Mark begins:

> 'I'm afraid medicine and marriage don't always mix well.' 'It doesn't have to be that way; my mother and father are good examples. He works all the time and she spends her days playing bridge and chairing committees. . . . It's a very satisfactory arrangement.' 'Perhaps that's why you are an only child.'[261]

Starkman's Dr 'Maury'[262] and his angry wife 'Nina' have been married for exactly 15 years. Their festering family problems continue to intensify.

> 'Has he remembered our anniversary this year? The year of . . . our son's running away, our daughter's school failure?'

Nina is sick of being a 'doctor's wife', and starts publishing poems in an 'obscure feminist university journal.' She is 'chipping away at his pedestal' but doesn't quite know how to tackle the job. Should she run away 'to live in a women's commune in Berkeley?' Or perhaps take a lover? In bed, Nina 'succumb[s] but [does not] surrender.' Instead of sharing 'his act of love', she fantasizes about some 'young Chicano . . . she met in the poetry stacks. . . . [Maury] falls asleep immediately . . . anesthetic on his fingers, spittle on his lips.' The situation is saved by the anaesthesiologists' strike. Maury, a surgeon, comes home early bearing a single rose and, for the time being, the status quo is maintained.[262]

Michael Crichton describes an entire cohort of doctors whose marriages disintegrate because of their work habits. One of them, 'Cameron Jackson . . . got divorced last spring,' muses Dr Berry in *A Case of Need*.[263]

> 'Cameron is a busy and dedicated orthopedist and he began missing meals at home, spending his life in the hospital. His wife couldn't take it after a while. She began by resenting Cameron. . . . I often think of Cameron Jackson and the dozen people I know like him. Usually I think of him late at night when I've been held up at the Lab, or when I've been so busy I haven't had time to call home and say I'll be late.'[263]

Boorish medical husbands and their well-educated wives

The demands of medical training and practice make it difficult for physicians (mostly men) to engage in non-medical pursuits, and may leave them poorly educated in comparison with their lay partners (mostly women). This educational discrepancy, which is discussed in detail in Chapter 4, may lead the 'high-tech cave man' to become resentful of his partner's intellectual achievements, while the civilized wife looks elsewhere for intellectual stimuli. Like many other problems that beset doctors' marriages, this theme transcends geographical boundaries.

Mary Braddon's *The Doctor's Wife*,[264] obviously inspired by *Madame Bovary*,[70] describes a sensitive, well-educated woman (Isabel Gilbert) who feels stifled by her virtuous but uninspiring husband (Dr George Gilbert). George, who is 'almost as innocent as a girl'[265] when he marries Isabel, cannot understand his wife's dislike of his ancestral home and his ancient furniture.[266] He has no idea that his physical appearance ('red and knobby hands'[267]), his conversation (schoolboy adventures[268]), his eating habits ('spring onions and Cheshire cheese'[267]) and his presumably clumsy sexual activities are distasteful to her. 'Spring onions! All-the-year-round onions.'[269] The inevitable flatus is not mentioned, but Isabel develops 'headaches',[270] which in nineteenth-century marital parlance means, among other things, 'not tonight, dear.' Dr Gilbert is completely unaware of his wife's dislikes and her frustrations. On one occasion when he finds her crying, he remarks inappropriately, 'I daresay it was the lobster salad . . . I ought to have told you not to eat it. I don't think there is anything more bilious than lobster salad dressed with cream.'[271] Isabel becomes infatuated with an idle, rich, disenchanted politician who writes mediocre poetry, but unlike Emma Bovary, Isabel Gilbert sins only in the spirit and not in the flesh. The book ends with the death of both the doctor and the lover, and with Isabel left as a rich widow.[264]

The story of Dr Osip Dymov[155] and his wife ('The Butterfly'; *see* pp. 17–18) is told from the point of view of the dedicated and cuckolded doctor. Had Chekhov been more sympathetic towards Olga, he might have mentioned her frustration at being married to a one-sided man who is unable to appreciate any of her various artistic activities. Olga paints, she acts and she plays the piano, but none of her accomplishments generates the slightest interest in the good, narrow husband. Is it any wonder that she seeks comfort from an artist who, she fancies, appreciates her talents?

Another medical boor, Proust's Professor Cottard,[218] does not have to worry about the impact of his ignorance on his marriage. His loyal wife, whose only aim in life is to please him (*see* p. 24), is not at all ashamed when, during her musical soirées, her tone-deaf husband departs for another room,[272,273] where he plays cards with a few kindred spirits (*see* Chapter 4).

Dr Will Kennicott, Sinclair Lewis's conscientious but unrefined general practitioner,[274] is unable to appreciate Carol, his librarian wife, and her literary endeavours (*see* Chapter 4). She reciprocates by trying to find intellectual satisfaction elsewhere, and there is a temporary separation. However, she ultimately comes to realize that her husband's medical and non-medical activities ('water pipes, goose hunting, Mrs Fagero's mastoid') are more genuine than the affectations of her literary set, and the two are reunited.[274]

The educational gap between Dr Andrew Manson, the medical hero in Cronin's *The Citadel*,[275] and his schoolteacher wife, Christine, is not the main reason for their estrangement, but it forms the basis of their first serious disagreement. The two are at a dinner party, where he feels humiliated by her ability to discuss literature and music, subjects about which he knows nothing (*see* p. 148). The subsequent marital strains are caused by Andrew's abandonment of his principles rather than by Christine's educational supremacy. His efforts to move upwards on the social scale, his greed and his infidelity almost wreck the marriage and although there is a reconciliation, Christine is killed soon afterwards, and the reader is left to wonder whether the euphoria would have continued.[276]

Dr Jim Ridgeley in *The Group*,[277] who had 'never read *Middlemarch*',[72] nevertheless imitates Tertius Lydgate and suddenly proposes to marry Polly Andrews, a lachrymose young woman who 'pressed her wet cheek against his stiff white coat.'[278] Like the Lydgates, the Ridgeleys are intellectually incompatible. Jim 'could not read novels', whereas Polly has had a superb education both at home and at Vassar College. However, unlike some of the other sad couples in *The Group*, the Ridgeleys are still together at the end of the book, and Polly, who is both highly educated and highly sexed, shows no signs of tiring of her 'good', illiterate and somewhat sexless medical husband.[277]

Brian Moore's *The Doctor's Wife*,[*][281] describes the disappearance of Sheila Redden, wife of Dr Kevin Redden, a Belfast surgeon. Unlike Charles Bovary[70] and George Gilbert,[264] Kevin is no simple poltroon.

> He had his FRCS and was on the staff of the Royal, the Protestant teaching hospital, which, when you considered that he was a Catholic, meant he knew his stuff.[282] [Sheila, who] had a restless side to her . . . had married very young at a time when she was unsure of herself and her prospects. . . . She was fond of reading and the theatre. Redden . . . [who] never opened a book, liked . . . golf and fishing.[282]

Like Dr George Gilbert 100 years earlier, Dr Redden is totally oblivious of his wife's discontent. 'Not one cross word' has passed between them.[282] Sheila and Kevin are planning a vacation in the south of France, but owing to a series of incidents related to his practice, the doctor has to stay in Belfast. He encourages Sheila to set out on her own, and within days she is in bed with a casual acquaintance whose genital organs are of gigantic proportions and with whom she is able to perform very explicit sexual acts in positions never attempted by the doctor.[283] The affair ends after a few weeks, but Sheila does not return to her family[281] (*see also* Chapter 4).

The mistrustful doctor

During their training, doctors acquire a logical approach to diagnostic problems, a detachment from the patient's emotions and a rational attitude to the human body. In the case of many doctors this analytical capacity goes out of the window during times of sexual excitement, and an incompatible marital partnership results (*see* p. 12). However, in a few individuals the trait of critical judgement is overexpressed. Such characters develop unwarranted suspicions, and wreck what might have become a perfect relationship. They turn into the antithesis of ardent lovers, and do their 'wooing with tongue depressors and Band-Aids.'[284]

Lilian Hellman's *The Children's Hour*[285] provides an example of a doctor who considers all diagnostic possibilities, and in the process shatters what is left of his engagement. Dr Joseph Cardin is engaged to Karen Wright, a teacher at a small boarding school for girls. Mary Tilford, a 14-year-old who is about to receive a well-deserved punishment, takes her revenge by spreading a malicious rumour about Karen, accusing her of a lesbian relationship with one of the other teachers. Dr Cardin who has previously made Mary's acquaintance after she staged a 'heart attack', knows her to be totally unreliable. Nevertheless he mulls over the possibility

---

* There are at least three other novels[198,245,264] and two short stories[279, 280] by that name. *See* Name Index.

that the child's story might be true. When Karen says to him 'Tell me what you want to know', Cardin replies 'I have nothing to ask. Nothing.' But then, very quickly, he changes his mind. 'Was it ever . . . ?' Karen decides that this element of doubt is not a good basis for a marriage and dismisses Cardin on the spot.[285]

The contrast between the family life of successful doctors and that of less 'fortunate' people

Several novels, short stories and plays contrast the miserable personal lives of successful medical men with those of lay people or undistinguished colleagues, implying that the greater the doctor's success, the less likely he is to find satisfaction in marriage. In *The Price*,[286] Arthur Miller presents two brothers – Dr Walter Franz, the 'successful' surgeon, and Victor Franz, the disgruntled police officer who supported their bankrupt father during the depression.[287] Both have marital problems, but those of the surgeon are much more severe. Victor's wife is discontented and drinks too much,[287] but the family is still intact, and the only son is at Massachusetts Institute of Technology (on a full scholarship).[288] Walter, the surgeon, has had to pay a heavy price for his professional success.

> '[Medicine is] a strange business. There's too much to learn and far too little time to learn it, and there's a price you have to pay for that. I tried awfully hard to kid myself, but there's simply no time for people. Not the way a woman expects, if she's any kind of woman.'[289]

After a bout of domestic violence[290] (*see* p. 220), Dr Franz's marriage falls apart. His daughter manages to become a successful designer,[287] but his estranged sons are not performing well academically. Victor asks about them.

> 'And the boys? They are in school?' 'They often are . . . I hardly see them. . . . With all the unsolved mysteries in the world, they're investigating the guitar.[287] But, what the hell. I've given up worrying about them.'

Busch's *Rise and Fall*[291] is another story contrasting the relationships of two brothers. Neither Jonas Reese, the lawyer, nor Jay Reese, the doctor, enjoys a happy personal life, but somehow the difficulties facing Jay seem more intractable than those facing Jonas. Dr Jay Reese, a native of Brooklyn (before the 'ethnic shift'), 'progresses' from the University of Pennsylvania Medical School via a residency in Syracuse to private paediatric practice in Poughkeepsie, New York. During his student days he marries a black woman, who stays for two years but then leaves him for another man. Now, many years after his wife's departure, Jay, aged 42, imagines that he has found a suitable mate – 'Nellie', a divorcee with a teenage daughter. The woman responds to Jay's advances with a distinct lack of eagerness: ' "Do you love me?" "No.". . . . "Do you like me?" "No.". . . . "Can you tolerate me in small doses?" "I don't think so. No." ' The precocious daughter's attitude is equally unpromising. Despite this bleak outlook, Jay continues to urge Nellie to come and live with him. A physical fight involving mother and daughter aggravates the tensions between Jay and Nellie, but Busch implies that the two will continue to see and traumatize one another.[291] While this drama is being acted out, Jay's young brother Jonas turns up. He has run away from his wife and children, whom he loves in theory but cannot abide at close quarters. The doctor's training enables him to analyze the mutually destructive, adolescent behaviour of family members who injure their loved ones 'just to make them react', but brother Jonas is unimpressed with Jay's analyses, his lectures on love or his advice. Indeed, he argues that he, Jonas, has at least experienced a 'normal' marriage, whereas Jay's prolonged bachelorhood suggests an irregular sexual orientation. Jonas enjoys Jay's discomfiture when Nellie's battered teenager has to be taken to hospital at the end of the story. His own marriage may be 'dying, dead, diseased, whatever you want to call it', but the doctor's personal life is a total wasteland where nothing will ever flourish.[291]

Gerald Green[292] also contrasts the domestic lives of two brothers; in his story both are physicians. Dr Kevin Derry, the 'successful' medical academic, has a rich wife and a dysfunctional marriage. 'Why aren't we more of a family?' asks Cynthia Derry. 'Where's all that togetherness?' 'Largely in women's magazines', replies her cynical husbamd.[293] Cynthia develops anorexia and bizarre sexual behaviour, and kills herself with an overdose of sleeping tablets.[292] Kevin's second marriage, to a medical researcher, ends in separation,[292] while his only son becomes a heroin addict (*see* p. 116). By contrast, Kevin's young brother, Dr Joe Derry, whose wife is a policeman's daughter, is reconciled to his tedious, poorly paid work in general practice (*see* pp. 182–3) by a genuinely happy family life, a rarity among fictional physicians.[292]

In *The Sunlight Dialogues*,[294] John Gardner adds an additional dimension to this litany of successful doctors who cannot manage their private lives. Dr Burns, a psychiatrist who is separated from his wife and taking care of their son, identifies his marital problems but seems incapable of solving them.

> 'We are separated. We cannot live together – a grotesque mismatch of slightly paranoid personalities. So we should stick together for the sake of the child and our arguments eating him alive? We should break up then and deprive him of love?'

Pathetically, this doctor, whose son 'loves me as much as he hates me', asks the Police Chief for help. 'Advise me! What should I do?'[294] The police officer, whose wife is blind, feels embarrassed by this request and decides to leave.

Clusters of doctors suffering from domestic discontent

Some authors portray an entire assembly of doctors who are incapable of achieving a harmonious relationship with their partners. None of the four physicians in Faulkner's *The Wild Palms*[235] give the remotest indication of enjoying a happy family life (*see also* Volume 1, Chapter 7). Dr Henry Wilbourne and Charlotte Rittenmeyer are infatuated with each other but evidently can see no future in their relationship, and literally destroy themselves.[235] The unnamed doctor/landlord who ultimately hands Henry over to the police sleeps 'in the stale bed of his childless wife.'[295] She wears a 'cotton nightgown shaped like a shroud . . . which . . . looked gray as if every garment she owned had partaken of that grim iron-color of her implacable and invincible morality.'[295] The doctor's wife, a metaphor for an unappetizing, inexhaustible dish, out of a sense of duty cooks some gumbo for her impoverished tenants.

> And when [the doctor] came home at noon she had the gumbo made, an enormous quantity of it, enough for a dozen people, made with that grim Samaritan . . . husbandry of good women as if she took a grim and vindictive and masochistic pleasure in the fact that the Samaritan deed would be performed at the price of its remainder, which would sit invincible and inexhaustible on the stove while days accumulated and passed, to be warmed and re-warmed and then re-warmed until consumed by two people who did not even like it.[295]

Doc Richardson, Faulkner's cold and competent surgeon,[296] shows no signs of being capable of love or affection, while even the sympathetically portrayed ship's doctor spends his time travelling up and down the Mississippi rather than attending to his family (if any).[297]

Another group of unhappily married doctors is to be found in Paige Mitchell's *A Wilderness of Monkeys*,[242] which tells the story of a saintly doctor set upon by three treacherous colleagues. The bad guys find the good doctor's work ethic threatening, and decide to destroy his reputation.[298] A court case ensues, the scoundrels are unmasked and the righteous doctor triumphs (*see also* pp. 81 and 130). Apart from having to pay their victim substantial damages,[299] the villainous doctors are also 'punished' by having to endure horrendous marital conditions. Dr Leighton Banning's beautiful but lazy, incompetent and frigid wife[300] hates and despises her husband. She stays with him only because of her determination to retain the title of Mrs Leighton Banning until she finds 'something better', and in the meantime she pays him back in kind for his marital infidelities.[301] Dr Harvey Frank, the instigator of the conspiracy, a man with an ambiguous sexual orientation, visits the local bisexual whorehouse[302] in order to satisfy his more unorthodox urges.[303] At home he is mothered by an unattractive middle-aged wife who provides culinary rather than sexual comfort.[299] Dr Benjamin Rogers, the founder of the clinic, is married to a woman who drinks in private, embarrasses him in public,[300] and finally kills herself with an overdose of sleeping tablets.[304] Their daughter secretly marries the son of Rogers' 'enemy.'

In the house of the righteous doctor, all is love and harmony. The wife is devoted to her husband,[305] while he rejects, with virtuous indignation,[306] the advances of a promiscuous nurse. The children are bright, charming and respectful.[301] The moral of *A Wilderness of Monkeys* is that the good are rewarded and the wicked punished. The majority of doctors are wicked and their marriages are appalling.

Similarly, the four partners and their spouses in Nourse's *The Practice*[243] are all trapped in disappointing marriages. Dr Isaacs' wife, a clone of Mrs Benjamin Rogers,[300,304] succumbs to her husband's constant bullying but takes her revenge by drinking alcohol, humiliating him at parties[307] and, after several unsuccessful suicide attempts,[308] hanging herself.[309] Dr Sonders' wife has to put up with his constant philandering.[310] Amy DeForrest, wife of the internist, becomes increasingly bitter at being trapped in a small town and, one suspects, in a stale relationship with an uninteresting husband.[310] Ellie Tanner, wife of Dr Rob Tanner, is so frustrated by her husband's gruelling work schedule, his uncommunicative behaviour and her total disconnection from his professional activities, that she even longs for scraps of medical gossip.[310] Rob, the crusader, is on the warpath against his colleagues' lackadaisical medical routines and some of their other perceived and real misdemeanours, and does not enjoy small talk. Ellie complains that she is being kept in the dark:

> 'I'm not sure what's happening and I feel so stupid and useless. Other people know things but not me.' 'Like what?' 'Oh, I know it's silly, but the whole town seems to know about Harry Sonders' . . . love life. The girls at the grocery have been tittering about it for weeks, and they assume that I know and I don't know anything. . . .' 'There's not a whole lot to know . . . Harry has got the hots for the local scrub nurse and they take off together after his surgery is finished. So what's to tell you about? Is this exciting dinner talk?' 'At least it's something,' Ellie said.[310]

The Tanners' marriage ends in a separation, although the possibility of a future reconciliation is not excluded.[242]

In Busch's *A History of Small Ideas*,[311] both the general practitioner father and the internist son have marital problems. Hank, the elderly general practitioner, and his wife, Edna, 'are not divorced because their dissatisfaction along with his . . . small medical practice, gave them what matrix they could find for their lives.' Their internist son Sidney, aged 41, has recently married a 38-year-old nurse with an angry, pimply, teenage son who tries 'to keep Sid away from . . . [his parents] in spite of the marriage.' The son's marriage may survive (like the father's), but it is going to be a hard struggle. [311]

Thomas's *Pictures at an Exhibition*[241] begins in the Auschwitz concentration camp where German doctors work as exterminators while the medical inmates assist their masters in their ghastly work with varying degrees of enthusiasm.[312] One of the physicians in the story, while serving in the British army, assists in the release of the prisoners and marries a Holocaust survivor.[313] In addition to this assortment of criminals, willing and unwilling helpers, and liberators, *Pictures at an Exhibition* describes a 'normal' British medical family, to whom the Holocaust is something that one reads about in newspapers or history books. However, neither Dr Alan James, a 'Harley Street' neurosurgeon[314] and experimental neurologist,[315–318] nor his son Christopher, an Oxford-trained psychiatrist, are able to lead a regular family life. Alan, an elderly Lothario (*see* p. 27), cannot keep his hands off Christopher's wife, whom he manages to impregnate. Christopher's mother (Alan's ex-wife) decamps when the boy, whose paternity is uncertain, is aged seven.[315] He grows up sufficiently masculine to play cricket,[315] but instead of enjoying a 'healthy' sex life, he has to content himself with groping fantasies,[315] voyeurism,[319] masturbation[319] and cross-dressing. His wife is portrayed as a shallow, sexually disinhibited woman (*see* 'The Wayward Wife', p. 17) who engages in multiple extramarital affairs[313,316] and denies her husband his 'conjugal rights,'[315] especially when he accompanies his feeble attempts with chatter about her other lovers. Remarkably, Christopher blames his profession rather than his own personality for his wretchedness, concluding that 'it's simply impossible to live a full professional life and be married.'[315]

Clusters of medical lechers continue to appear in contemporary novels. Cuthbert's *The Silent Cradle*,[320] a medical conspiracy* novel, contains accounts of two prowling physicians who regard their marriages as 'a minor complication.'[321] Various other medical characters in *The Silent Cradle*[320] have been through broken

---

* The central theme of medical conspiracy novels almost invariably involves the deliberate mismanagement of patients.

marriages and relationships. The book ends with the union of a 38-year-old female obstetrician and a 46-year-old anaesthesiologist.

The priestly doctor

Workaholic habits, intellectual incompatibility and a work atmosphere that encourages philandering are obviously not conducive to successful family relationships. In addition, there is in operation a more profound mechanism that makes it difficult to imagine doctors 'naked or married.'[322] 'Many patients . . . [don't] want their doctors to have a sex life at all; they need . . . an unthreatening comforting priest-father.'[323,324] Sylvia Plath's Esther Greenwood[325] is furious at the family photograph on Dr Gordon's desk, which is half-turned towards the patient's side.

> 'How could this Doctor Gordon help me . . . with a beautiful wife and beautiful children and a beautiful dog haloing him like the angels on a Christmas card?'[325]

Arnold Bennett[326] expresses very similar sentiments. According to Bennett, before a physician can 'serve at the altar of Asclepios' he must divest himself of his monetary affairs, his racial and religious prejudices and his family ties. After his lunch, Bennett's Dr Raste[326] acts like a normal father, discussing the family dog with his little girl, but this charming scene comes to an end when he has to go to his office to see the afternoon patients. 'He had no child nor dog now. He was the medico, chemically pure.'[326]

The notion that his doctor could be leading a normal family life seems so outlandish to Thomas Wolfe's Monk Webber[327] that at first he totally refuses to entertain the idea. Monk has sustained some head injuries during a fight, and is being treated by Dr ('Geheimrat[*]') Becker, a prominent but not particularly skilful Munich surgeon.[328] When Monk, who is spending the night in Becker's establishment, discovers an unsutured scalp laceration, he wants to see the doctor at once and becomes furious when the orderly tells him that the doctor is not available.

> 'At home?' Monk stared at him. 'He has a home! You mean to tell me Becker has a home?' 'But ja. Naturlich,' he said in a tone of patient weariness. 'And wife, and kinder.' 'A wife!' Monk looked blank. 'And children! You mean to tell me he has children?' 'But naturally, of course. Four of them!' That this creature had any existence apart from the life of the hospital had never occurred to Monk, and now it seemed fantastic. His presence possessed and dominated the place; he seemed an organism that was constantly buttoned to its thick, strong neck in a butcher's robe of starched white, and no more to be imagined without this garment in the ordinary clothing of citizenship than one of the nuns in the high heels and trimmed skirts of a worldly woman.[327]

Arnold Bennett,[326] Thomas Wolfe[327] and Sylvia Plath[325] all articulate the same concept – the bustling wife, the brood of children and the family pet do not fit into the picture of the healer/philosopher/confessor, whether skilful or otherwise. These distractions exist, but they distort the image.

---

[*] The title 'Geheimrat' (= confidential councillor) was bestowed on prominent citizens including physicians by various German Governments before 1918.

Happy marriages: subservient but contented wives

Some nineteenth-century writers do not see the doctor's family life as an unmitigated disaster. Charles Dickens, for instance, has no problems with Mrs Esther Wood-court, wife of Dr Allan Woodcourt in *Bleak House*.[329] She is quite happy to bask in the reflected glory of her wonderful husband, who is universally admired and praised.

> 'The people even praise me as the doctor's wife. The people even like me as I go about, and make so much of me that I am quite abashed. I owe it all to him, my love, my pride. They like me for his sake as I do everything I do in life for his sake.'[329]

Similarly, Charlotte Yonge evidently regards the marriage of Dr and Mrs Richard May[7] as perfect. 'Papa' is a respected and kindly professional man, although sardonic and somewhat overbearing towards his 11 children. 'Mamma' is saintly and submissive. Like many of his fictional colleagues, Dr May is a widower. Within the first few pages of the book, the doctor's carriage overturns, and Mrs May dies from head injuries.

Charles Reade is a little more subtle. His hypomanic and somewhat paranoid Dr Sampson,[330] whose colleagues regard him as a crank (but whose theories are ultimately proved correct), has a charming wife who tactfully controls her husband's boisterous behaviour. She is able to keep her 'lion' house-trained so that he does not bore the guests at a wedding party with his multiple grievances and long lists of conspirators who are plotting against him.[330]

> Whenever he got racy, she put a hand gently on his shoulder and by some mesmeric effect it moderated him.

Lucy Snowe, in Charlotte Bronte's *Villette*,[331] supplies a detailed chronicle of the relationships between Dr John Graham Bretton and his various women. As Lucy is herself a half-hearted aspirant to the doctor's favours, her testimony, favourable or otherwise, must be considered somewhat unreliable. However, in the end all turns out for the best and Bretton becomes a member of that relatively rare species – a happily married medical man. Lucy initially imagines that Bretton is conducting a furtive liaison with one of the domestics at her boarding school. The lady in question is a genuine bimbo, 'a pretty little French grisette, airy, fickle, dressy, vain and mercenary.'[332] Lucy then suspects Dr Bretton (probably unjustly) of harbouring designs on the school principal, who is 'dishonest, rich and fourteen years his senior.'[332] Next the doctor becomes attached to Ginevra Fanshawe,[333] a beautiful, selfish, 'featherbrained' teenage student, 'neither girlish nor innocent',[334] who annoys Lucy in a variety of ways, in particular by her inability or her unwillingness to mend her own underwear.[333] Ginevra, who is aware that the doctor 'loves her to distraction', declares that he 'amuses' her and that she would be 'shocked and disappointed' if she did not 'break his heart.' Lucy asks Ginevra 'I wonder whether [Bretton] is a fool?' Ginevra replies 'He is about me, but he is wise in other things (so they say) . . . I can wind him around my little finger.'[333] Dr Bretton's infatuation with Ginevra evaporates in an instant when she sneers at his mother, who, he declares, is 'better to me than ten wives.'[334]

After these real or imagined false starts, Bretton's quest for a suitable mate concludes with his marriage to Paulina, a childhood sweetheart who at the age of six was an 'officious, fidgety little body'[335] but who is now no longer subject to 'naughtiness and whims.'[336] Lucy's endorsement of Dr Bretton's marriage to this child-wife is fulsome:

> Bright . . . was the destiny of [the doctor's] sweet wife. She kept her husband's love, she aided in his progress – of his happiness she was the cornerstone. [Their] children he reared with a suave, yet a firm hand.[337]

Peter Harding, MD, whose letters make up *The Corner of Harley Street*,[338] is a smug, Polonius-like character, but he enjoys an almost ideal family life. His wife worships him,[339] and his children respect their father and value his opinions. All of them seem 'successful.' The older son, who has a degree in classics,[340] is now a medical student[341] with a Scottish fiancée from a 'suitable' background. Like his father he plays 'rugger' football,[340] and he is about to add grouse shooting to his other accomplishments.[342] Neither the doctor nor his wife seem uneasy when their 23-year-old daughter exchanges her 'progressive' ideas[343] and her young boyfriend[344] for a balding army colonel[345] more than twice her age. The younger daughter has just discovered boys,[346] but gives her parents no cause for concern. The only cloud on the horizon is young Tom, who expresses a desire to become a lay evangelist.[347] The doctor father has to use all his diplomatic skills to discourage his teenage son from making rash and potentially disastrous career changes,[348] and in his last letter Harding hints that he may be succeeding.[349]

In addition to his wife and children, Dr Harding has several other relatives, who are fond of him and come to him for advice. 'Aunt Josephine,' who is prone to hypochondriasis and excursions into 'alternative' medicine,[350] and 'Uncle Jacob,' who has reached the age of 76 despite his insobriety,[351] are treated with amused tolerance. Young Dr John Summers, a nephew, is advised not to worry too much about his youthful appearance even though some of his patients believe in a positive correlation between age and ability.[352] (*See* p. 225.) Even in late middle age, the doctor seems slightly afraid of his older sister and her sharp tongue, so that his letters to her are factual and free from advice.[353] A cousin, the Reverend Bruce Harding, is instructed by the doctor on the relevance of the Anglican Church to the twentieth century[354] and on its attitude towards other denominations.[355]

Harding is the epitome of an urbane Edwardian English gentleman who happens to be a successful physician. He cultivates idleness, and would feel particularly ill at ease with uncouth, single-minded medical heroes like Howard Sommers[356] or Martin Arrowsmith.[48] Indeed, Harding warns his medical-student son against becoming too dedicated: 'Never, never, never pack technical books in your holiday trunk.'[341] Young Horace Harding will no doubt develop into a copy of his father and turn into a fine family man and a mediocre physician.

Dreiser's flawless Dr Gridley[357] has a wife and children, but they are colourless individuals who do little more than provide a background for the wonderful physician. We hear almost nothing about the doctor's sons other than their fondness for birds. His wife reproaches him gently about his indifference to money, while his daughter 'lovingly humoured his every whim.' Naturally, when this philosopher-priest dies, he leaves his family destitute.

Several unexciting twentieth-century fictional physicians manage to combine medical practice with a reasonable family life. In Arnold Bennett's *Riceyman*

Steps, Dr Raste, who has recently returned from military service,[358] takes 'a passionate pride' in his daughter,[359] he escorts her and the family dog on regular walks[326] (*see* p. 38), and his occasional support of the little girl against her mother[326] does not seem to cause any major marital disharmony.

Dr Thomas, the physician of Auden's 'Miss Gee',[360] also seems to enjoy a harmonious family life. We see him at dinner, sharing his food and his hare-brained theories with his wife, asserting that, in his view, sexual frustration causes uterine cancer and implying that she suffers neither from sexual deprivation nor from any malignant disorders. Mrs Thomas responds with what is probably her stock phrase when the table conversation turns to clinical topics: 'Don't be so morbid, dear.'[360]

Dr Frank Gibbs in Wilder's *Our Town*,[361] an 'earthy' physician, practises a recognizable type of monotonous medicine, delivering babies, 'tapping people and making them say "ah".'[362] (*See also* p. 176.) The doctor's wife is a competent cook and housekeeper with no intellectual pretensions. When the two were married the doctor was anxious that 'we wouldn't have material for conversation [to last more than] . . . a few weeks . . . I was afraid we'd . . . eat our meals in silence.'[363] It turns out that the conversation is indeed not particularly scintillating, 'good weather, bad weather,' but it evidently suffices, the two stay together and the family dynamics are satisfactory.

The two undistinguished but conscientious doctors in Barbara Pym's *A Few Green Leaves*[364] practise as family physicians in a small English village. They are both married to 'bossy' wives,[364,365] but the marriages are intact and the two women enjoy participating in the social life of the community.[364,366] Similarly, the three anachronistic 'solo' general practitioners in *While You're Here Doctor*[367] enjoy old-fashioned happy marriages that last a lifetime, although a young trainee family doctor is less fortunate. He is married to an Irish nurse who cannot hold her liquor and who becomes inappropriately exuberant at a dinner party.[368]

John Irving's Dr Nicholas Zajac manages to establish a satisfactory family life on his second attempt. At the beginning of the story, Zajac, an outstanding hand surgeon 'in his advancing forties' is 'first and foremost a divorced dad.'[369] He worships Rudy, his six-year-old son, whose mother 'had nearly succeeded in poisoning Rudy's feelings for his father.' Surprisingly, Rudy Zajac has so far acquired only one of his father's multiple eccentricities and behavioural abnormalities. The boy, like his father and the family dog, has an eating disorder.[369] Despite his impressive penis,[369] the doctor is not particularly interested in casual sex. He leads a celibate existence until he marries Irma, his housekeeper, an uneducated, socially awkward, but athletic and 'well-built' woman in her twenties who adores him[369] (*see* p. 108). The last description of Dr Zajac's home life suggests an atmosphere of absolute domestic bliss enveloping the doctor, his very pregnant second wife, his son and Medea, the dog with the dietary indiscretions.[370] If, at some future stage, Zajac will tire of Irma, who is considered by his colleagues to be 'too coarse to be [his] . . . housekeeper' or, more likely, she will tire of him, there is no hint of any impending decline in conjugal devotion in *The Fourth Hand*.

Happy marriages: negative medical role models

Sinclair Lewis[48] goes out of his way to ridicule two of Dr Arrowsmith's colleagues and to demonstrate that these men, despite their exemplary family life, are very inferior physicians. Dr Coughlin, a general practitioner in 'Leopolis, North Dakota', takes his wife and children on a motoring vacation round the state.[371] During the trip, he drops in on some fellow country doctors, with whom he discusses the collection of fees and the treatment of jaundice, employing as much intellectual rigour as does his wife when she chats about the cost of laundry soap and her recipe for pickled peaches. The most important part of the professional conversation revolves around the perceived shortcomings of medical colleagues. During one particular visit and after the usual preliminaries ('I don't like to knock my fellow practitioner and I suppose he's well intentioned') two of these 'great healers', sitting in judgment on their colleagues, come to the conclusion that one of them is an ignoramus, one a great hand holder, one a loudmouth and one [Arrowsmith] an alcoholic atheist.

Another negative role model from *Arrowsmith* is Dr Almus Pickerbaugh, the Director of Public Health in 'Nautilus', Iowa. Pickerbaugh, a politician rather than a physician (*see* Volume 3), lives in a 'Real Old-fashioned Home' called 'Uneedar-est.'[372] His eight daughters, who bear floral names such as Orchid, Verbena and Jonquil, 'were all bouncing, all blond, all pretty, all eager, all musical and not merely pure but clamorously clean-minded.' They had been trained to sing together as the 'Healthette Octette', and their repertoire included the 'famous health hymn (written by Dr Almus Pickerbaugh) extolling traditional feminine virtues and condemning boozers, spitters and gamblers.' The family played word games, including charades, 'at which Pickerbaugh was tremendous. The sight of him on the floor in his wife's fur coat, being a seal on an ice floe was incomparable.'[372] Throughout the lengthy description of Pickerbaugh, his migrainous wife and his eight bouncing 'chick-abiddees', one is conscious of the childless Arrowsmith wincing at the antics of this 'ideal' family. In the end Pickerbaugh is shipped off to Washington as a newly elected Congressman,[373] while Arrowsmith (who lacks Pickerbaugh's political skills) soldiers on in medicine.

Dr Meade's marriage in *Gone With the Wind* not only survives the war and the loss of two sons, but Mrs Meade also remains genuinely fond of her husband.[374] However, the ubiquitous doctor is hardly a typical medical practitioner, even for the 1860s. His main role is that of a small-town politician ('Atlanta's root of all strength and all wisdom'[375]), he writes patriotic letters to the press and he repeats standard confederacy nonsense at public and semi-public gatherings. He is extraordinarily pretentious, even in the privacy of his bedroom.[374] His medical activities obtrude only occasionally. He offers (inappropriately) to mix his wife a sedative, and he declares (one suspects equally inappropriately) after a cursory inspection that a wounded soldier's hand must be amputated.[376] When Melanie Wilkes bleeds to death after a miscarriage, Dr Meade acts as stage manager, ushering various friends and relatives in and out of the dying woman's room and instructing them in what to say. Rhett Butler sums him up in two words – 'pompous goat.'[377]

Happy marriages: true companionship

Guterson's Dr Ben Givens, a cardiothoracic surgeon, and his wife, Rachel, a burns-unit nurse, are married during the Second World War and remain happy together until her death 50 years later.[378] Givens, 'a restrained, particular man',[379] 'does not take [marital harmony] for granted, even after fifty years',[380] and attributes 'what he had been granted' to the personality of his late wife: 'She was a better person than I am. . . . She gave everything.'[381]

> When they had argued or carried some silent grievance or were divided temporarily by ill-chosen words, still Ben had clung to her. She'd carried a tranquil grace at her center. A poise he could not limn . . . which had kept him turned toward her.[380]

Rachel Givens' poise and serenity are transmitted to her daughter and grandson, who obviously love and admire the old doctor and take care of him during the last few months of his life.[379]

Also reviewed in retrospect, the marriage of Dr Benito Zamora, a Mexican, and his late 'fair' American wife had been a happy one despite their different ethnic backgrounds and their childlessness.[382] Since her death he has become desperately lonely, and he now plans to leave California and return to Mexico to take care of his demented mother and to work in the free clinics he has endowed.

Things are different in the house of *The Last Angry Man*.[383] Sarah Abelman, the placid, loyal wife of Dr Samuel Abelman, watches helplessly as her husband's misguided idealism, his unprofessional attitudes and his recurrent, violent rages gradually destroy his practice.[384] However, she does not consider him a failure, she rarely reproaches him and she remains content to live with him in their Brooklyn slum. The doctor in turn shows no signs of marital infidelity, and he appears happy in Sarah's company despite her obsessive attention to unimportant details and her grating voice.[383]

Three Nobel laureates grapple with the apparent incongruity of the stable medical family, and solve the problem in three different ways. Martin Arrowsmith's marriage to Leora Tozer is almost perfect.[48] Sinclair Lewis makes no attempt to hide the flaws of this restless, argumentative, undisciplined medical researcher or those of Leora, his bright but poorly educated and somewhat lazy spouse. The occasional arguments and tensions between Martin and Leora[385,386] make the 'lasting solidity'[386] of the Arrowsmith marriage all the more credible. Martin commits all the blunders that wreck medical marriages. After an evening at the movies, he sends Leora home in a taxi and goes back to his laboratory where he works all night.[387] He criticizes her 'sloppiness' in diction and dress.[386] He is even tempted by a flirtatious teenager[385] and a lonely, rich widow,[388] although the thought of his loyal wife makes him desist on each occasion. Leora lives totally for Martin.[389] She reminds him of his ideals,[390] particularly when he shows signs of 'turning into a megaphone',[391] but in general she is conscious of having been 'absorbed'[389] by her husband and is content to have no independent existence. There are just two problems with the Arrowsmith marriage. It is childless,[392] and it comes to a premature end when Leora dies in her thirties.[393]

The stormy 50-year marriage between Dr Juvenal Urbino and his wife, Fermina, forms the central theme of Garcia-Marquez's *Love in The Time of Cholera*.[394] The initial omens look dreadful. The two come from totally different cultural and social backgrounds: Juvenal belongs to one of the old colonial families,[395] whereas Fermina's father, an illiterate mule-trader and cattle-gelder,[396] becomes rich as a result of a variety of criminal activities.[397] The doctor has been educated at the University of Paris[398] and pursues many cultural and civic interests,[399] whereas Fermina's scholastic limitations restrict her to domestic affairs and shopping expeditions. Juvenal is a devout and 'militant'[400] Catholic (*see also* Chapter 3, pp. 129–30), whereas Fermina has become 'convinced that the men and women of the Church lacked any virtue inspired by God.'[401] The doctor marries her not for love but 'because he liked her haughtiness, her seriousness and her strength.'[402] After they return from their honeymoon she feels imprisoned and desperately unhappy in the stuffy colonial environment of the Urbino family.[403] Juvenal's behaviour is that of a 'perfect' macho husband. 'He never picked up anything from the floor, or turned out a light or closed a door,' while Fermina's role is that of a 'deluxe servant.'[404] Their sex life is unsatisfactory.

> She always had a headache, or it was too hot, . . . or she pretended to be asleep, or she had her period again, her period, her period, always her period. So much so that Dr Urbino had dared to say in class, . . . that after ten years of marriage women had their periods as often as three times a week.[405]

Juvenal's infidelity leads to a two-year separation. Remarkably, the union recovers and even thrives despite the multiple unfavourable predictive factors. It also produces a mediocre medical son. Juvenal and Fermina navigate their way through 'the arduous calvary of conjugal life',[406] he comes to recognize that 'without her I would be nothing',[407] while in his declining years she assumes the role of the loving carer.[408] Towards the end 'They were not capable of living for even an instant without the other.'[408]

A unique allegorical medical marriage is described in Saramago's *Blindness*.[409] Before the catastrophe, the relationship between the doctor and his wife seems excellent in every respect.[410] Children are not mentioned, but the two are 'close . . . in everything'[410] and they 'still greeted each other with words of affection after all these years of marriage.' She takes an intelligent interest in the clinical problems of his patients, and the physical bond between husband and wife is active and healthy.[410] When the disaster occurs and the doctor succumbs to an epidemic of blindness, his wife, who retains her sight, accompanies him to the quarantine station (a disused mental hospital) because she cannot bear the thought of a separation.[411] As soon as the gates are locked behind them, she turns into a fortress of dignity and common sense, while the doctor loses not only his profession but also his manhood. When the vicious gangsters who tyrannize the inmates use the threat of starvation to obtain sexual favours, he becomes a dispirited consenting cuckold.[412] By contrast, his wife comforts and avenges the violated women. She liberates, guides and nourishes her little group, while he turns into one of her passive and helpless followers.[413] When the mysterious affliction has run its course and the doctor begins to plan a cataract operation, 'when life gets back to normal and everything is working again',[414] this wonderfully resourceful woman seems content to resume her former role as 'the doctor's wife.' Indeed, throughout her brief career as leader she never seeks or receives any other title.*

---

* See footnote on p. 205.

A recent addition to the list of atypical doctors who enjoy an exemplary family life is McEwan's Dr Henry Perowne,[415] the neurosurgical hero of *Saturday*. Perowne, aged 49 and at the height of his career, remains deeply in love with his wife of 24 years. He has confidence in his children and remains remarkably unfazed by his unmarried daughter's pregnancy (which is discovered under unusual circumstances) and his son's exchange of a high-school education for a career in guitar playing. Dr Perowne's love for his wife is reciprocated, and the trust in his children seems justified.[415]

The doctor and his children

In the majority of fictional works, the doctor's relationships with his sons and daughters appear as unsatisfactory as his marriage, with his medical background exacerbating rather than relieving the inevitable tensions between parents and children. He is frequently away from home, but when he does put in an appearance, his presence overwhelms or antagonizes the teenagers. They reject his clinical and rational advice which is accepted by most of his patients. He has been taught to prognosticate and he is better at predicting the consequences of non-compliance than 'lay' parents, but his forceful arguments may produce an equally forceful reaction. Tensions may end in tragedy regardless of whether he prevails or not.

Henry James' classical account of the conflict between Dr Austin Sloper and his daughter Catherine[416] shows what may happen if the doctor has his way. Sloper disapproves of Morris Townsend, a charming but unreliable young man who wants to marry Catherine, the widower-doctor's only surviving child. Sloper's professional analysis of Townsend's motives[417] turns out to be entirely correct – Townsend is indeed an idle and selfish money-chaser.[418] However, in the process of getting rid of Catherine's undesirable lover, Dr Sloper traumatizes her to such an extent with his lack of sympathy and his sarcasm that he leaves her 'deeply and incurably wounded.'[419] She becomes convinced that her father does not love her; she turns into an old maid and entirely loses her capacity for love and affection. Parental disapproval of their children's potential spouses is obviously not confined to medical families, but Dr Sloper's cold, clinical analysis of Townsend's motives clearly aggravates matters.

Maud Thornton, the daughter of Dr Jarvis Thornton in Herrick's *The Man Who Wins*,[420] is younger and more demanding than Catherine Sloper,[416] and the doctor is still in the planning stage. During a dispassionate analysis of his family's clinical problems, Thornton, who wants to do more than simply react to difficulties as they arise, considers a variety of 'preventive measures.' His wife, a chronic invalid, will presumably continue to enjoy ill health and is beyond any meaningful treatment. However, Maud, whose state of health is not much better than her mother's, requires some 'intervention.'

> 'Her nerves are morbid, her egotism is excessive, her restlessness abnormal. She is rather a brilliant girl, I think, and to me a very dear one. . . . As a mother [Maud] would be atrocious.'

After studying his daughter for two years the doctor comes up with what he thinks is an ideal solution to a difficult problem. Maud needs

> 'a certain kind of husband. He must be rich, for Maud had inherited . . . [her mother's] dependency upon luxury. And he must be able to devote

himself pretty steadily to her whims, subordinate himself good-naturedly and obtain for her whatever she might fancy at the time. . . . The desirable husband must be able to place her well socially, for she had already shown herself keen in making distinctions.' Dr Thornton concludes that he needs 'an acquiescent fool for a son-in-law, a kind of gentlemanly valet!'[420]

In the case of Francis Brett Young's Dr John Bradley,[421] the widowed doctor-father is quite incapable of solving his only son's behavioural problems, and cannot even communicate with the young man.[422] Bradley Junior enters medical school but either cannot or will not study. He becomes addicted to opiates (initially prescribed by his father) and dies of an overdose.[423]

Likewise, Dr Emanuel Hain, a respected and overworked surgeon, is unable to exchange even a few significant words with his only child, a teenage son who is going through a sexual identity crisis.[424] The boy adopts a sarcastic attitude towards his father, whom he addresses as 'the professor.' He inquires 'How is the professor feeling tonight? How many corpses has the professor pickled today?' He spends most of his time producing abstract drawings and, predictably, his performance at school deteriorates. Dr Hain, who is quite unable to deal with this predicament, declares that 'The boy gives me the creeps.' He purloins two 'artistic creations' which he shows to his psychiatric colleagues, but they are unable to come up with a specific diagnosis or any meaningful advice. In the end Hain, the Jew, sees his son, a half-Jew, drift off towards the homosexual elements of the Nazi party, where the boy is murdered at the age of 19.[424]

Dr Joshua Randall, a member of a distinguished Boston medical dynasty, has similar problems.[425] Randall, a prominent cardiac surgeon, is unaware or pretends to be unaware of his neglected daughter's dangerous emotional problems. He describes her as 'sweet and beautiful . . . [without] a malicious or dirty thought in her head.'[426] In fact, this 'sweet' girl hates her domineering father so intensely that she ritually throws darts at his picture 'every night before going to sleep.'[427] She has her first abortion at the age of 15,[428] and then continues to become pregnant on a yearly basis. Karen obviously wants to use 'the shame and trouble of an illegitimate child' to punish and humiliate her medical father, and she dies at the age of 17 from a perforated uterus,[429] after yet another attempted abortion.[430]

We do not have many medical details about Joyce Carol Oates' prosperous physician,[431] who lives in a genteel suburb of Detroit, treats the 'slightly sick' and presents papers at medical conventions. On the other hand, we are provided with plenty of information about his 16-year-old kleptomaniac daughter, who 'escapes' from the Country Club atmosphere of Bloomfield Hills to the slums of Detroit. There she is 'befriended' by drug addicts and prostitutes, who use her and then turn her over to the police when they get tired of her. Her father re-enters the story briefly to bail his daughter out of jail and take her back to their 'classic contemporary' home with its high ceilings and its chandeliers. The girl recalls:

'Father. Tying a necktie. In a hurry. On my first evening home he put his hand on my arm and said "Honey, we're going to forget all about this."'[431]

The story of the doctor's daughter who runs off to live in utmost squalor with a group of diseased drug addicts is retold in greater detail in Oates' *Wonderland*.[432]

Michele Ellen ('Shelley') Vogel, daughter of Dr Jesse Vogel, a neurosurgeon, has an IQ of 144 but fails to relate to her parents, her sister or her peers, and performs poorly in high school.[433] Shelley evidently resents her father's power and knowledge to such a degree that she leaves the prosperous family home for the stinking, purulent pigsties inhabited by fellow dropouts and drug addicts. Admittedly, with her family history of major psychoses, Shelley is particularly vulnerable to developing deviant behaviour. Her paternal grandfather kills most of his family and himself in a fit of rage and depression,[434] while her medical father, who barely escapes this mass slaughter, becomes permanently warped through his experiences. Dr Vogel, a highly successful professional man, is described by his colleagues as 'elusive, ambitious, hard-working, brilliant', but to his wife and daughters he remains totally incomprehensible.[435] He wants to possess and protect his family, particularly his favourite daughter, Shelley, who writes to him (from her self-imposed exile):

> You were never home but when you were home you wanted us there. Before you. Humbled before you.[435]

In her letters, Shelley hints at odd sexual fantasies about her father and herself:

> I did not dare stand straight, did not dare let you see how my body was growing. I did not dare risk your eyes on me. Your nervousness. Love lapping onto me like waves, like the warm waves of the pool you built for me.[435]

Shelley's mother, the daughter of a Nobel laureate in physiology[436] who has sexual problems of her own,[437] and does not become a beautiful woman until 'she grew free of [her husband]',[435] is of no help in improving the relationship between Shelley and her father.[438]

On top of all this is Oates' perception that doctors, because of their training, find it particularly difficult to provide love and affection for their families. They feel that they must 'straighten the crooked and plane the rough places', with the result that their wives and children long for the crooked and the rough. One of Shelley's roommates, a dropout from medical school and a drug addict, acts as Shelley's spokesman when the doctor at last finds his daughter, ravaged in body and mind:

> 'I can feel it in you, the desire to do something – to dissect us or operate on us – to snip our nerves – to clean us out with a scouring pad. . . . I know you are a surgeon. But have mercy.'[439]

Dr Carl Pedersen, another medical character from *Wonderland,* is described by Trautmann and Pollard[440] as an 'evil' physician, but the evidence for his misdeeds rests on the testimony of his wife, who is an unreliable witness.[441] Pedersen probably does no more harm than other pompous, domineering and arrogant medical men of his generation.[442] His children do not become drug addicts or run away from home, but his family life is nonetheless a grotesque parody. His daughter Hilda, a mathematical genius,[443] suffers from morbid obesity.[444] His son Frederich, also grossly obese, is considered to be a musical genius, although one gathers that his compositions will never amount to anything.[445] Pedersen's wife is totally dominated by her husband, but comforts herself by drinking alcohol.[446] On at least one occasion she stages a symbolic flight, but within days she is back with her husband, whom she says she detests.[441]

One of the most detailed accounts of the physician as an unsatisfactory family man is to be found in Bellow's *Seize The Day*.[447] The story is that of a prodigal son, 'Tommy Wilhelm', who returns to his father (old Dr Adler) asking for help and comfort. The retired physician, who is not at all pleased by his son's arrival,[448] gives him a lecture on the subject of his ongoing self-destructive behaviour. 'I don't know how many times you have to be burned in order to learn something. The same mistake, over and over.'[449] The final interview ends with Dr Adler crying out 'Go away. . . . It's torture for me to look at you, you slob.'[449]

To some extent Dr Adler is simply a selfish old miser without a shred of generosity. He rejects his only son, of whom he feels ashamed and whose dirty personal habits the fastidious doctor finds repulsive.[450] The old skinflint also declines to help his daughter, whose artistic work he cannot appreciate.[451] He is unable to remember the year of his wife's death,[452] and he refuses to pay for a new stone bench at her grave in the local cemetery.[453]

Bellow suggests several times that the tensions between Tommy Wilhelm and his father are due, at least in part, to Dr Adler's former profession. There is the ever-recurring theme of the lack of time.

> Dad never was a pal to me when I was young, he reflected. He was at the office or the hospital or lecturing. He expected me to look out for myself and never gave me much thought. Now he looks down on me.[454]

Dr Adler is almost 80 years old, he has retired from practice, and shortage of time is no longer a problem for him. However, his medical habits persist. When Tommy, who sees himself as a failure, wants to unburden himself to his father, the old man reacts by 'behaving towards his son as he had formerly done to his patients.'[455] Over many years of practice Dr Adler has learned to ration his sympathy (*see* Volume 1, Chapter 7) and not to waste it on individuals who do not have 'real ailments.'[456] When Tommy persists in discussing his personal and financial problems, the old doctor subjects his son's 'complaints' to close scrutiny and tries to disentangle the truth from the falsehoods.

> 'Why did you lose your job with Rojax?' 'I didn't, I've told you.' 'You're lying. You wouldn't have ended the connection. You need the money too badly. . . . Since you have to talk and can't let it alone, tell the truth. Was there a scandal – a woman?'[456]

Dr Adler provides medical advice: 'Take a swim and get a massage'[449] and 'Cut down on drugs.'[451] Above all, he warns his son not to become involved with an unscrupulous dealer in commodities who will (and does) swindle Tommy out of his last few dollars.[457] When it becomes clear once again that Tommy's condition is not amenable to 'medical' or even common-sense advice, the old doctor removes himself 'from the danger of contagion'[449] and informs his son that he is unable to help him.

Drs David and Angela Wilson, the childlike medical couple in Robin Cook's *Fatal Cure*,[458] have decided, somewhat impulsively, to leave the rarefied medical atmosphere of Boston and to relocate to a community hospital in 'Bartlet', Vermont. They phone their parents to share their excitement. David's mother and father, simple folk who have retired to New Hampshire, are delighted. David and Angela will be almost neighbours of theirs, and there will be plenty of opportunities for visits. Angela's father, a New York physician, is cold and judgemental.

'It's easy to drop out of the academic big leagues,' Dr Walter Christopher said. 'But it's hard getting back in. I think you should have asked my opinion before you made such a foolish move. Here's your mother.'

Dr Christopher is quite right – the move to Vermont is an absolute disaster. However, his correct analysis of the situation does not endear him to his daughter and son-in-law.[458]

Summary

There is no simple explanation for the perception that the male doctor's family life, if it exists at all, is disappointing. The demands of the profession inevitably turn physicians into one-sided individuals. 'Earthy' physical temptations and the 'priestly' nature of his calling pull the doctor in opposite directions, but neither is conducive to a close family relationship. Despite the doctor's training, which enables him to elicit facts and to foresee the future, some members of the profession, almost perversely, choose completely inappropriate partners. Most importantly, the doctor's ability to detach himself emotionally from disasters is inappropriate when applied to feelings such as love and generosity.

References

1 Mitchell SW (1888) *Doctor and Patient*. Arno Press, New York, 1972, p. 99.
2 Rinehart MR (1935) *The Doctor*. Farrar and Rinehart, New York, p. 141.
3 Ibid., p. 75.
4 Williams WC (1952) *The Build-Up*. Random House, New York, pp. 77–81.
5 Green G (1979) *The Healers*. Melbourne House, London, pp. 236–7.
6 Leavitt D (1989) *Equal Affections*. Penguin, Harmondsworth, p. 175.
7 Yonge C (1856) *The Daisy Chain*. Macmillan, London, 1911, pp. 1–24.
8 Lewis S (1924) *Arrowsmith*. Signet Books, New York, 1961, p. 194.
9 Balzac H de (1833) *The Country Doctor* (translated by Marriage E). Dent, London, 1923, pp. 36–7.
10 Shaw GB (1906) The Doctor's Dilemma. In: *The Bodley Head Bernard Shaw: Collected Plays with their Prefaces. Volume 3*. The Bodley Head, London, 1971, p. 351.
11 Söderberg H (1905) *Doctor Glas* (translated by Austin PB). Chatto and Windus, London, 1963.
12 Chekhov AP (1900–1901) Three Sisters. In: *The Oxford Chekhov* (translated by Hingley R). *Volume 3*. Oxford University Press, London, 1964, p. 106.
13 Chekhov AP (1887–1889) Ivanov. In: *The Oxford Chekhov* (translated by Hingley R). *Volume 2*. Oxford University Press, London, 1967, pp. 163–227.
14 Chekhov AP (1888) An Awkward Business. In: *The Oxford Chekhov* (translated by Hingley R). *Volume 4*. Oxford University Press, London, 1980, pp. 99–115.
15 Chekhov AP (1892) Ward Number Six. In: *The Oxford Chekhov* (translated by Hingley R). *Volume 6*. Oxford University Press, London, 1971, pp. 121–67.
16 Chekhov AP (1898) Doctor Startsev. In: *The Oxford Chekhov* (translated by Hingley R). *Volume 9*. Oxford University Press, London, 1975, pp. 51–66.
17 Chekhov AP (1897) Uncle Vanya. In: *The Oxford Chekhov* (translated by Hingley R). *Volume 3*. Oxford University Press, London, 1964, pp. 15–67.
18 Ibid., p. 27.
19 Ibid., pp. 38–40.

20 Ibid., p. 62.

21 Ibid., p. 66.

22 Chekhov AP (1896) The Seagull. In: *The Oxford Chekhov* (translated by Hingley R). *Volume 2*. Oxford University Press, London, 1967, pp. 231–81.

23 Ibid., p. 270.

24 Ibid., p. 239.

25 Ibid., p. 252.

26 Grecco S (1980) A Physician Healing Himself: Chekhov's treatment of doctors in the major plays. In: Peschel ER (ed.) *Medicine and Literature*. Neale Watson Academic Publications, New York, pp. 3–10.

27 Dostoyevsky F (1880) *The Brothers Karamazov* (translated by Magarshack D). *Volume 2*. Penguin, Harmondsworth, 1978, p. 791.

28 Young FB (1919) *The Young Physician*. Heinemann, London, 1934, p. 184.

29 Young FB (1928) *My Brother Jonathan*. Heinemann, London, p. 83.

30 Ibid., p. 553.

31 Ibid., p. 568.

32 Remarque EM (1945) *Arch of Triumph* (translated by Sorell W and Lindley D). Appleton Century, New York, pp. 170–92.

33 Ibid., pp. 41–4.

34 Ibid., p. 252.

35 Faulkner W (1933) Doctor Martino. In: *Dr Martino and Other Stories*. Chatto and Windus, London, 1968, pp. 163–83.

36 Sobel IP (1973) *The Hospital Makers*. Doubleday, Garden City, NY, p. 79.

37 Warren RP (1946) *All the King's Men*. Modern Library, New York, 1953.

38 Norris CB (1969) *The Image of the Physician in Modern American Literature*. PhD Dissertation, University of Maryland, Baltimore, MD, p. 93.

39 Irving J (1985) *Cider House Rules*. Bantam Books, New York, 1986, p. 59.

40 Jewett SO (1884) *A Country Doctor*. Houghton Mifflin Company, Boston, MA, p. 43.

41 Ibid., p. 56.

42 Maugham WS (1915) *Of Human Bondage*. Signet Classics, New York, 1991, p. 652.

43 Marquis DRP (1939) Country Doctor. In: *The Best of Don Marquis*. Garden City Books, Garden City, NY, pp. 444–63.

44 Metalious G (1956) *Peyton Place*. Dell, New York, 1958, p. 33.

45 Ashton H (1930) *Doctor Serocold*. Penguin, London, 1936, pp. 76–80.

46 Ibid., pp. 11–12.

47 Stoker B (1897) *Dracula*. Penguin, London, 1993, pp. 227–8.

48 Lewis S (1924) *Arrowsmith*. Signet Books, New York, 1961.

49 Ibid., p. 374.

50 Ibid., p. 416.

51 Ibid., p. 430.

52 Rollman BL, Mead LA, Wang NY and Klag MJ (1997) Medical specialty and the incidence of divorce. *NEJM*. **336**: 800–3.

53 Kundera M (1984) *The Unbearable Lightness of Being* (translated by Heim MH). Faber and Faber, London, 1988, p. 10.

54 Wilner H (1966) *All the Little Heroes*. Bobbs-Merrill, Indianapolis, IN.

55 Ibid., pp. 42–50.

56 Ibid., pp. 200–10.

57 Ibid., p. 251.

58 Ibid., p. 145.

59 Ibid., p. 311.

60 Grisham J (1995) *The Rainmaker*. Island Books (Dell Publishing), New York, 1996.

61 Ross L (1961) The ordeal of Dr Blauberman. *The New Yorker*. 13 May, p. 13.

62 Galgut D (2003) *The Good Doctor*. Atlantic, London.

63 Ibid., pp. 130–9.
64 Cook R (1981) *Brain*. Pan Books, London, pp. 108–9.
65 Rinehart MR, op. cit., p. 308.
66 Doctor X (Nourse AE) (1965) *Intern*. Harper and Row, New York, p. 241.
67 Cook R (1993) *Fatal Cure*. Pan Books, London, 1995, pp. 114–15.
68 Williams WC (1948) A Dream of Love. In: *The Collected Plays of William Carlos Williams*. New Directions, Norfolk, VA, 1961, p. 156.
69 Williams WC (1932) Old Doc Rivers. In: *The Doctor Stories*. New Directions, New York, 1984, pp. 16–17.
70 Flaubert G (1857) *Madame Bovary* (translated by Steegmuller F). Modern Library, New York, 1982.
71 Gaskell E (1864–1866) *Wives and Daughters*. Oxford University Press, Oxford, 1987.
72 Eliot G (1871–1872) *Middlemarch*. Penguin, Harmondsworth, 1988.
73 Flaubert G, op. cit., p. 12.
74 Ibid., p. 360.
75 Ibid., pp. 13–23.
76 Ibid., pp. 39–49.
77 Ibid., p. 328.
78 Ibid., pp. 394–6.
79 Gaskell E, op. cit., pp. 36–7.
80 Ibid., p. 547.
81 Ibid., p. 32.
82 Ibid., p. 59.
83 Ibid., pp. 147–8.
84 Ibid., p. 114.
85 Ibid., p. 125.
86 Ibid., p. 98.
87 Ibid., p. 337.
88 Ibid., p. 341.
89 Ibid., pp. 398–405.
90 Ibid., pp. 184–5.
91 Ibid., p. 131.
92 Ibid., pp. 683–4.
93 Eliot G, op. cit., pp. 335–6.
94 Ibid., p. 475.
95 Ibid., p. 497.
96 Rothfield L (1992) *Vital Signs: medical realism in nineteenth-century fiction*. Princeton University Press, Princeton, NJ, p. 114.
97 Eliot G, op. cit., p. 854.
98 Ibid., p. 825.
99 Ibid., p. 850.
100 Ibid., p. 861.
101 Ibid., p. 893.
102 Ibid., p. 858.
103 Diogenes Laertius (*c.* AD 200) Socrates. In: *The Lives of Eminent Philosophers* (translated by Hicks RD). *Volume 1*. Harvard University Press, Cambridge, MA, 1972, p. 167.
104 Sayers D (1923) *Whose Body*. Gollancz, London, 1971, pp. 70–1.
105 James H (1884) Lady Barberina. In: *The New York Edition of Henry James. Volume 14*. Augustus Kelley, Fairfield, NJ, 1976, pp. 79–81.
106 Ibid., p. 142.
107 Norris CB, op. cit., p. 155.

108 Danby F (Frankau J) (1887) *Dr Phillips: a Maida Vale idyll*. Garland Publishing, New York, 1984.
109 Ibid., pp. 340–1.
110 Ibid., p. 52.
111 Ibid., pp. 27–30.
112 Ibid., p. 250.
113 Ibid., pp. 316–21.
114 Mauriac F (1925) *The Desert of Love* (translated by Hopkins G). Eyre and Spottiswoode, London, 1949.
115 Ibid., p. 68.
116 Ibid., p. 55.
117 Ibid., pp. 35–6.
118 Ibid., p. 92.
119 Ibid., p. 82.
120 Ibid., pp. 154–8.
121 Rinehart MR, op. cit.
122 Ibid., pp. 247–9.
123 Ibid., p. 465.
124 Ibid., pp. 500–6.
125 Blodgett R (1932) *Home is the Sailor*. Harcourt Brace, New York, pp. 84–92.
126 Ibid., p. 325.
127 Ibid., pp. 258–66.
128 Ibid., p. 239.
129 Ibid., pp. 337–48.
130 Ibid., p. 287.
131 Bellaman H and Bellaman K (1948) *Parris Mitchell of King's Row*. Simon and Schuster, New York, pp. 187–8.
132 Ibid., p. 292.
133 Thompson M (1955) *Not as a Stranger*. Michael Joseph, London, pp. 237–9.
134 Ibid., p. 429.
135 Ibid., pp. 509–10.
136 Ibid., pp. 693–4.
137 Ellison H (1957) Wanted in Surgery. In: *Paingod and Other Delusions*. Pyramid Books, New York, 1965, pp. 106–35.
138 Sava G (1979) *No Man is Perfect*. Robert Hale, London.
139 The Bible, Revised Standard Version. Oxford University Press, New York, 1977, Genesis, 30: 16–18.
140 The Bible, Revised Standard Version. Oxford University Press, New York, 1977, Luke, 10: 38–40.
141 Martineau H (1839) *Deerbrook*. Virago Press, London, 1983, p. 212.
142 Morgan J (1956) *Doctor Jo*. Samuel French, London, p. 45.
143 Baldwin F (1939) *Medical Centre*. Horwitz, Sydney, 1962, p. 24.
144 Ibid., pp. 41–7.
145 Ibid., p. 61.
146 Seifert E (1977) *Doctor Tuck*. Collins, London, 1979, pp. 4–20.
147 Ibid., pp. 81–2.
148 Fisher H (1982) *The Tender Heart*. Mills and Boon, London.
149 Dooling R (1991) *Critical Care*. William Morrow, New York, p. 126.
150 The Bible, Revised Standard Version, Oxford University Press, New York, 1977, Hosea, 1: 2.
151 Boccaccio G (1348–1353) *The Decameron* (translated by McWilliam GH). Penguin, Harmondsworth, 1980, pp. 392–401.
152 Miller A (1997) *Ingenious Pain*. Harcourt Brace, New York, pp. 177–9.

153 Chellis MD (1870) *The Old Doctor's Son*. Henry A Young, Boston, MA, p. 14.

154 Doyle AC (1894) A Physiologist's Wife. In: *Round the Red Lamp*. John Murray, London, 1934, pp. 120–55.

155 Chekhov AP (1892) The Butterfly. In: *The Oxford Chekhov* (translated by Hingley R). *Volume 6*. Oxford University Press, London, 1971, pp. 61–82.

156 Chekhov AP (1892) My Wife. In: *The Oxford Chekhov* (translated by Hingley R). *Volume 6*. Oxford University Press, London, 1971, pp. 19–58.

157 Mitchell SW (1901) *Circumstance*. The Century Company, New York, 1902, pp. 51–2.

158 Ibid., pp. 444–52.

159 Malamud B (1973) In Retirement. In: *Rembrandt's Hat*. Farrar Straus Giroux, New York, pp. 109–24.

160 Schnitzler A (1917) *Dr Graesler* (translated by Slade EC). Thomas Seltzer, New York, 1923, pp. 71–5.

161 Ibid., pp. 116–23.

162 Ibid., p. 178.

163 Maugham WS, op. cit.

164 Ibid., pp. 674–9.

165 Ibid., p. 491.

166 Ibid., pp. 346–51.

167 Ibid., pp. 534–9.

168 Ibid., p. 476.

169 Deeping W (1925) *Sorrell and Son*. Cassell, London, 1927.

170 Ibid., pp. 252–3.

171 Ibid., pp. 299–307.

172 Ibid., p. 312.

173 Ibid., pp. 341–2.

174 Ibid., pp. 350–5.

175 Ibid., p. 357.

176 Ibid., pp. 361–8.

177 Bashford HH (1911) *The Corner of Harley Street: being some familiar correspondence of Peter Harding MD*. Constable, London, 1913, pp. 204–10.

178 Young FB (1928) *My Brother Jonathan*. Heinemann, London, pp. 575–95.

179 Miller CJ (1931) The doctors of fiction. *Surg Gynecol Obstet*. 52: 493–7.

180 Goldsworthy P (2003) *Three Dog Night*. Penguin, Melbourne.

181 Young FB (1919) *The Young Physician*. Heinemann, London, 1935, pp. 466–7.

182 Young FB (1928) *My Brother Jonathan*. Heinemann, London, pp. 203–11.

183 Collier J (1931) De Mortuis. In: *Fancies and Goodnights*. Time Life Books, Alexandria, VA, 1980, pp. 11–19.

184 Williams T (1948) Summer and Smoke. In: *The Theatre of Tennessee Williams*. *Volume 2*. New Directions, New York, 1971, p. 130.

185 Ibid., pp. 132–4.

186 Ibid., p. 154.

187 Ibid., p. 227.

188 Ibid., p. 221.

189 Ibid., p. 211.

190 Ibid., pp. 248–50.

191 Caldwell T (1968) *Testimony of Two Men*. Collins, London, 1990, pp. 13–15.

192 Ibid., pp. 53–7.

193 Ibid., pp. 141–4.

194 Ibid., p. 107.

195 Ibid., p. 278.

196 Lewis S, op. cit., pp. 390–1.

197 Ibid., p. 429.

198 Cave H (1951) The Doctor's Wife. In: *The Witching Lands*. Alvin Redman, London, 1962, pp. 62–80.

199 Tucker A (1939) *Miss Susan Slagle's*. Heinemann, London, 1940.

200 Crichton M (Hudson J, pseudonym) (1968) *A Case of Need*. Signet, New York, 1969, pp. 215–16.

201 Percy W (1987) *The Thanatos Syndrome*. Ivy Books, New York, 1991, p. 106.

202 Fitzgerald FS (1934) *Tender is the Night*. Penguin, Harmondsworth, 1998, pp. 129–30.

203 Ibid., p. 169.

204 Ibid., pp. 206–11.

205 Ibid., p. 182.

206 Ibid., pp. 273–4.

207 Ibid., p. 325.

208 Barnes D (1921) The Doctors (also titled Katrina Silverstaff). In: Herring P (ed.) *Djuna Barnes: collected stories*. Sun and Moon Press, Los Angeles, CA, 1996, pp. 319–26.

209 Watson R (1977) Tale of a Physician. In: *Lily Lang*. St Martin's Press, New York, pp. 161–72.

210 Miller A, op. cit.

211 Ibid., pp. 31–2.

212 Ibid., pp. 138–40.

213 Ibid., pp. 196–7.

214 Ibid., pp. 287–9.

215 Rinehart MR, op. cit., pp. 161–6.

216 Richardson HH (Robertson EFL) (1917–1929) *The Fortunes of Richard Mahony*. Penguin, Harmondsworth, 1990.

217 Woolf V (1925) *Mrs Dalloway*. Zodiac Press, London, 1947.

218 Proust M (1913–1922) *Remembrance of Things Past* (translated by Scott-Moncrieff CK and Kilmartin T). *Volume 2*. Penguin, Harmondsworth, 1987, p. 995.

219 Richardson HH, op. cit., pp. 488–97.

220 Ibid., pp. 321–31.

221 Ibid., pp. 819–31.

222 Woolf V, op. cit., pp. 110–12.

223 Hemingway E (1925) The Doctor and the Doctor's Wife. In: *The Complete Short Stories of Ernest Hemingway*. Scribner Paperback Edition, Simon and Schuster, New York, 1998, pp. 73–6.

224 Mauriac F (1927–1935) *Thérèse* (translated by Hopkins G). Penguin, Harmondsworth, 1959.

225 Ibid., pp. 119–38.

226 Chandler R (1953) *The Long Goodbye*. Pan, London, 1979, pp. 131–5.

227 Ibid., p. 257.

228 Weldon F (1976) *Remember Me*. Coronet, London, 1983.

229 Ibid., p. 177.

230 Ibid., p. 98.

231 Ibid., p. 118.

232 James PD (1971) *Shroud for a Nightingale*. Sphere Books, London, 1988, pp. 250–1.

233 Ibid., p. 275.

234 Ibid., p. 178.

235 Faulkner W (1939) *The Wild Palms*. Random House, New York.

236 Ibid., p. 300.

237 Slaughter FG (1974) Women in White. In: *Four Complete Novels*. Avenel Books, New York, 1980, pp. 438–46.

238 Green G, op. cit., pp. 179–81.

239 Hardy T (1886–1887) *The Woodlanders*. Oxford University Press, Oxford, 1988, p. 274.

240 Singer IB (1964) A Wedding in Brownsville. In: *Short Friday and Other Stories* (translated by Faerstein C and Polley E). Farrar Straus and Giroux, New York, pp. 190–206.

241 Thomas DM (1993) *Pictures at an Exhibition*. Bloomsbury, London.

242 Mitchell P (1965) *A Wilderness of Monkeys*. Arthur Barker, London.

243 Nourse AE (1978) *The Practice*. Futura Publications, London, 1979.

244 Straub P (1988) *Koko*. Penguin, Harmondsworth, 1989, pp. 90–5.

245 Ariyoshi S (1967) *The Doctor's Wife* (translated by Hironaka W and Kostant AS). Kodansha, Tokyo, 1989, p. 68.

246 Nitzberg EM (1991) *Hippocrates' Handmaidens: women married to physicians*. Haworth Press, New York, pp. 62–8.

247 Ibid., pp. 194–8.

248 Ibid., pp. 177–83.

249 Ibid., pp. 72–3.

250 Slaughter FG (1972) *Convention MD*. Hutchinson, London, 1973, p. 160.

251 Le Sage AR (1715) *The Adventures of Gil Blas de Santillana* (translated by Smollett T). Oxford University Press, London, 1907, pp. 127–44.

252 Rinehart MR, op. cit., p. 136.

253 Ibid., p. 293.

254 McCullers C (1943) *The Heart is a Lonely Hunter*. Cresset Press, London, 1953, pp. 77–8.

255 Camus A (1947) *The Plague* (translated by Gilbert S). Penguin, Harmondsworth, 1960, p. 11.

256 Ibid., pp. 237–8.

257 Slaughter FG (1969) Surgeon's Choice. In: *Four Complete Novels*. Avenel Press, New York, 1980, p. 241.

258 Slaughter FG (1972) *Convention MD*. Hutchinson, London, 1973, p. 32.

259 Ibid., pp. 191–4.

260 Ibid., p. 275.

261 Slaughter FG (1983) *Doctors at Risk*. Hutchinson, London, p. 37.

262 Starkman EM (1980) Anniversary. In: Mazow JW (ed.) *The Woman Who Lost Her Names*. Harper and Row, San Francisco, CA, pp. 168–76.

263 Crichton M (Hudson J, pseudonym), op. cit., p. 54.

264 Braddon ME (1864) *The Doctor's Wife*. Oxford University Press, Oxford, 1998.

265 Ibid., p. 6.

266 Ibid., p. 114.

267 Ibid., p. 199.

268 Ibid., p. 108.

269 Ibid., p. 183.

270 Ibid., p. 221.

271 Ibid., p. 224.

272 Proust M, op. cit., volume 1, p. 218.

273 Ibid., p. 467.

274 Lewis S (1920) *Main Street*. Harcourt Brace and Company, New York, 1948.

275 Cronin AJ (1937) *The Citadel*. Gollancz, London, p. 156.

276 Ibid., pp. 390–411.

277 McCarthy M (1954) *The Group*. Signet, New York, 1964.

278 Ibid., pp. 311–22.

279 Updike J (1961) The Doctor's Wife. In: *Pigeon Feathers and Other Stories*. Andre Deutsch, London, 1963, pp. 197–210.

280 Ozick C (1971) The Doctor's Wife. In: *The Pagan Rabbi and Other Stories*. Penguin, New York, 1983, p. 181.

281 Moore B (1976) *The Doctor's Wife*. Jonathan Cape, London.

282 Ibid., pp. 145–7.
283 Ibid., pp. 80–2.
284 Busch F (1979) *Rounds*. Farrar Straus and Giroux, New York, p. 90.
285 Hellman L (1934) *The Children's Hour*. Dramatists Play Service, New York, 1981, p. 63.
286 Miller A (1968) *The Price*. Secker and Warburg, London.
287 Ibid., pp. 16–21.
288 Ibid., pp. 53–4.
289 Ibid., p. 74.
290 Ibid., p. 82.
291 Busch F (1984) Rise and Fall. In: *Too Late American Boyhood Blues*. David R Godine, Boston, MA, pp. 17–51.
292 Green G (1979) *The Healers*. Melbourne House, London.
293 Ibid., p. 227.
294 Gardner J (1972) *The Sunlight Dialogues*. Ballantine Books, New York, 1973, p. 665.
295 Faulkner W (1939) *The Wild Palms*. Random House, New York, pp. 4–16.
296 Ibid., pp. 274–306.
297 Ibid., pp. 241–9.
298 Mitchell P, op. cit., pp. 78–81.
299 Ibid., pp. 366–7.
300 Ibid., pp. 198–206.
301 Ibid., pp. 158–63.
302 Ibid., p. 185.
303 Ibid., p. 255.
304 Ibid., pp. 247–8.
305 Ibid., p. 128.
306 Ibid., p. 63.
307 Nourse AE, op. cit., pp. 157–8.
308 Ibid., p. 423.
309 Ibid., p. 454.
310 Ibid., pp. 309–10.
311 Busch F (1984) A History of Small Ideas. In: *Too Late American Boyhood Blues*. David R Godine, Boston, MA, pp. 150–70.
312 Thomas DM, op. cit., pp. 28–9.
313 Ibid., pp. 195–7.
314 Ibid., p. 181.
315 Ibid., pp. 79–84.
316 Ibid., pp. 121–3.
317 Ibid., p. 165.
318 Ibid., p. 219.
319 Ibid., pp. 110–11.
320 Cuthbert M (1998) *The Silent Cradle*. Simon and Schuster, London.
321 Ibid., p. 140.
322 Auden WH (1972) The Art of Healing: in memoriam David Protetch, MD. In: *Epistle to a Godson and Other Poems*. Faber and Faber, London, pp. 13–15.
323 Haseltine F and Yaw Y (1976) *Woman Doctor*. Houghton Mifflin, Boston, MA, p. 80.
324 Posen S (2005) *The Doctor in Literature. Volume 1. Satisfaction or resentment?* Radcliffe Publishing, Oxford, p. 60.
325 Plath S (1963) *The Bell Jar*. Bantam Books, New York, 1972, p. 106.
326 Bennett A (1923) *Riceyman Steps*. Cassell, London, 1947, p. 178–80.
327 Wolfe T (1939) *The Web and the Rock*. Heinemann, London, 1969, p. 627.
328 Posen S, op. cit., p. 155.
329 Dickens C (1852–1853) *Bleak House*. Collins, London, 1953, p. 796.

330 Reade C (1863) *Hard Cash*. Chatto and Windus, London, 1894, p. 468.
331 Brontë C (1853) *Villette*. Penguin, Harmondsworth, 1983.
332 Ibid., pp. 167–9.
333 Ibid., pp. 148–52.
334 Ibid., pp. 296–302.
335 Ibid., p. 82.
336 Ibid., p. 463.
337 Ibid., pp. 532–3.
338 Bashford HH (1911) *The Corner of Harley Street: being some familiar correspondence of Peter Harding, MD*. Constable, London, 1913.
339 Ibid., p. 270.
340 Ibid., pp. 21–2.
341 Ibid., pp. 168–9.
342 Ibid., pp. 174–5.
343 Ibid., pp. 39–40.
344 Ibid., p. 246.
345 Ibid., p. 254.
346 Ibid., p. 265.
347 Ibid., p. 41.
348 Ibid., pp. 93–4.
349 Ibid., p. 268.
350 Ibid., pp. 32–3.
351 Ibid., p. 63.
352 Ibid., p. 237.
353 Ibid., pp. 242–5.
354 Ibid., pp. 212–16.
355 Ibid., p. 253.
356 Herrick R (1900) *The Web of Life*. Macmillan, London.
357 Dreiser T (1919) The Country Doctor. In: *Twelve Men*. Constable, London, 1930, pp. 102–22.
358 Bennett A, op. cit., p. 12.
359 Ibid, p. 314.
360 Auden WH (1936) Miss Gee. In: *Selections by the Author*. Penguin, Harmondsworth, 1970, pp. 43–5.
361 Wilder T (1938) *Our Town*. Longmans, London, 1965, p. 8.
362 Ibid., p. 26.
363 Ibid., p. 59.
364 Pym B (1980) *A Few Green Leaves*. EP Dutton, New York, p. 2.
365 Ibid., p. 18.
366 Ibid., p. 242.
367 Russell R (1985) *While You're Here, Doctor*. Souvenir Press, London.
368 Ibid., pp. 177–84.
369 Irving J (2001) *The Fourth Hand*. Bloomsbury, London, pp. 29–42.
370 Ibid., pp. 162–5.
371 Lewis S (1924) *Arrowsmith*. Signet Books, New York, 1961, pp. 168–72.
372 Ibid., pp. 193–7.
373 Ibid., p. 244.
374 Mitchell M (1936) *Gone With the Wind*. Avon Books, New York, 1973, p. 807.
375 Ibid., p. 150.
376 Ibid., p. 296.
377 Ibid., p. 184.
378 Guterson D (1999) *East of the Mountains*. Bloomsbury, London, p. 147.
379 Ibid., pp. 3–11.

380 Ibid., p. 256.
381 Ibid., p. 274.
382 Adams A (1991) The Last Lovely City. In: Stone R and Kenison K (eds) *The Best American Short Stories 1992*. Houghton Mifflin, Boston, MA, 1992, pp. 1–14.
383 Green G (1956) *The Last Angry Man*. Charles Scribner's Sons, New York.
384 Ibid., pp. 324–9.
385 Lewis S (1924) *Arrowsmith*. Signet Books, New York, 1961, pp. 211–12.
386 Ibid., p. 262.
387 Ibid., p. 294.
388 Ibid., p. 371.
389 Ibid., p. 336.
390 Ibid., pp. 208–9.
391 Ibid., p. 309.
392 Ibid., p. 167.
393 Ibid., p. 395.
394 Garcia-Marquez G (1985) *Love in the Time of Cholera* (translated by Grossman E). Jonathan Cape, London, 1988.
395 Ibid., p. 21.
396 Ibid., p. 90.
397 Ibid., pp. 322–4.
398 Ibid., p. 109.
399 Ibid., p. 47.
400 Ibid., p. 42.
401 Ibid., pp. 253–4.
402 Ibid., p. 126.
403 Ibid., pp. 210–14.
404 Ibid., pp. 225–6.
405 Ibid., pp. 239–40.
406 Ibid., p. 349.
407 Ibid., p. 195.
408 Ibid., p. 30.
409 Saramago J (1995) *Blindness* (translated by Pontiero G). Harvill Press, London, 1997.
410 Ibid., pp. 21–30.
411 Ibid., p. 39.
412 Ibid., p. 169.
413 Ibid., pp. 201–23.
414 Ibid., p. 309.
415 McEwan I (2005) *Saturday*. Jonathan Cape, London.
416 James H (1881) *Washington Square*. Bantam Books, New York, 1959.
417 Ibid., pp. 52–6.
418 Ibid., pp. 127–32.
419 Ibid., p. 144.
420 Herrick R (1897) *The Man Who Wins*. Charles Scribner's Sons, New York, pp. 98–109.
421 Young FB (1938) *Dr Bradley Remembers*. Heinemann, London.
422 Ibid., p. 631.
423 Ibid., p. 670.
424 Baum V (1939) *Nanking Road* (translated by Creighton B). Geoffrey Bles, London, pp. 73–6.
425 Crichton M, op. cit., p. 60.
426 Ibid., pp. 124–5.
427 Ibid., p. 146.
428 Ibid., pp. 315–16.
429 Ibid., pp. 76–7.

430 Ibid., p. 379.

431 Oates JC (1969) How I Contemplated the World from the Detroit House of Correction and Began My Life Over Again. In: *The Wheel of Love*. Vanguard Press, New York, 1970, pp. 170–89.

432 Oates JC (1971) *Wonderland*. Vanguard Press, New York.

433 Ibid., pp. 505–12.

434 Ibid., pp. 50–71.

435 Ibid., pp. 430–4.

436 Ibid., pp. 264–7.

437 Ibid., pp. 297–300.

438 Ibid., p. 455.

439 Ibid., pp. 485–6.

440 Trautmann J and Pollard C (1982) *Literature and Medicine: an annotated bibliography*. University of Pittsburgh Press, Pittsburgh, PA.

441 Oates JC (1971) *Wonderland*. Vanguard Press, New York, pp. 185–97.

442 Ibid., pp. 123–4.

443 Ibid., p. 148.

444 Ibid., pp. 138–44.

445 Ibid., p. 162.

446 Ibid., p. 172.

447 Bellow S (1956) *Seize The Day*. Penguin, New York, 1996.

448 Ibid., p. 42.

449 Ibid., pp. 108–10.

450 Ibid., p. 36.

451 Ibid., pp. 45–6.

452 Ibid., p. 27.

453 Ibid., p. 34.

454 Ibid., p. 14.

455 Ibid., p. 11.

456 Ibid., p. 51.

457 Ibid., p. 104.

458 Cook R (1993) *Fatal Cure*. Pan Books, London, 1995, p. 80.

CHAPTER 2

The physician and his colleagues

Individuals practising the craft of healing have, since ancient times, enjoyed the status of an elite with inherent privileges and obligations.[1] The term 'elitism,' in this context, does not necessarily contain pejorative overtones, but it is by definition exclusive, and carries with it certain responsibilities such as a 'collegiate' behaviour towards other members of the profession. The interaction between medical colleagues, especially when not governed by the rules of etiquette, continues to fascinate writers of fiction regardless of whether or not they have received any formal medical training.

There is a widespread, deeply entrenched (and to a large extent false) perception that interpersonal relationships within the medical profession are uneasy if not hostile, and that infighting is endemic both inside and outside hospitals. The male doctor is portrayed not only as a friendless individual, but also as incapable of relating to his colleagues and subordinates. Instead of cooperating with each other in the interests of their patients, doctors are continually fighting among themselves over status, money and personal prejudices. These tensions and quarrels become particularly unpleasant when two physicians share the management of a patient.

Are physicians socially segregated from the lay population?

'Are all your friends doctors?' 'No – some of them are in other businesses.'[2]

Except in the context of transgressions of sexual boundaries,[3] social interaction between the doctor and his patient is rarely discussed in the medical literature. How often do patients turn into personal friends and how often do friends become patients? Are such role combinations desirable?

Writers of fiction are divided on the subject. *Clarissa Harlowe*[4] takes it for granted that 'friendship and physician' are incompatible. More recent writers also assume that close familiarity between a doctor and his patient is undesirable, and that the professional relationship works best when it is unencumbered by personal considerations. 'One should never know doctors personally,' declares one of Remarque's characters in *Arch of Triumph*[5] to his close friend Dr Ravic.

'I have been drunk with you – how could I have you operate on me? I might be sure that you were a better surgeon than someone else I didn't know – nevertheless I'd take the other. Confidence in the unknown [is] a deep-rooted human quality. Doctors should live in hospitals and never be let out into the world of the uninitiated.'[5]

WH Auden disagrees.[6] He insists on making the acquaintance of his physicians in a bar before he will allow them into his bedroom.

> The healer I faith is someone I've gossiped
> and drunk with before I call him to touch me.[6]

In general, twentieth-century fiction writers agree with Remarque[5] rather than with Auden.[6] The physician is portrayed as a solitary, priestly[7] and self-sufficient character who does not enjoy a satisfactory family life (*see* Chapter 1) and who has few or no social contacts among his non-medical acquaintances, especially among patients or potential patients. The notion of a social division between doctors and lay persons is expressed by both parties with Mary Rinehart's young Dr Arden[8] representing the medical side. Arden, an idealistic, celibate character, feels ill at ease and out of place trying to relax at a party with some non-medical contemporaries.* The sound of talk and laughter and the cheerful tinkle of ice in glasses makes him feel like 'a worker among the drones.'[8]

> When they found out what he was, they affected to find it slightly humorous. 'My God, a doctor! You don't look like one.' 'Why not?' 'Well, where's the good old beard or whatever it is?'[8]

The non-medical point of view is expressed by Eugene O'Neill's Sam Evans when he is asked whether Dr Edmund Darrell is a close friend of his:

> 'I wouldn't say Ned was close to anyone. He's a dyed-in-the-wool doc. He's only close to whatever's the matter with you.'[8a]

The doctor's social isolation is a relatively recent phenomenon. As late as the end of the nineteenth century, upper-middle-class physicians were still portrayed as forming an integral part of their local communities. Dawson's Dr John Selkirk[9] and Weir Mitchell's Dr Sydney Archer[10] feel very much at home among the more prosperous of their fellow citizens of London[9] and Philadelphia,[10] who make up their circles of friends as well as their lists of patients. Archer regularly dines with members of the Fairthorne family, he attends them when they are ill, and he warns off a scheming adventuress who has made old John Fairthorne change his will[10] (*see* p. 157). Selkirk acts as moral guardian and marriage guidance counsellor of his acquaintances as well as their medical adviser[9] (*see also* pp. 128–9).

In small rural communities where social contacts between the doctor and the local people are almost inevitable, the degree of the doctor's integration depends to some extent on his 'priestly' or 'earthy' status.[7] Dr Robert Gibson in Elizabeth Gaskell's *Wives and Daughters*[11] and Dr Richard Mahony in Richardson's *The Fortunes of Richard Mahony*[12] are both priestly figures. Although not totally set apart from the non-medical population, they always remain a little aloof, Gibson because of

---

* Arden is a particularly earnest young man, while the other party guests seem exceptionally frivolous,[8] so that he feels 'as if he belonged to a class apart.' While Rinehart exaggerates the gulf between the physician and his non-medical contemporaries, many doctors to this day experience feelings of isolation at totally non-medical social events and experience a sense of relief when called away to attend to a patient.

pressure of work and his ambiguous social status, and Mahony because of his odd personality.

Earthy small-town physicians like Will Kennicott in *Main Street*,[13] George Bull in *The Last Adam*[14] and 'Ray' in *Passing the Ball*[15] go deer hunting,[13] snake catching[14] and riding to hounds[15] with their non-medical friends. Faulkner's Dr Peabody [16] may be too fat for such strenuous activities, but his banter with a group of local residents suggests that there is little or no professional segregation. The subject of conversation on this occasion[16] is the collapse of an old bridge as a result of a flood. One of the older citizens remembers that Dr Peabody was the first man to cross it after it was built, 'coming to my house when Jody was born.' 'If I'd crossed it every time your wife littered since, it'd a been wore out long before this, Billy',[16] Peabody replies, amidst general laughter. Dr Jethro Forbes of 'Revere, Kansas'[17] is hardly earthy but, as the lone doctor in the town, he has only the local undertaker (who is also the mayor) as his daily breakfast companion and confidant. Similarly, Dr Edward Burleigh, an isolated, unmarried general practitioner in rural Nebraska, has a special relationship with the Rosicky family, and calls in at their homestead for breakfast after delivering a baby at another property several miles away.[18] Naturally, the Rosickys want to hear what happened at the confinement, and the doctor, despite his priestly status, becomes involved in gossip. Other rural physicians use their spare cash to buy properties in the area[19,20] and to turn themselves into gentlemen farmers. Their wives join (or are expected to join) other locally prominent women on various committees.[13]

On a much lower socio-economic level, 'Doctor' Iannis in *Captain Corelli's Mandolin*[21] is totally at ease with and part of the village population on his Greek island. His entire clientele consists of individuals whom he has known all his life, and many of his patients are also his regular boon companions at the local coffee-drinking establishment.

In addition, a few marginalized doctors in contemporary 'Western' settings try to combine the mutually exclusive roles of friend and medical adviser. Green's Dr Samuel Abelman, whose practice has largely disintegrated,[22] still tries, against the specific advice of his colleagues, 'to make friends out of patients.'[23] The dual relationship works well for a while but then there is a blazing fight, with the doctor losing both patient and friend.[24]

Another 'physician–friend', also low-ranking in the medical hierarchy, is Peter Corris's Dr Ian Sangster,[25] who

> was noted for his complete refusal to follow what he called 'medical correctness.' He ate fast food, smoked, drank a lot, imbibed a dozen cups of coffee every day and didn't exercise.[25]

Dr Sangster is equally unconventional in his dealings with medical colleagues. Accepted professional behaviour requires that a doctor does not conspire with a patient to withhold information from medical colleagues or, worse still, to provide colleagues with false information. Sangster has no such compunctions. He is quite prepared to 'confirm any lie' that his friend, Detective Cliff Hardy, proposes to tell the doctor at an impotence clinic.[25] When Hardy asks Dr Sangster for information about another medical practitioner, Sangster's loyalty to his friend completely overrides his feelings of professional solidarity, and he describes his medical colleague in the most unflattering terms as a 'slave to the health funds, a collaborator with plastic surgeons, a pill pusher, a quack for hire.'[25]

By contrast, the 'mainstream' contemporary doctor, especially the hospital doctor, is socially segregated in a medical ghetto so that both at work and during his brief moments of relaxation he interacts largely with his peers. It is this interaction that forms the basis of most of this chapter.

The practitioner and the consultant: the view from the top

The arrival at the bedside of a second doctor (for whatever reason) obviously has the potential to cause considerable disharmony between the medical parties concerned. Hippocrates issued a specific warning that 'physicians who meet in consultation must never quarrel or jeer at one another.'[26] Molière[27] lampoons the two physicians who almost come to blows when arguing for or against venesection in a young girl. Each tries to reinforce his own position by reminding the other of past therapeutic failures. 'Do you remember the lady you sent into the next world three days ago?'[27]

More recent fictional consultants continue to humiliate, disparage or patronize their primary care colleagues who, if present, regress to the role of medical students cowering before their teachers. The following representative passages come from six different countries and were written over a period of almost two centuries.

> A doctor from Yvetot with whom [Charles Bovary] had recently held a consultation had humiliated him right at the bedside in front of the assembled relatives.[28]

Dostoyevsky's consultant does not insult the local family practitioner to his face but he is quite happy to make disparaging remarks about his colleague's competence behind his back.

> The famous Moscow doctor had delivered himself of several exceedingly offensive remarks about Dr Herzenstube's medical ability.[29] For although the Moscow doctor charged no less than twenty-five roubles for a visit, several people in our town were overjoyed at his arrival, did not grudge the expense and rushed to consult him. All these patients, of course, had been previously treated by Dr Herzenstube [the kindly old 'Skotoprigonyevsk' family physician], and the famous doctor had criticized his treatment with extreme harshness. . . . The first thing he asked a patient as soon as he entered his room was: 'Well, who has been messing about with you? Herzenstube? Ha ha.'[29]

According to Dr Cutler Walpole, Bernard Shaw's prominent London surgeon,

> 'these damned general practitioners ought never to be allowed to touch a patient except under the orders of a consultant.'[30]

Virginia Woolf's Sir William Bradshaw,[31] another prominent London consultant, agrees wholeheartedly with this view.

> How long had Dr Holmes been attending him? Six weeks. Prescribed a little bromide? Said there was nothing the matter? Ah yes [these general practitioners], thought Sir William. It took half his time to undo their blunders. Some were irreparable.[31]

When the angelic child in Thomas Mann's *Doctor Faustus*[32] is suspected of suffering from tuberculous meningitis, the distinguished Munich consultant 'confirmed the diagnosis of his obsequious rural colleague.'

Lawrence Sanders' Barbara Delaney[33] has kidney stones complicated by a *Proteus* infection, and requires an operation.

> The surgeon introduced by Dr Bernardi . . . was a brusque no-nonsense man without warmth, but he had impressed Delaney with his direct questions, quick decisions [and] his sharp interruptions of Bernardi's effusions.[33]

Even at the end of the twentieth century, Dr Fred Dixon, an elderly non-hospital physician, is treated with thinly disguised contempt by a 'Boston Heart Institute' colleague. It is Sunday afternoon and Dixon is visiting his patient, Violet Corcoran, who almost dies in thyrotoxic crisis.[34] One of the faculty cardiologists introduces him to Dr Brian Holbrook in a tone of voice that suggests 'merely having Dr Dixon as one's physician carried with it certain health risks.' The brilliant Dr Holbrook feels slightly ill at ease with Dr Dixon's treatment. Dixon's knowledge of thyroid physiology may indeed be rudimentary, but he shows sufficient interest to visit his patient at the weekend, and deserves at least a semblance of politeness.[34]

Dr Chang, the scholarly physician in *The Dream of the Red Chamber*,[35] practises traditional Chinese medicine, but his comments on his fellow practitioners are very similar to remarks that might have been made, under similar circumstances, in the West: 'I'm afraid my colleagues have allowed her condition to deteriorate.'[35]

All of these passages convey the same message: consultants* entertain and at times express a profound contempt for their less well-qualified brethren. The primary care physicians are distinguished by their ignorance, their obsequiousness and their loquaciousness, while the proud and knowledgeable consultant says little, solves problems with effortless ease and defecates on his less-specialized colleagues from a great height and at every opportunity.

Interns and residents in large hospitals readily imbibe this attitude (*see also* pp. 76 and 79) and sneer at the perceived incompetence of colleagues who are not attached to their particular institution. Nourse's *Intern*[36] refers to 'some backwoods jerk' performing a breast biopsy because 'he was too stupid or too greedy to send her where the job could have been done right in the first place.'

Another general practitioner incurs this young man's derision for ligating the femoral artery during a varicose vein procedure.[36] The youthful firebrand is tempted to advise the patient to sue this 'jackass [who] couldn't tell the saphenous vein from the femoral artery', but more prudent counsel prevails.

In due course, the consultant himself may fall from his pedestal. Virginia Woolf's Dr Holmes,[31] the general practitioner who is shown to be an incompetent fool and is held in contempt by Sir William Bradshaw,[31] actually does less harm than Sir William with his string of fashionable and expensive 'rest homes.' Barbara Delaney[33] does not die under the care of the 'oily and effusive' family physician, but after a nephrectomy performed by the 'brusque no-nonsense' surgeon.[33]

---

* Since the second decade of the twentieth century the term 'consultant' has become almost synonymous with 'specialist.' The change in the relative status of generalists and specialists around that time forms the background to Green's *The Last Angry Man*.[22]

Flaubert's *Madame Bovary*[28,37–39] provides a veritable pecking order of physicians humiliating one another. Charles Bovary, the stupid and incompetent general practitioner, is at the bottom of the heap. He is incapable of recognizing and treating a faint,[37] let alone operating on a clubfoot. Dr Canivet, 'of considerable standing and equal self-assurance laughed with unconcealed scorn when he saw Hippolyte's leg', which had become gangrenous as a result of Bovary's surgical efforts.[38] Canivet himself is subsequently rebuked (in private) for his incompetent treatment of Emma Bovary, who had taken a lethal dose of arsenic.[39]

> Today he was as meek as he had been arrogant the day he had operated on Hippolyte; his face was fixed in a continual approving smile.[39]

The practitioner and the consultant: the view from below

The 'lower orders' in this hierarchy understandably resent the doctors of the upper strata, whom they regard with suspicion and hostility. Obsequiousness towards a senior consultant does not necessarily denote respect. On the contrary, various arguments are employed to denigrate the specialists, usually behind their backs. One of these is the cliché that 'the specialist is only interested in one orifice', which implies that the general practitioner treats his patients as human beings. Dr Matthew Swain, the small-town general practitioner in *Peyton Place*,[40] detests specialists.

> 'Yes. I'm a specialist', he had once roared at a famous ear, eye, nose and throat man. 'I specialize in sick people. What do you do?'[40]

Dr Raste, the English general practitioner in Arnold Bennett's *Riceyman Steps*,[41] expresses similar sentiments, although with a little more subtlety. Raste, who is unable to diagnose the cause of Henry Earlforward's dysphagia, proposes to have him admitted to hospital where he can be X-rayed and seen by specialists.

> 'I'm not a specialist', declared Dr Raste. He uttered the phrase with a peculiar intonation, not entirely condemning specialists but putting them in their place, regarding them very critically and rather condescendingly as befitting one whose field of work and knowledge was the whole boundless realm of human pathology.[41]

In the slums of Brooklyn, Dr Samuel Abelman, a fossilized general practitioner, spends his life fulminating against 'specialist professors, fancy internists and pediatricians'[42] who refuse to make night calls, and who work out of luxurious offices, charge exorbitant fees and steal his gullible patients.[24]

Doc Cathey, the old, earthy general practitioner in John Gardner's *Nickel Mountain*,[43] uses a slightly different tactic. According to Dr Cathey, family physicians have a long-term commitment to their patients, whereas specialists 'don't know one damn patient from another.'[43] Dr Cathey is paying a hospital visit to Callie Soames, who is having a long and difficult labour with her first child. Callie and her husband Henry Soames (not the baby's natural father) are both rhesus-negative.

Callie leaned up on one elbow and said, 'Anyway, it doesn't matter on the first one. The doctor said so.' Doc Cathey peeked at her over the rims of his glasses, then at Henry. 'Maybe', he said. 'That may be. They know everything, these fancy city doctors.' . . . [Doc Cathey] looked at Henry. 'You told Costard she's a bleeder?' Henry nodded. 'He said he'd give her some kind of vitamin.' Doc Cathey scowled and looked at the door again. 'He will, if he remembers.'[43]

The clownish 'boondocks' doctor in *Arrowsmith*[44] declares himself unimpressed by specialists' qualifications and their 'evidence-based medicine.' The general practitioner, this doctor implies, sees real medicine and his observations are infinitely more precious than the pseudoscientific rubbish that comes out of university medical centres. This character, who uses foxes' lungs for the treatment of asthma and TB, is telling another general practitioner about a conversation with a respiratory specialist who had laughed at this 'therapeutic innovation.'

> '[He] said it wasn't scientific – and I said to him, "Hell!" I said, "scientific," I said, "I don't know if it's the latest fad and wrinkle in science or not", I said, "but I get results" . . . I tell you a plug GP may not have a lot of letters after his name but he sees a slew of mysterious things that he can't explain and I swear I believe most of these damn alleged scientists could learn a whale of a lot from plain country practitioners.'[44]

The need for a specialist opinion undermines the general practitioner's self-confidence, which, like the stethoscope, is part of the medical mystique. A doctor makes his patients feel at ease by his delusion or his pretence that he can deliver a cure, and that if he cannot, no one else can. Against this background, a consultation with another physician becomes, by definition, an admission of defeat.

Mrs Louise Maynard, a patient who has been transferred by the diffident and incompetent Dr Grace Breen to the care of the supremely confident Dr Rufus Mulbridge,[45] explains her perception of the two doctors after her recovery.

> 'You're not fit to be a doctor, Grace', she said. 'You're too nervous and too conscientious. . . . If you saw a case go wrong in your hands you'd want to call in someone else. . . . Do you suppose Dr Mulbridge would have given me up to another doctor because he was afraid he couldn't cure me? No indeed. He'd have let me die first and I shouldn't have blamed him.'[45]

Even Jewett's Dr Leslie,[46] despite his 'scholarly habits' and his 'great repute among his professional brethren', considers that to a country doctor 'a consultation is more or less a downfall of pride.'[46]

Mauriac's Dr Pédemay[47] only narrowly escapes this 'downfall' when his patient's condition suddenly improves. Pédemay is the family doctor taking care of Bernard Desqueyroux, whose wife is poisoning him with arsenic from time to time. The patient's fluctuating symptoms and signs mystify Pédemay, and Bernard's mother

> played with the idea of calling in a well-known consultant, but she did not wish to affront the doctor, who was an old friend. . . . About the middle of August . . . after a more than usually alarming crisis, Pédemay himself suggested a second opinion. Fortunately, however, next day Bernard began to show signs of improvement, and three weeks later he

was said to be well on the way to convalescence. 'That was a narrow escape for me', said Pédemay. 'If the great man had got here in time, all the credit for the cure would have gone to him.'[47]

One of the clearest expressions of the ambivalence of general practitioners towards specialists comes from Dr Richard Mahony, whose financial difficulties force him to resume general practice in a Melbourne suburb.[48] After a few weeks in practice he suddenly realized that

> since putting up his plate he had treated none but the simplest cases. Only the ABC of doctoring had been required of him. The fact was specialists were all too easy to get at. But no! That wouldn't hold water either. Was it not rather he himself who, at first hint of a complication, was ready to refer a patient . . . [so as] to shirk undue worry and responsibility?[48]

Elizabeth Seifert's medical romances of the 1940s, which read as if they had been written or at least approved by the then governing body of the American Medical Association, nevertheless contain occasional realistic passages. Dr Jim Wyatt, a general practitioner in a small Missouri town, who has surgical aspirations, expresses deep resentment of patients with hernias who go off to the Mayo Clinic or the Barnes Hospital rather than letting him operate on them.[49]

The general practitioner's resentment of specialists may express itself in the form of grudging and ungracious referrals, as in the case of Donna Stubbs in Walker Percy's *The Thanatos Syndrome*.[50] Donna is sent to a psychiatrist on account of her obesity.

> She was referred to me by more successful physicians who'd finally thrown up their hands. What do I want with her, they'd tell me, the only trouble with her is she eats too damn much, I've got people in real trouble, and so on – as a surgeon might refer a low back pain to a chiropractor. He may be a quack but he can't do you any harm.[50]

Town versus gown

Frank Slaughter, writing in the 1960s, repeatedly mentions the resentment felt by the 'town' doctors towards their academic colleagues.[51] Despite the prestige that may accrue to members of a medical community through the establishment of a teaching hospital in their area, the arrival of alien faculty members can hardly be expected to elicit outbursts of joy from the established physicians.

> A lot of doctors in the area had no love for the Medical School at Weston and even less for the Faculty Clinic that had taken away some of their most prosperous patients.[51]

This dislike of academics is particularly well developed among practising surgeons, who openly declare that their university colleagues ought to confine their surgical activities to cats and dogs, and leave 'real' surgery to 'real' surgeons.[52]

Many years before Slaughter[51] and Roe[52], 'Doctor Leslie', who might have become an academic physician himself,[46] expresses very similar sentiments. Leslie, who has decided to work as a general practitioner in 'Oldfields' rather than 'transplant himself to some more prominent position of the medical world', has little time for university types 'who have not had the experience which alone can make their advice reliable.' These 'medical scholars' may know a lot of 'anatomy and physiology', but when it comes to 'practical matters' they are inferior to country practitioners.[46] Dr Leslie expresses some nostalgia for the time when, under the apprenticeship system, aspiring young doctors were taught by real physicians and not by physiology professors.[46]

Naturally, academic doctors hold a different point of view. They regard themselves as the leaders of the profession and consider 'merchant' physicians to be ignorant hacks, interested only in their cash registers. Jim Morelle, a surgeon, and Stanley Levinson, a paediatrician, both of Sobel's 'McKinley Hospital', a self-perceived 'centre of excellence',[53] have cultivated this attitude to a highly developed degree. Here they are discussing Dr Hettrick, a suburban paediatrician who has been persuaded to call in Jim for a consultation. Jim and Stanley suspect, although neither of them has met either the suburban doctor or the patient, that Hettrick has 'pulled a terrible boner.' They proceed to make unfavourable comparisons between physicians who have teaching hospital appointments and those who do not.

> Wouldn't you say that half my time has been spent in the free wards and clinics of McKinley? And a good hunk of the rest devoted to teaching. . . . Throw in the innumerable conferences and medical meetings . . . and you've got a lot of effort put into not making money. Now you really don't think the suburban doc goes through this? . . . He doesn't set foot in a free ward or a free clinic; he does no teaching and he's a stranger to research. If [he] feels a little education would make him look good, he takes a few days off to go to a convention – income tax deductible. . . . These things don't bother the parents at all. He's busy and they long ago decided the busiest doctor is the best doctor.[53]

The conversation goes on in this vein for a while. When Jim finally gets to examine the patient, he finds signs of an appendix abscess, which the suburban doctor had failed to diagnose. The boy is transferred to Jim's large city-based institution, and after a successful operation he makes a full recovery.[53]

Dr Morelle and Dr Levinson disparage their suburban colleagues in private.[53] Dr Laj Randa, the aggressive chief of cardiac surgery at a major Boston institution, has no such inhibitions. He is quite happy to sneer at a non-academic surgical colleague (Dr Clarkin) in the presence of his fellows, nurses and one of Dr Clarkin's patients,[54] whose coronary artery grafts had become blocked after six years: ' "Typical result for Clarkin", . . . Randa said to his sycophants.'

Dr Giovanis, an academic researcher, becomes very sarcastic when discussing the 'rewards' of private practice with Brendan O'Brien, one of his fellows.[55] Researchers, Giovanis implies, are unrecognized and underpaid, but they are the true leaders of the profession, the chosen few, who lead a monastic existence in the wilderness while their colleagues in practice gorge themselves at the fleshpots.

> 'What is it you want from life, O'Brien? You want to spend twenty years driving fancy cars, spending your weekends in your big place in the country and throwing tax deductible parties catered by little men in black tuxedos for all the guys who trade patients with you?'[55] (*see also* p. 71)

Corrupt and inappropriate choices of consultant

Some referrals from one physician to another are of dubious clinical value, while others are unethical if not illegal. The 'second opinion' at the deathbed of Samuel Richardson's whorehouse proprietress[56] clearly involves collusion between two doctors, with additional costs but no further benefit to the patient. When the first surgeon informs 'the infamous Sinclair', who has a fractured femur, that 'it was impossible to save her', the old wretch begins howling like a wolf, so that for the sake of noise reduction a second surgeon, 'a friend of the other', is sent for. He agrees with his colleague that the prognosis is hopeless, but tries to deceive the old harlot into believing that the first doctor is too pessimistic and 'that if she would be patient she might recover.' The ruse fails and the animal noises continue.[56]

The 'ceremonious consultation' between the Surgeon of the Fleet and his 'brother surgeons' in Melville's *White Jacket*[57] is a farce from beginning to end. The senior man, who presumably controls or at least has a say in the promotion of the others, begins: 'You have seen there is no resource but amputation', and having indicated that his mind is made up, he goes on to ask 'Gentlemen, what do you say?' Surprisingly, one of his subordinates actually dares to disagree. The others are less courageous, the amputation goes ahead and the patient dies.[57]

The London referral pattern of the 1930s is described in most unfavourable terms in Cronin's *The Citadel*.[58] Dr Freddie Hamson, an empty-headed fool but a socially successful consultant, meets his old classmate, Dr Andrew Manson, a small-town general practitioner, at a medical convention.[58] Hamson is affable and patronizing, while Manson, before he becomes corrupted, is idealistic and politically naive.

> 'What do you think of the conference?' 'I suppose', Andrew answered doubtfully, 'it's a useful way of keeping up to date.' 'Up to date, my uncle! I haven't been to one of their . . . sectional meetings all week. No, no, old man, it's the contacts you make that matter, the fellows you meet. . . . That's why I'm here. When I get back to town, I'll ring them up, go out and play golf with them. Later on – . . . that means business.' 'I don't quite follow you, Freddie', Manson said. 'Why, it's as simple as falling off a log . . . I've got my eye on a nice little room up west where a smart little brass plate . . . would look dashed well. When the plate does go up, these fellows, my pals, will send me cases. . . . Reciprocity. You scratch my back and I'll scratch yours. . . . And apart from that it pays to push in with the small suburban fellows. Sometimes they can send you stuff . . .'[58]

Simenon[59] presents a similar referral pattern with French variations. Dr Elie Bergelon, an obscure family practitioner in a lower-middle-class district, meets

> Doctor Mandalin in the street. . . . Mandalin was a respected public figure. He lived in a magnificent period house in the most affluent district of Bugle. He had built his own sumptuously equipped clinic. 'I say, Bergelon, old man. . . . Don't for one moment imagine that I'm complaining, but you don't seem to refer many of your patients to me.' . . . 'Well, you know . . . most of my patients come from the one district.' 'My charges aren't as high as people say. I don't charge more

than the patients can afford. And as for yourself . . . the entire fee for the first operation I perform on one of your patients will be made over to you. Thereafter, you will receive half the fee for each patient. Au revoir, old man, see you soon.'[59]

Mandalin follows up with an invitation to a dinner party where

> they were waited on by a butler in white gloves. All the male guests were doctors who . . . referred their patients to the master of the house.[59]

Mandalin's dinner invitation is a success. Bergelon refers a maternity case but, because of Mandalin's incompetence and drunkenness, the pregnancy ends in disaster. Both mother and infant die, and the husband lodges an official complaint, claiming 'that his wife's confinement was scandalously mishandled' (*see also* Volume 1, Chapter 11).

> [Bergelon] was not in the least put out by this news [of impending litigation]. . . . He . . . was relishing the sight of Mandalin writhing on the hook. By contrast, his consulting room, shabby and dingy as it was, seemed a haven of unpretentious tranquility.[59]

A similar catastrophe occurs in *Bodies and Souls*[60] when a medical consultant is selected on the basis of non-medical considerations. This particular incident involves Professor Jean Doutreval, his son-in-law, Associate Professor Ludovic Vallorge, and Doutreval's pregnant daughter, Mariette Vallorge (née Doutreval). The two professors, who are attending a conference in Amsterdam, receive a telephone call from the University Hospital in Angers, France, where Mariette has gone into labour. The obstetricians in Angers believe that a Caesarean section is necessary, and want Mariette's father and husband to decide who should perform the operation.[60] Doutreval, who wants his colleagues' support for a psychiatric institute, and Vallorge, who is after a full chair, decide to bypass the most skilful surgeon (who is not a full professor) so as not to offend Professor Géraudin, the politically powerful chief of surgery. Despite specific warnings that Géraudin is well past his surgical prime, they ask him to perform the Caesarean section, and Mariette bleeds to death on the operating table[60] (*see also* p. 230).

According to Hemingway,[61] the bond between the referring doctor and the consultant depends not only on their social and political connections, but also on a shared lack of ability. Mediocrities, says Hemingway, tend to patronize each other, because incompetent doctors feel more comfortable with incompetent consultants than with leaders of the profession.

> I have noticed that doctors who fail in the practice of medicine have a tendency to seek one another's company and aid in consultation. A doctor who cannot take out your appendix properly will recommend to you a doctor who will be unable to remove your tonsils with success.[61]

Fierce rivalry between competitors: the survival of the 'fittest'

Multiple nineteenth- and twentieth-century authors describe professional jealousies and mutual animosities between physicians who fail to recognize that they are (or should be) 'on the same side.' In private practice, tensions and arguments usually involve doctors who are in financial competition with one another, while in hospitals and university departments, infighting is likely to concern status and power, although money may also be involved.[62]

Balzac[63] and Harriet Martineau[64] writing in the 1830s, Sinclair Lewis[13] and Francis Brett Young[65-67] in the 1920s, Céline[68] and Cronin[69] in the 1930s, Frank Slaughter[70] in the 1960s and Alan Nourse[71-73] in the 1970s all imply that there is constant and ferocious competition between physicians, who use every possible trick to hinder and denigrate each other. Balzac's Dr Desplein,[63] who has become an eminent surgeon despite unbelievable obstacles, has this to say about his colleagues and the 'help' he has received from them:

> When certain people see you ready to set your foot in the stirrup, some pull your coat tails, others loosen the buckle of the strap that you may fall and crack your skull. One wrenches off your horse's shoes, another steals your whip, and the least treacherous of them all is the man whom you see coming to fire his pistol at you point blank.[63]

Balzac's equestrian metaphors would clearly be out of place in 1969, but Slaughter's physician[70] conveys very similar paranoid messages about his hostile colleagues:

> Out in practice all the doctors are busy climbing over the others to get ahead, and kicking the other fellow in the face for good measure while they're going up.[70]

Similarly, throughout Francis Brett Young's *My Brother Jonathan*[65] runs the implicit assumption that ongoing antagonism between medical practitioners constitutes a normal state of affairs. As soon as Dr Jonathan Dakers leaves 'Prince's Hospital'[65] in order to go into practice in a small industrial town, he becomes embroiled in a bitter dispute between two former medical partners. Dakers willingly participates in a 'war to the knife'[66] between himself and Dr Craig, a war that is terminated only by Craig's illness and Dakers' death.[66] Similarly, among the multiple plots and subplots of Nourse's *The Practice*[71] the theme of medical infighting recurs with predictable regularity. Dr Isaacs has been 'locked in from the first in bitter conflict with an older, better established doctor practicing down the valley.' The two fight mainly over the 'ownership' of patients, although the 'other' practice's treatment methods and fees are frequently scrutinized and criticized.[72] Dr Rob Tanner, the newest member of Isaacs' practice, who is not averse to a good fight, becomes an involuntary participant in this ongoing dispute.[73]

Dr Edward Hope of *Deerbrook*,[64] whose political views are considered 'incorrect', watches helplessly as his practice virtually disintegrates when his enemies import a second medical man into the town. He maintains a remarkably philosophical attitude towards his seemingly inevitable financial ruin, but eventually goes into partnership with his erstwhile competitor, Edwards appreciates that this 'new' doctor will never 'make a striking figure in the world, yet . . . [he] might sustain a fair portion of respectability and usefulness in a country station.'[64]

In Sinclair Lewis's *Main Street*,[13] Dr Will Kennicott, whose financial position is not as precarious as that of Dr Hope,[64] nevertheless waxes very eloquent when discussing the other local practitioners, whom he considers charlatans with a propensity for extracting money from credulous patients.

> Westlake got hold of Ma Dawson and scared her to death and made her think the kid had appendicitis, and by golly if he and McGanum didn't operate and holler their heads off about the terrible adhesions they found and what a regular Charley and Will Mayo they were for classy surgery. They let on that if they'd waited two hours the kid would have developed peritonitis and God knows what all; and then they collected a nice fat hundred and fifty dollars.[13]

Sordid bedside quarrels between physicians such as those mentioned by Hippocrates[26] and described in detail by Molière[27] seem to have given way to 'Doctor, would you mind stepping over here',[74] so that the subsequent venomous arguments are not overheard by nurses or patients. However, instances of doctors abusing one another at the bedside are still described in early twentieth-century literature. Richardson's Dr Richard Mahony[75] has his medical qualifications questioned. 'Make him turn out his credentials', his rival calls out, among other insults.[75] Céline's two doctors are both practising in a squalid industrial suburb of Paris, both have been corrupted by their poverty, and a fight erupts when each of them believes that he is entitled to a 20-franc fee for attending a dying man.[68]

Patients are regarded as valuable possessions, so that a doctor who deliberately or unwittingly attracts them away from a colleague and into his own practice commits an act of theft. In James' *Two Doctors*,[76] which dates from the early twentieth century but is set in eighteenth-century England, one general practitioner complains that his rival '*embezzled* four of my best patients this month.'

Perceived 'patient pilfering' is a major source of discord between two doctors in a Welsh mining town,[69] much to the distress of the young and idealistic Dr Andrew Manson, who had expected to find 'unity, peace and concord.'

> [There was] no unity, no sense of co-operation and little friendliness. They were simply set up, one against the other . . . each trying to secure as many patients for himself as he could. Downright suspicion and bad feeling were often the result. . . . [Dr] Urquhart, for instance, when a patient of [Dr] Oxborrow transferred . . . to him [would] take the half-finished bottle of medicine from the man's hand . . . uncork it, smell it with contempt and explode: 'So this is what Oxborrow has been givin' ye! Damn it to hell! He's been slowly poisoning ye!'[69]

Manson, who believes that he can achieve some cooperation between his colleagues, calls a meeting of all the doctors of 'Aberalaw' to discuss common problems. Refreshments are served.

> The beer was increasing Dr Urquhart's natural belligerence; after glancing steadily at [Dr] Oxborrow for some minutes, he shot out: 'Now I find myself in your company, Doctor Oxborrow, maybe you'll find it convenient to explain how Tudor Evans, Seventeen Glyn Terrace,

came off my list on to yours.' 'I don't remember the case', said Oxborrow. . . . 'But I do!' Urquhart exploded. 'It was one of the cases you *stole* from me.'[69]

After this potentially explosive situation has been defused, Manson mentions the possibility of a night roster system.

'Wouldn't work', Urquhart snapped. 'Dammit to hell! I'd sooner stay up every night of the month than trust old Foxborrow with one of my cases. Hee hee! When he borrows he doesn't pay back.'[69]

Protectiveness; treatment policies; general cantankerousness

Although money is the major source of friction between medical colleagues, doctors also become protective about 'their' patients and cannot bear the thought of someone else taking charge. The physicians' well-developed powers of observation are used with great effect to study their competitors' frailties, with distrust persisting even when one of them is on his deathbed. However, non-financial rivalries generally remain latent and open hostilities are avoided.

In Braddon's *The Doctor's Wife*,[77] Dr George Gilbert has been looking after a number of patients with typhoid fever and is now himself suffering from the disease. He consults his colleague and rival, Mr Pawlkatt, who advises rest, but Dr Gilbert cannot bear the idea of lying in bed while his poor patients require attention.

True, Mr Pawlkatt had promised to attend to George's patients, but then unhappily George did not believe in Mr Pawlkatt . . . and the idea of Mr Pawlkatt attending the sick people in the lanes and seizing with delight on the opportunity of reversing his rival's treatment was almost harder to bear than the thought of the same sufferers being altogether unattended.[77]

Dr Gilbert disregards Pawlkatt's orders, continues to visit 'his' patients and eventually dies of the disease.[78]

Simone de Beauvoir's *A Very Easy Death*[79] contains descriptions of multiple medical characters. One of these appears only briefly, but long enough to illustrate his sense of 'ownership.' Dr D, Madame de Beauvoir's regular physician, who is not a brilliant diagnostician, has told the old lady that she is suffering from 'an upset liver and sluggish bowels' when in fact she has cancer of the colon. Dr D's lack of clinical acumen is combined with a perception of 'tenure' and a sense of intolerance towards his colleagues. When Simone's mother breaks her hip and the neighbours call in a woman doctor from the same apartment block, Doctor D becomes annoyed at this 'intrusion' and refuses to have anything further to do with his former patient.[79]

In a more modern setting, Doctor Nick, a suburban general practitioner and political conservative in Goldsworthy's *The Nice Chinese Doctor*,[80] normally advocates the operation of 'free-market forces'. However, he expresses (to his receptionist) a sense of outrage when Dr Thomas Ng sets up his office on the other side of the street, even though Nick has more patients than he can handle. Nick's resentment is due not so much to financial insecurity as to his possessiveness.

'You're like a jealous lover', comments his brother Paul, 'you don't want anyone else touching your patients.'[80]

The doctor's lack of confidence in the ability of his colleagues is a medical trait that transcends time and place. The two senior physicians in *Middlemarch*,[81] who share a dislike of newcomers and innovators, 'concealed with much etiquette their contempt for each other's skill.' Daudet's doctors[82] show less reticence and openly disparage one another, even though they work on the imaginary island of the 'Morticoles', which is controlled by doctors for the benefit of doctors. Felix Canelon, the shipwrecked sailor whose injured ankle has previously been 'examined' by Dr Tabard, ends up in hospital under the care of Dr Malasvon. After examining the patient, Malasvon 'burst into peals of laughter. "You are lucky Tabard didn't cripple you for life."' (Encore une chance qu'il ne vous ait pas estropi pour votre vie, le collègue Tabard.[82])

The critical faculties of Dr Benjamin Abrams, a young attending endocrinologist at Washington's 'St George' Hospital,[83] are so finely honed that he expresses contempt for almost all of his medical colleagues. Senior faculty members are 'old tenured farts who crawl out of their holes once a month hoping to see a young smart-ass' foul up a case at a clinico-pathological conference. The younger members of the staff are castigated because they rely on CT scans rather than their clinical acumen. Physicians with 'glamour practices' are resented when they 'just happen . . . to mention the Supreme Court justice or senator they number amongst their patients.'[83] The Chairman of the Department of Medicine, whose office is 'a little smaller than Madison Square Gardens', has no doubt engaged in 'vicious . . . faculty politics' in order to obtain his current position. At the other end of the academic spectrum is the overseas-trained medical graduate who can barely speak English and does not quite understand the difference between hyper- and hypoglycaemia.[83]

Dr Abrams shows signs of growing up and developing occasional twinges of humility. He had planned to score a few points off the psychiatrists during a clinico-pathological conference, because they had been describing a patient as 'paranoid and bipolar manic depressive, when in fact she had a real disease' (an insulinoma). Abrams manages to resist this temptation.[83]

> Ever since I opened my own office I've been eating humble pie. It's astonishing how the guy with the real tumor is indistinguishable from the legions of walking worried who cross my threshold complaining of . . . feeling pins and needles all over. . . . Nothing looks so clear in the office as it does in the auditorium. So I couldn't be too smug about [the] . . . psychiatrists.[83]

Finally, there is the physician who, perversely and irrationally, resents all members of his profession. William Carlos Williams' Doctor Dev Evans[84] 'detests his profession in the herd [and] had no intimates among its members.'[84] The doctor-father in Bernhard's *Gargoyles*[85] holds all his former classmates in contempt. He describes them as 'life-long dilettantes' who long ago abandoned their idealism and their intellectuality and who have turned into 'well-dressed quacks, who travelled much, hurriedly said hello . . . and talked about their family problems, about the houses they were building and obsessively about their cars.'[85]

The generation gap

Much latent and overt medical strife is attributable to age differences between the participants. The younger man wants to introduce 'scientific' methods and 'newer' treatment modalities, while the long-established physician has become rigid and mistrustful of innovations. The older man is conscious of his waning clinical and political power, and harbours the age-old resentment of the incumbent against the would-be successor. Conan Doyle's Dr Archer is one of the 'carbolic acid men, Hayes is the leader of the cleanliness and cold water school, and they all hate each other like poison.'[86]

Rider Haggard's medical adversaries[87] fight one another over a perceived insult. The older of the two doctors, who has become casual in his approach, diagnoses 'rheumatism' without examining the patient, while young Dr Therne, who inspects and palpates the painful leg, realizes that he is dealing with a case of venous thrombosis. The patient goes on to die of a pulmonary embolus, and there is a scene in the autopsy room where the young man is accused of attempting to humiliate his older colleague,[87] who subsequently revenges himself by giving evidence against Therne in a manslaughter trial.[88]

One of the best descriptions of the medical generation gap syndrome appears in Somerset Maugham's *Of Human Bondage*.[89] The story begins with old Dr South expressing his derision for the young 'up-to-date' graduates of university hospitals[89] who come to work as his assistants. South, who has been in general practice for 30 years, feels nothing but contempt for these arrogant young men, whose heads are filled with 'useless' book learning but who are unable to apply a simple bandage.

> They came with the unconcealed scorn for the general practitioner which they had absorbed in the air at the hospital; but they had seen only the complicated cases which appeared in the wards; they knew how to treat an obscure disease of the suprarenal bodies, but were hopeless when consulted for a cold in the head. Their knowledge was theoretical and their self-assurance unbounded.[89]

Then comes the traumatic moment of truth,[89] when a patient whom Dr South has known and treated all of her life decides that she prefers Dr Philip Carey, a recent graduate. Carey has by now acquired some of the art of medicine, his bookishness turns out to have its uses, and he is presumably better looking than his older colleague.

> One evening when Philip had reached his last week with Doctor South, a child came to the surgery door while the old doctor and Philip were making up prescriptions. It was a little ragged girl with a dirty face and bare feet. Philip opened the door. 'Please sir, will you come to Mrs Fletcher's in Ivy Lane at once.' 'What's the matter with Mrs Fletcher?' called out Dr South in his rasping voice. The child took no notice of him but addressed herself again to Philip. 'Please, sir, her little boy has had an accident and will you come at once?' 'Tell Mrs Fletcher I'm coming', called out Dr South. The little girl hesitated for a moment, and putting a dirty finger in a dirty mouth stood still and looked at Philip. 'What's the matter, kid?' said Philip, smiling. 'Please, sir, Mrs Fletcher says will the new doctor come?'

The old doctor, widowed and estranged from his only child (*see* p. 7), reacts with rage against the patient: 'Aren't I good enough to attend her filthy brat?'. However, he then accepts the inevitable: 'What's the good of my going? They want you.'[89]

Helen Ashton[90] also takes up the theme of the age gap between doctors. Dr Luke Serocold, an elderly English general practitioner, and his 'modern' colleague, Dr Jevons, manage not to fight openly. The two speak politely to one another, and when one of them operates, the other gives the anaesthetic. However, Serocold harbours 'a great deal of unconfessed dislike' of the popular, cheerful and competent Jevons, who is almost 30 years his junior, and eager to buy his practice.[90]

Serocold, a morose and solitary figure, prone to long bouts of rumination, dislikes his young colleague,

> a big, well-fed, muscular man [who] obviously ate and slept well [and who] liked the broad jokes that offended Doctor Serocold's fastidious taste.

When Serocold's partner dies, Jevons offers to help out.

> 'See you in hell first', thought Doctor Serocold ungratefully, and replied, in a tone which he vainly tried to keep natural, 'thanks, we can manage for the present.'[90]

Serocold detests Jevons' smoking habits, his clothes, his 'loud laugh and noisy affability,' his relaxed way with women, and even his car,

> that vulgar aluminium thing, like a Thermos flask. He says he can get sixty out of her . . . I hope she spills him into a ditch one of these days.[90]

Remarkably, it is the cantankerous, suspicious old Serocold who is portrayed as the priestly disciple of St Luke, while the cheerful, well-organized and good-natured Jevons is made to play the part of the earthy physician.[7]

In Cozzens' *The Last Adam*[91] it is the older of the two doctors who is cast in the role of the 'earthy' character. Dr George Bull is almost the prototype of Carolyn Norris's 'Pan' physician.[7] 'Ill-educated, unscientific, anti-intellectual . . . obese, dirty, noisy and overpowering, he is a man sprung from the soil rather than an antiseptic hospital.'[7] By contrast, Dr Verney, who received his training at Harvard, Johns Hopkins* and Vienna,[92] is well groomed and well spoken.[93] He spends a long time with his patients, taking a thorough history and performing a full physical examination so that 'when he's through, he has a four-page record.'[94] Unlike Dr Bull, he harbours no lecherous thoughts, and also unlike Dr Bull he 'wouldn't make you feel . . . that he regarded your life or death as a matter of no importance, and considered you a fool to be roared at for bothering him about it.'[93]

Dr Verney practises 'scientific' medicine using all the latest drugs[95] and equipment. 'Nurses . . . in uniform making urinalyses. Half a ton of fluoroscopic machines.'[94] Naturally, the two doctors are suspicious of each other's methods. Dr Bull, the old 'horse doctor', believes that a full physical examination is put on to impress the patients, especially the female patients.

---

* *See* footnote on pp. 21–2.

> 'Nine cases out of ten he doesn't know a thing he couldn't have found out by feeling a pulse and asking a couple of questions. . . . But everybody thinks when he's written down so much he must know something.'[94]

Dr Verney does not comment openly on the old doctor's primitive methods, but he hears plenty of adverse comments from disgruntled patients who used to consult Dr Bull but now see him.[96] Cozzens resists the temptation to weave the potential antagonism between the two physicians into a plot. Despite their different ages, backgrounds and prejudices the two doctors are polite to one another, discuss their patients, and collaborate when a typhoid epidemic hits 'New Winton, Connecticut.'[97]

Differences in age are used as an argument at Proust's dinner party,[98] where a plot is being hatched to promote the career of Dr Cottard, an up-and-coming young physician. One of the guests mentions that a well-known musician is seriously ill and that Dr Potain expects him to die.

> 'What!' cried Mme Verdurin, 'do people still call in Potain?' 'Ah, Mme Verdurin', [Dr] Cottard simpered, 'you forget that you are speaking of one of my colleagues. I should say one of my masters.' . . . 'Don't speak to me about your masters; you know ten times as much as he does!' . . . 'But Madame, he is in the Academy', replied the doctor with heavy irony.[98]

Weir Mitchell's decisive young interventionist, Dr Sydney Archer, does not fight openly with Dr Thomas Soper, but he is bored by the old man, who ruminates over his cases and whose tendency to 'yield to a colleague's opinion'[99] is considered a sign of weakness. Archer is impatient with Soper's chatter, especially his medical chatter.[100]

> 'Old Soper stopped me . . . just for a moment, to describe an interesting case. It took ten minutes. . . . Then he reported a case at length as if insomnia was as rare as Morvan's disease. . . . He said at last he might have to ask my counsel (*sic*). He never will.'[100]

Archer, the former army surgeon[101] who now engages in 'research'[102] as well as hospital and private practice,[101] disapproves of his older colleague, who is unable to distinguish between important and unimportant clinical features and who makes heavy weather of non-specific symptoms. Soper is bewildered by the 'confusing inrush of novel ideas'[102] which he cannot 'digest or assimilate.' Naturally, this diffident and out-of-date physician, who has no teaching hospital appointment,[100] and who is dimly conscious of his limitations, seeks free advice from his more recently trained colleague. He will obviously not ask Archer to see his patients, who might draw unfavourable comparisons between the knowledgeable younger man and the 'soporific' old windbag.

Yet another difference between traditional and modern doctors lies in their use of sales techniques. Shirley Jackson's Dr Victor Wright,[103] an old-fashioned 'hypnotist', expresses outrage at his more modern psychiatric colleagues who use 'all kinds of names for nothing and all kinds of cures for ailments that don't exist.' Wright is particularly incensed by the younger generation's attitude towards publicity and advertising. He ruminates:

> 'I believe I am an honest man and there aren't many of us left. The young flashy fellows, just starting out, who do everything except put their

names in neon lights and run bingo games in their waiting room, are my particular detestation.'[103]

Dr Samuel Abelman, Green's *Last Angry Man*,[22] who graduated in 1912[104] and spent many years trying unsuccessfully 'to make friends out of patients' (*see* p. 63) and to prevent the encroachments of 'fancy specialists' on his practice[24,42] (*see* p. 66), now has to face a new danger. A young generation of doctors is joining the ranks. When Dr Seymour Baumgart (class of 1940) sets up an office next door to Abelman, the older man finds himself up against a most unscrupulous competitor.[105] The entire Baumgart clan roam the street, acting like 'pullers-in' at old-fashioned New York clothing stores, accosting potential patients, warning them 'that Dr Abelman would kill them sooner or later' and advising them that 'the young doctors [have] got all the new machines.'[105] Samuel Abelman is too proud to complain, and predicts that his old-timers will not be taken in by the Baumgarts' trickery. He is wrong: 'The gullible, the frightened, the ignorant [were] ready to believe the worst about the stiff, moralizing old man who had thrown so many frauds (*sic*) out of his office, had delivered so many lost lectures.' They take themselves off to young Baumgart and find him 'neat and professional'[105] (*see also* Volume 1, pp. 176–7).

Dr Martin Isaacs, the coarse, old-fashioned but capable general practitioner who looks 'like an old-time senator from Texas',[106] holds views on the medical 'generation gap' very similar to those of Somerset Maugham's old Dr South[89] (*see* p. 76), but expresses them in more contemporary terminology.

> 'These smart young punks just out of training give me a pain in the crotch. . . . They think they know everything there is to know about medicine and they don't mind telling you about it loud and clear. . . . Of course it's still kind of nice to have an old Stone Age muddler like me . . . to bail 'em out when they get in trouble.'[107]

The 'smart young punks' have equally uncomplimentary opinions of their seniors. The junior doctors looking after Franz Biberkopf's 'catatonia' feel nothing but contempt for the clinical experience of their older colleagues, which they describe as the wisdom of arteriosclerotic graybeards waiting for their pension – 'intellectual content: zero'.[107a] Nourse's *Intern*[108] regards old Dr Donald MacDuff as 'one of these doddering eighty-year-old herb and root specialists who are still practicing medicine on a license granted fifty years ago and haven't read a medical journal since'.[108]

A senior position on the staff of an institution does not protect the incumbent from this syndrome. On the contrary, in the confined space of a hospital unit the younger doctors are constantly speculating about the possible retirement of their seniors and reminding each other of the proverb 'where there is death there is hope.'

In Van der Meersch's *Bodies and Souls*,[60] Professor Géraudin, whose surgical skills are on the decline (*see* pp. 71 and 228–9), is terrified of his younger colleagues.[109]

> That was Géraudin's great worry. . . . He must not grow old. . . . The whisper circulated that he was over sixty. . . . Residents and friends began to observe him, watching and scrutinizing with a doctor's pitiless eye whenever he was operating. . . . That was why Géraudin . . . surrounded by a little group of younger men greedy for his downfall . . . became more and more jealous of his prestige . . . as he aged.[109]

Dr Joseph Pearson, the old pathologist in Hailey's *The Final Diagnosis*,[110] whose judgment is impaired (*see also* p. 230), becomes needlessly belligerent at a mortality meeting where he accuses one of the surgeons of negligence.[110] In his own department he is absurdly jealous of his young assistant, who is told 'I'm still in charge'[111] and 'you'll get whatever [responsibility] I choose to give you.'[111] In due course both Géraudin[109] and Pearson[110,111] have to retire, but not before each of them has been responsible for a patient's death.

The crusader

Fights between older and younger generations of doctors become particularly savage when personality clashes or disagreements over treatment policies assume idealistic overtones. When young Dr Juvenal Urbino in *Love in the Time of Cholera*[112] returns from Paris to backward South America in the late 1870s, and attempts to introduce 'modern' ideas and treatment methods, he finds himself in conflict with the entire hospital staff. His colleagues

> could not tolerate the young newcomer's tasting a patient's urine to determine the presence of sugar, quoting Charcot and Trousseau as if they were his roommates, . . . [and] maintaining a suspicious faith in the recent invention of suppositories. . . . His renovating spirit, his maniacal sense of civic duty . . . provoked the resentment of his older colleagues and the sly jokes of the younger ones.[112]

(Ultimately, Urbino becomes the respected doyen of the city's medical community, and his 'advanced' medical views turn into inappropriate suspicions of all further innovations.[113])

Self-appointed messiahs such as Dr Robinson Tanner,[114–116] Dr Jonathan Ferrier[117–128] and Dr Lucas Marsh,[129] whose stated aim in life is the 'perfection' of the medical profession, may cause a great deal of harm before they discover that their holy grail is unattainable. Tanner manages to get rid of some of the more dangerous entrenched customs he discovers upon his arrival at 'Twin Forks, Montana',[114,115] but in the process the practice is 'smashed from top to bottom',[116] while the geographical problems of the isolated town remain insoluble.

Dr Jonathan Ferrier of 'Hambledon, Pennsylvania' the omniscient hero of Caldwell's romance, *Testimony of Two Men*,[19] is able to make a spot diagnosis of ovarian cancer,[123] acute leukaemia[118] and leprosy[122] without having to consult with other colleagues. He can deal successfully with attempted suicide,[120] pelvic sepsis[121] and cardiogenic shock.[126] This medical paragon is constantly searching for imperfections among his senior colleagues. He specializes in sniffing out incompetent and drug-addicted doctors[19] and bringing about the dismissal of these contemptible individuals[120] after first subjecting them to a great deal of verbal abuse. The Chief of Staff of the hospital is referred to as a 'cloaca.'[119] Dr Emil Schaefer 'isn't fit to deliver a sow'[127] and is called a criminal fool to his face.[127] Another 'evil' colleague, Dr Claude Brinkerman, is considered 'unfit to clip . . . dogs' nails.'[124] Ferrier finds his way into the operating room, where Brinkerman is in the process of performing a salpingectomy (for an ectopic pregnancy) and makes extraordinary threats against the older man in front of the resident and nursing staff. 'I shall watch every move you make, so you don't do the girl a sly mischief. . . .

You have a reputation for that.'[128] This medical Sir Galahad is of course detested by the established doctors of the town, although he has a few loyal supporters.[19] Jonathan Ferrier maintains this arrogant attitude throughout *Testimony of Two Men*, and at the end of the book he looks forward to his new role as chief of surgery, which will allow him to judge and dismiss 'incompetent' colleagues.[126] Caldwell's fanciful account of Dr Ferrier's one-man crusade is full of unbelievable details even for a story set at the beginning of the twentieth century. However, the general messages are very similar to those found in other works of fiction. First, old and young doctors detest one another. Second, doctors constantly gossip about their colleagues' misdiagnoses[19] and other medical failings. Third, when the inevitable happens and a doctor is forced, by the relevant regulatory body, to give up practice, the rest are secretly or overtly pleased to see one of their number crucified.[19]

Thompson's Dr Lucas Marsh[129] is another fanatic who believes in an abstract concept of 'medicine' as something 'fine, pure and maybe holy.' However, Marsh, who is more junior and more modest than Ferrier,[117] realizes on the last page of *Not as a Stranger*[129] that the practice of medicine is incompatible with lofty criticism and persecution of other doctors. Dr Ignac Semmelweis's single-minded hand-washing campaign in Thompson's *The Cry and the Covenant*[130] constitutes a source of weakness as well as an inspiration. A less messianic approach might have avoided a great deal of friction with senior and powerful colleagues and achieved a more successful outcome.

Dr Sagiura, in Paige Mitchell's *A Wilderness of Monkeys*,[131] is an evangelist of the meek and saintly rather than one of the fire-and-brimstone variety.[132] Sagiura, a deeply religious man (*see also* p. 130), has received a 'call' to set up a first-rate diagnostic clinic. He informs his colleagues at a business meeting that 'God willing' he will fulfill his 'destiny' with or without their assistance.[132] Sagiura's three partners, who are portrayed as villainous, weak or incompetent, feel uncomfortable with this display of 'religiosity.'[133] They are also concerned about a financial threat. For many years Sagiura has been carrying more than his fair share of the workload at the 'Stuartsville Clinic',[134] and his associates are afraid that an independent practice under his direction will bankrupt them. Instead of simply terminating the partnership and paying him an appropriate consideration as an inducement to relocate in a different town, they spread the rumour that he is insane and persuade the local hospital board to withdraw his admitting privileges.[133] A trial ensues and the jury find in favour of Dr Sagiura, who receives substantial damages.[135] We do not hear whether he subsequently succeeds in finding partners who share his lofty ideals.

Collegiate relations within hospitals

Francis Brett Young, a physician-author, gives a very pleasant account of the camaraderie at 'Prince's Hospital',[65] where the residents live

> in a tired but good-natured atmosphere of small talk, bridge and medical shop. . . . [The residents] were undistinguished [but] they were also, on the whole, homogeneous. Their interests were so narrowed that all could share them; their quarters so close that anything in the nature of dissension was avoided at all costs.[65]

This sense of solidarity becomes particularly compelling during and after shared traumatic experiences. Abby DiMatteo, the heroine of Gerritsen's *Harvest*,[136] who is subjected to an almost sadistic inquisition as part of a residents' round, retrieves the situation after some awkward moments and gives the Chairman of the Surgical Residency Program an answer that elicits a 'curt nod' rather than a sarcastic broadside.[137] Other members of the group share her sense of relief.

> One of the other residents gave Abby's arm a squeeze. 'Hey, DiMatteo', he whispered. 'Flying colors.'[137]

Cooperation between members of the hospital staff is almost perfect during major emergencies such as cardiac arrests. Writers of 'medical thrillers'[136,138,139] like to describe these 'battlefield' situations, during which the most senior member of the resuscitation team issues crisp orders such as 'let's shock', '400 joules', 'keep pumping' or 'ten milliequivalents of potassium.' There is no time for arguments, the participants obey willingly and the drama is over (one way or the other) within a few minutes. The sense of togetherness may last a little longer.

However, institutional settings by no means ensure unity and concord among physicians. On the contrary, the constant proximity of the protagonists aggravates antipathies and professional jealousies, which do not always remain latent. In the days when diagnosis was a kind of a crossword puzzle or bridge problem,[140] with a few scanty clues (and the answer provided in the post-mortem room the next day[141,142]), and when treatment options consisted of 'taking the waters' at this or that health resort,[142a] personal or factional rivalries might express themselves as learned and acrimonious disputations around the bedside with congratulations or recriminations after the autopsy. For instance, Dr Ebenwald in *Professor Bernhardi*[143] talks of the 'opposition' having 'triumphed' because an autopsy had shown a circumscribed renal cell carcinoma that might have been operable.[144] Such uncouth remarks are not made in the more genteel atmosphere of a London teaching hospital,[141] but even here the clinic chief feels so apprehensive about his colleagues' reactions that he uses terminology more appropriate to a battlefield than to a hospital. When, in the post-mortem room, the 'uncompromising knife of the pathologist' proves his diagnosis incorrect, Dr Peter Harding 'accepts defeat' and attempts to 'retire strategically.' However, his mistake does not go entirely unnoticed. 'I caught young Martyn . . . smiling significantly across at [another student] . . . who was very tactfully endeavouring to appear oblivious.' The chief considers that his retreat was made 'in fair order . . . with baggage intact and a minimum of casualties.'[141]

In recent times mainstream medicine has become more precise and more standardized. Differential diagnosis has overcome the 'hit-and-miss' aspects of a guessing game, and professional disagreements are now likely to involve points of emphasis rather than basic principles. However, personal prejudices and dislikes persist. Richard Selzer's plastic surgeon, Dr Hugh Franciscus,[145] has plenty of detractors but

> no close friends on the staff. There was something a little sad in that. As though long ago he had been flayed by friendship and now the slightest breeze would hurt. Confidences resulted in dishonor. Perhaps the person in whom one confided would scorn him, betray. . . . Franciscus seemed aware of an air of personal harshness in his environment to which he reacted by keeping his own counsel.[145]

On a more prosaic level, Straub's Dr Michael Poole,[146] a paediatrician on the staff of a large suburban hospital, figured that 'about a quarter of Westerholm's seventy doctors were not presently talking to him. . . . This was just normal medicine.'[147]

When Tomas, the neurosurgeon in Kundera's *The Unbearable Lightness of Being*,[148] is fired from his position on the hospital staff because of a dispute with the authorities, he receives no support at all from his colleagues. They smile at him hypocritically, they treat him to 'sincere handshakes' and they let him go without a word of protest.[148] Later, when Tomas, now a window cleaner, meets up with 'Doctor S', one of his former colleagues who has kept his job, he is assured that 'everything at the hospital is the same.'[149] In other words, 'your enforced departure has not made the slightest difference to the rest of us.' Although the story is set in Communist Czechoslovakia, the reader is left with the strong impression that collegiate support might be equally unforthcoming in a democratic country.

Partnership practices

Successful partnership practices depend on harmony and trust between the associates, at least at a superficial level. In *The Practice*,[150] the relationships between the four medical doctors in 'Twin Forks', Montana, are far from harmonious, but they suddenly improve in the face of a disaster. Dr Martin Isaacs, the experienced, dictatorial head of the practice, abuses and bullies his colleagues, who, he believes, are ineffectual,[151] dishonest,[152] or both. He regards his new assistant, Dr Rob Tanner, as an ignorant upstart[107] (*see* p. 79), but when this young man lands himself (and his patient) in serious trouble, Isaacs not only saves the situation, but also covers up the inexperienced doctor's serious lapse of judgement and persuades an orthopaedic surgeon to do likewise.[153] Tanner tries unsuccessfully and against the advice of a senior nurse to treat a forearm fracture by closed reduction. He is unable to align the fragments, and his efforts result in a haematoma with a compromised circulation in the hand.

> The boy's hand was suddenly a pasty yellow color, noticeably cool to the touch. What was more, the middle of the forearm was beginning to bulge like an overstuffed sausage. . . . At that point Martin Isaacs walked in the door, wet X-rays in his hand. 'Rob, what in the hell do you think you are doing, fooling around with a fracture like this?'

Isaacs takes in the complications at a glance and proceeds to tidy up the mess and cover his tracks. On the telephone to an orthopaedic surgeon in Missoula he is brief and efficient.

> 'Charlie? Martin Isaacs in Twin Forks. I'm afraid I've got a mean one for you out here. Eight-year-old boy with a double fracture of the right forearm. I – ah – tried a closed reduction, and I shouldn't have. May have nicked the radial; we've got a big hematoma in there all of a sudden. . . . Yes, I've got it wrapped. . . . No, no, I'll ship him on in; you're obviously going to have to open it up. He'll be on his way in a few minutes. . . . Oh, and Charlie this is a little bit embarrassing to me, what with the parents and all, if you take my meaning. . . . Right, right. A little leg up would help a lot. I'd take that very kindly.'[153]

The boy makes a full recovery, the parents are grateful for the skilled treatment provided by Tanner and Isaacs, and the partners come out of the potential disaster 'smelling like a rose.'

Cooperation and respect between partners become essential in highly specialized practices, especially those with pretensions to excellence. In *The Fourth Hand*,[154] Irving describes in some detail the complex relationship between the stuffy old partners in 'the leading center for hand care in Boston' and their overachieving but eccentric associate, Dr Nicholas Zajac. They need him but they envy him. Fortunately for the firm, their envy is tempered by pity for Zajac's personal problems.

> [Zajac's colleagues at] Schatzman, Gingeleskie, Mengerink and Associates . . . were woefully behind his surgical skills[147] . . . it was only a matter of time before Dr Zajac, although he was still in his forties, would have to be included in the *title* of Boston's foremost surgical associates in hand treatment. Soon it would have to be Schatzman, Gingeleskie, Mengerink, *Zajac* and Associates.[154]

The prospect of having to share their letterhead with this nonentity is less than pleasing to Schatzman and colleagues, whose distress becomes even more acute at the thought that 'Harvard* would soon make Zajac an associate professor.' The senior partners console themselves by contemplating Zajac's 'bizarre eating habits, his collapsed family life and his desperate love for his unhappy six-year-old son.'[154] They react with sly malice when Zajac's star patient rejects his transplanted hand.[155] Zajac, in turn, declares privately that 'he doubted Dr Mengerink could cure a hangnail.'[154] Relations between the partners improve when Zajac marries his housekeeper and replaces the photographs of his famous patients with those of his pregnant wife.[156]

Capricious behaviour; ritual humiliations; the hospital as a boot camp

The great strength of hospitals – their hierarchical structure – also constitutes a significant source of friction. The chiefs and the senior staff exercise such a decisive influence over the future careers of the younger doctors, that the juniors are at their mercy to an even greater extent than the patients. This power structure may lead to bad-mannered, capricious or dogmatic behaviour on the part of the seniors. Dr William Tick,

> Professor of Medicine at a great Eastern medical school . . . had favored the education-by-insult theory of pedagogy. There were eminent doctors who still winced when they recalled some of Tick's appraisals of their budding talents.[157]

Professor Prader, the chief of haematology in *Ward 402*,[158] is renowned for his capricious behaviour. He

---

* *See* footnote on pp. 21–2.

could get angry with you for not having all the red blood cell indices ready when you were treating a patient with iron-deficient anemia when the day before he'd lectured that in most cases of this type of anemia the smear itself was enough for the diagnosis.[159]

Dubious physical signs become important when discovered by a senior staff member. A 'Grade I' heart murmur is audible 'only if the Professor of Medicine insists that it's there.'[160]

The relative weakness of the junior staff also encourages a particular type of bullying – the verbal abuse of the weak by the strong under the pretext of 'professional training.' Ellis[161] provides a brilliant illustration of this syndrome when he describes, in considerable detail, how Dr Vernet, the chief physician, publicly and repeatedly humiliates young Dr Florent in front of a patient (Paul Davenant) and members of the nursing staff.[161]

> Dr Bruneau left the room to return shortly with a young doctor of most timid aspect. 'Come Florent', said Dr Vernet, giving Paul the smile of a confederate, 'come and give us your opinion of the condition of Monsieur Davenant.' And still smiling he seated himself on the corner of his desk whilst Dr Florent ran his stethoscope over Paul's chest, telling him at the same time to breathe deeply, to cough and to say trente-trois. . . . 'A little quicker, Florent, Monsieur Davenant is getting tired', said Dr Vernet, and as Dr Florent started to stammer a diagnosis [he interrupts and announces his own verdict].[162]

The performance is repeated during a subsequent episode when an old-fashioned laryngoscopy is being performed.[163]

> Then in order that Dr Florent might gain some practical experience, Dr Vernet told him to continue in his stead. An exchange of seats. Dr Vernet gazed laconically at his young assistant as the latter nervously affixed a reflector to his forehead. In his anxiety to cause Paul as little discomfort as possible, Dr Florent inserted and withdrew the instrument before it had wholly performed its function. Dr Vernet watched, advised, and criticized; at last losing his patience . . . he flicked on the lights.[163]

Vernet also makes fun of his senior assistant, Dr Bruneau, whose knowledge of English is limited.[164] Florent, who inadvertently unsterilizes a glass table is told (wearily and in public) 'Florent, you're ruining my life' (vous m'empoisonnez l'existence).[164]

Bedside teaching frequently degenerates into a smorgasbord of truisms, half-truths, untruths and insults (*see also* Volume 1, p. 207). The most important message is that the trainee is the epitome of laziness and ignorance. 'Didn't they teach you *anything* in medical school?'[165]

Dr Watson Kreck,* Associate Clinical Professor of Neurology at the Paradiso Veterans Affairs Hospital, is making rounds with Dr Redshield, the new resident.[166]

---

* Several of Schneiderman's characters bear 'catchy' names of major and minor medical pioneers such as 'Henderson', 'Hasselbalch' and 'Klippelfeil', with or without slight variations from the original (*see also* Volume 1, p. 207).

'Well, Redshield', snapped Kreck, jabbing out his hand, 'what have you got to show me?'. . . . 'Nothing very much.' 'What? Nothing? You mean to say in this whole ward full of fantastic neurological specimens you've got nothing to show me? What do you take me for, Redshield?' He twitched his shoulders two or three times as though preparing to spring. Kreck had made his name in micturition syncope and took no shit from neurological residents. Redshield twitched one or two times himself and aimed what he hoped was an appealing smile at Kreck. 'I arrived just yesterday'. . . . 'Yesterday? Then what have you been doing since then? When I was a resident I didn't eat. I didn't sleep. I didn't do anything until I had every patient memorized, memorized right down to the last detail. A doctor has to dedicate himself.'[166]

The chief obstetric resident in Frede's *The Interns*[167] uses the same 'boot-camp' approach. 'Tell me, Parelli', he says to one of the junior members of the staff, 'is there any reason why I should assume you've had the benefit of a medical education?'[168] An intern in Robin Cook's *Coma*[169] is crudely and unnecessarily abused on a ward round because the ENT team had not arrived to perform a tracheostomy on a comatose patient.

Bullying is particularly intense in surgical units. The chiefs throw instruments on the floor or hurl them against a wall to indicate their displeasure. They harass surgical residents, who are constantly insulted, accused of incompetence and threatened with dismissal.[170] The entire tortuous plot of Lloyd Douglas's *Green Light*[171] is based on the behaviour of the senior surgeon who, instead of acknowledging his responsibility for an operative disaster, shifts the blame on to his assistant.[171]

Like a battered youngster who, if he survives, goes on to batter his own children, the harassed residents who are unable to retaliate take their revenge by tyrannizing the more junior staff.[168,170] The senior surgical resident in *Coma*[169] waxes sarcastic when his juniors are a little slow in draping a patient on the operating table, and inquires 'What are you trying to do, make this your life's work?' A little later he yells 'Are you here to help me or hinder me?'[169] Dr George Newman, the chief resident in neurosurgery in *Brain*,[170] abuses one of his junior residents using the same expression.

Examiners of candidates for admission to surgical bodies enjoy the power structure inherent in the situation, and may use it to ask tricky questions on the pretext that the answer (or the lack of it) may provide some insight into the young doctor's personality. A classic account of such an examination is found in Smollett's *Roderick Random*.[172] After one of the censors at 'Surgeon's Hall' has subjected Roderick to a great deal of bullying, the wit of the group asks the 'crunch' question:

'If . . . during an engagement at sea, a man should be brought to you with his head shot off, how would you behave?' After some hesitation, I owned such a case had never come under my observation, neither did I remember to have seen any method of cure proposed for such an accident in any of the systems of surgery I had perused.[172]

The answer evidently shows the 'right' mixture of confidence and humility, and Roderick receives his qualification.[172]

Bullying of junior staff is more subtle in internal medicine, where it may take the form of one-upmanship. Some prominent physicians acquire their reputation by dogmatic diagnoses, quotations and misquotations from the latest medical journals and, occasionally, by straightforward dishonesty. Dr Rintman, the 'great' New York diagnostician, is conducting rounds in 'McKinley Hospital.'[173] The year is 1933, 'when diagnosis was the giant, treatment the dwarf and he the greatest consultant in the City.' Dr Rintman, about to begin a round,

> raised his head and inhaled deeply a few times as if to show that the air he was now sampling would lead him to something that would confound them all. 'There's scurvy in this room!' he announced softly. 'The scent is clear.' Turning to the House Physician he said 'You smell it of course.' Too flabbergasted to answer, the Chief Intern just shook his head. . . . He was unaware of Rintman's secret custom. Every afternoon, about fifteen minutes before rounds, he would drop into the admitting office . . . and study the names of all the patients who had entered the hospital. . . . Today he had pounced on the fact that a man with scurvy had gone to Male One. Although the head clerk knew the purpose of Rintman's visits, she . . . never . . . betrayed him. Whatever increased his prestige added luster to the hospital.[173]

Cooperation under pressure from outside

The 'negative co-operativity' between physicians rapidly changes to positive in the face of 'external' enemies such as politicians, regulatory bodies, administrators and lawyers. Dr Paul Rice, from a medical family, and Dr Jerry Warren, an African-American, are colleagues at the 'Danton Clinic' when Dr Danton, the dictatorial founder and head of the institution, throws both of them out.[174] The two become firm friends, they transfer together to the cardiothoracic unit at a university hospital, and despite their different backgrounds and positions (Paul is Jerry's chief) there is very little tension between them. Indeed, Paul takes up 'progressive' causes, he starts dating a Mexican American girl from a poor immigrant family, and at the banquet of the medical convention he sits at a multi-cultural table rather than with the power brokers.[175]

The tendency for doctors to support each other becomes particularly strong when there is a threat of a malpractice suit. Doctors share a fear of 'ambulance-chasing lawyers on fat contingency fees'[176] and 'ridiculous multi-million-dollar settle-ments'[176] so that, when such dangers loom, even sworn enemies keep silent. 'Whistleblowers' are not appreciated in any organization, and are particularly unwelcome in the medical profession (*see also* p. 223).

When Dr Sagiura in Paige Mitchell's *A Wilderness of Monkeys*[132-135] approaches two partners in a law firm because he wants to sue his former associates (*see also* p. 81), the lawyers express surprise and speculate that the doctor may not be quite sane.

> Doctors don't usually go around suing each other. [In the presence of the Law] they stick together like glue even if they hate each other's guts.[177]

Reed in *The Verdict*[178] goes even further.

> With doctors it's worse than the Mafia. They have a conspiracy of
> silence. [A doctor] can saw the wrong leg off the Pope and everyone gets
> deaf, dumb and blind. He can leave Kelley clamps inside a guy's stomach
> and the College of Surgeons will swear that it's accepted medical practice
> to store a little hardware inside the abdomen. They really stick together
> these guys. The medical Mafia.[179]

Mitchell[177] and Reed[179] are, of course, exaggerating, but every practising physician
who is confronted with a colleague's mistake is acutely aware that 'but for the grace
of God' he might have committed a similar error of judgement.

Warwick Deeping[180] narrates the story of a consultation involving two former
classmates – Dr Christopher Sorrell, a successful London surgeon, and Dr Maurice
Pentreath, a chronic loser who is now vegetating in a general practice in 'Mill-
chester.'[181] Pentreath is a pathetic figure. He neglects to take a post-reduction X-ray
of a little girl's forearm fracture, because 'he is afraid of what [he] might see.' Sorrell,
who is not particularly impressed with Pentreath's clinical skills, nonetheless agrees
to make a special trip and to prevent any kind of litigation that the child's family
might be contemplating.[180,181] (*See also* Volume 1, p. 231.)

In Michael Crichton's *A Case of Need*,[182] a doctor's daughter dies as a result of
perforation of the uterus after a bungled abortion. Suspicion falls first on one doctor
and then on another, but the amateur investigator, a pathologist, believes that
neither of the two is guilty. The lawyer defending one of the doctors disagrees.[182]

> 'The trouble with you . . . is that you're like all doctors. You can't believe
> that one of your own is rotten. What you'd really like to see is an ex-army
> medical orderly or a nurse on trial. Or a nice little old midwife. That's
> who you'd like to stick with this rap. Not a doctor.'[182]

(The pathologist is right. The perpetrator was a drug-addicted nurse.)

Dr Parris Mitchell of *King's Row*,[183] a psychiatrist on the staff of the state
asylum, finds himself at the centre of a political storm over the sale of some land to
the institution. He is gratified when

> various members of the staff, some of whom he had not thought of as
> being particularly friendly, had come to him with jocular or sympathetic
> comments. Parris did not know how much of this was spontaneous and
> how much of it might have been inspired by [his friend] Dr Nolan.[183]

However, there is no doubt regarding the genuine support for Parris and the real
dislike of his 'external enemies'.

Medical practitioners may detest some of their colleagues and criticize them
among themselves, but they become uncomfortable if 'lay' individuals, especially
patients, express adverse opinions about fellow doctors and their professional
abilities. They have been taught Osler's precept* in medical school and behave
accordingly, even in fiction.

Gavin Prescott, a hospital orderly in Havard's *Coming of Age*[185] who has a
somewhat unusual relationship with his half-sister Linda, believes that she has a

---

* 'Never listen to a patient who begins with a story about the carelessness and inefficiency of Doctor
Blank. Shut him or her up with a snap knowing full well that the same tale may be told of you a few
months later. Fully half of the quarrels of physicians are fomented by the tittle-tattle of patients, and the
only safeguard is not to listen.'[184]

lump in her breast and wants Dr Jonathan Brookes, a young surgical trainee, to examine her. Linda refuses to see her general practitioner.

> 'Who is your GP?' 'Old Dr O'Connor.' 'Can't say I've heard of him' Jonathan admitted. 'Doesn't know his arse from his elbow.'[185]

The medical profession closes ranks.

> 'Come on, Gavin, I'm sure that's not true.' 'Don't get me wrong, Dr Brooks. O'Connor's great; never too busy to see you, never gives you the impression you're wasting his time; his older patients worship him, the Catholics especially. . . . But he's knocking eighty and not much good on lumps in the breast, I shouldn't think.'[185]

When John Tremont in Wharton's *Dad*[186] complains to Dr Ethridge, his father's regular physician, about the insensitive behaviour of Dr Santana, the hospital urologist, he gets a very unsympathetic hearing. Instead of enquiring about the details, Dr Ethridge describes Dr Santana as one of the hospital's 'bright young men.'[187]

Consultations with former chiefs

Not all consultations result in a breakdown of collegiate relationships. Recently graduated physicians who call in their former teachers are content to bask in the great man's reflected glory, and there is no friction between the junior and senior doctor.

When, at the age of 29, Dr John Seward in Stoker's *Dracula*[188] finds himself the superintendent of an 'immense lunatic asylum', he remains a very junior medical student to his consultant and former teacher, Professor Abraham Van Helsing. The professor refuses to reveal his hypotheses to his disciple,[189] he sends Seward out of the room while he examines one of the vampire's victims, and he pulls Seward's ear 'playfully as he used . . . to do . . . long ago.'[189] Van Helsing, who combines the roles of detective, technician, philosopher and priest (*see also* pp. 8 and 156–7), is also a remarkably versatile physician. He is a hypnotist,[190] a neurosurgeon,[191] a haematologist[189] and a dispenser of intensive care,[189] as well as an authority on 'obscure diseases.'[189] Throughout the lengthy investigation into the activities of Count Dracula, there is not even a hint that Seward resents either Van Helsing's role as team leader or his own subservient status.

Dawson's Dr John Selkirk, who has called in Dr Carson, his surgical father figure, to perform a life-saving operation, also reveres his former mentor.[192] As a student, he resented Carson on account of his sarcasm and his 'grim ironic smile.' Now that Selkirk is in practice, his attitude has changed. At the end of a difficult surgical procedure, neither he nor any of the other former students are offended by Dr Carson's behaviour: 'We knew quite well that we were poor creatures beside him and we did not mind knowing it.'[192]

Similarly, Dr Antoine Thibault,[193] who brings along his former chief from the Children's Hospital to see the retarded daughter of a colleague, is very much aware of the Professor's superior status and its effect on the stricken family. The little girl is dying from some intracranial infection, and the mere presence of the senior physician helps to relieve the parents' anguish and guilt.[193]

Yet another consultation between a recent graduate and his former professor is described in Eric Ambler's *Doctor Frigo*.[194] Dr Ernesto Castillo, aged 31, has under his care, in one of the Caribbean islands, a prominent politician who suffers from an undiagnosed neurological disease. The professor, who has been specially flown out from Paris, 'a slim imposing old man, very well preserved . . . proved to be in a vile temper. . . . [Castillo] offered to carry the instrument bag he had with him. He ignored the offer.'[194] Castillo, who is telling the story in the first person, continues to be terrified of his former teacher.

> He stared at me. 'Is it your case, Doctor?' 'Yes.' 'Very well' he said grimly. 'We shall see.' The crack of doom would have sounded more reassuring. Going up in the lift, I made efforts to stop moistening my lips repeatedly and to pull myself together. I saw him noting both efforts with bleak satisfaction. . . . 'And what do you think is the matter with the man?' I told him the tentative diagnosis I had made. [Amyotrophic lateral sclerosis.] He snorted. 'What do you know about that? Ever seen a . . . case?' 'No, Professor. What I know about it I learned from listening to your lecture on the subject.'[194]

The professor subsequently agrees with Ernesto's diagnosis.

Consultations with the local expert

When a senior physician is asked to confirm or refute a colleague's recommendations, the 'second opinion' does not necessarily lead to a confrontation. On the contrary, as Charles Reade[195] points out, when a particular management option has already been advocated, a consultant is likely, for diplomatic and psychological reasons, to confirm the approach suggested by his colleague even though he might have chosen a different method. So long as the treatment advised by the first doctor is not totally outlandish, the provider of the second opinion will be strongly tempted to back his colleague, although he will refuse to cooperate with what he considers overt quackery. The fact that the quack may be 'right' is irrelevant.

David Dodd, the central character in *Hard Cash*,[196] has had an epileptic seizure and is carried home, unconscious, to his wife. Mr Osmond, the local surgeon,

> came softly into the room, examined Dodd's eye, felt his pulse, and said he must be bled at once. Mrs Dodd was averse to this. 'Oh, let us try everything else first', said she; but Osmond told her there was no other remedy. . . . Dr Short now drove up and was ushered in. Mrs Dodd asked him imploringly whether it was necessary to bleed. But Dr Short knew his business too well to be entrapped into an independent opinion where a surgeon had been before him. He drew Mr Osmond apart, and inquired what he had recommended; this ascertained, he turned to Mrs Dodd and said, 'I advise venesection. . . . The case is simple . . . I leave it in competent hands.' And he retired, leaving the inferior practitioner well pleased with him and with himself; no insignificant part of the physician's art.[196]

Dr Short's tolerance does not extend to Dr Sampson, an eccentric physician whose views are far ahead of his time and who does not believe in bleeding at all.[196]

Sampson retaliates by referring to his colleagues as 'vagabonds . . . who would starve Cupid and venesect Venus.'[197]

The relationship between Dr Miles, a family practitioner, and Dr John Pritchard, a consultant obstetrician, in Conan Doyle's *The Curse of Eve*[198] is described factually and without any adversarial overtones. Lucy Johnson's home confinement has turned out more troublesome than Dr Miles anticipated, and he suggests a second opinion. He gives the husband a choice of consultants, but intimates that he would prefer Dr Pritchard, despite his high charges. The two doctors meet outside Lucy's bedroom and Miles apologizes for getting Pritchard out of bed – 'nasty case – decent people.'[198] After the baby has been safely delivered and the senior man has been paid, the two doctors talk briefly on their way out.

> 'Looked nasty at one time.' 'Very glad to have your help.' 'Delighted I'm sure. Won't you step round to have a cup of coffee?' 'No thanks, I'm expecting another case.'[198]

Miles is obviously the less influential of the two. He apologizes to Pritchard, he is praised for his skilful assistance (possibly administering the anaesthetic while Pritchard performs a forceps delivery) and he issues an invitation for coffee, which is declined. However, there is not even a hint of patronization on the part of Pritchard or resentment by Miles of his own apparently inferior status.[198]

The brief appearance of Dr Dieulafoy at the deathbed of Marcel's grandmother (*see* Volume 1, p. 30) causes no ill feelings among her regular medical attendants.[199]

> [Dieulafoy] a great physician, a marvelous teacher . . . had been sent for not to cure but to certify . . . that . . . [the] patient was in extremis.[199]

His ritual examination and his few murmured words constitute no threat to the 'doctor in charge of the case', who cheerfully goes on with his useless therapeutic efforts.

Similarly, once Parris Mitchell has gained the confidence of his colleagues in *King's Row*,[200] they refer patients to him without any sign of resentment. One patient declares 'Dr Waring has been our physician for years and he says you're the only person who can . . . help me.'

A particularly dramatic consultation is described by Sobel in *The Hospital Makers*.[201] Dr Emmerich, the Chief of Surgery at 'McKinley Hospital', has been asked by Dr Jake Morelle, a general practitioner, to see a case in consultation. The patient, a 45-year-old furrier, has lost 50 pounds in weight and a hard mass is palpable in his epigastrium. While the patient is getting dressed, the two doctors discuss the problem.

> The surgeon said 'I'll operate on him, but you know the outlook in carcinoma of the stomach, especially one as far advanced as this.' Jake said nothing. After a moment Emmerich glanced at him sharply. 'You agree, of course.' 'No, I don't.' Emmerich gave him the eagle stare. 'Every patient is entitled to an exploratory laparotomy if only on the remote chance that it might not be cancer.' 'Oh, I think he should be operated on all right. It's just that I don't think he has cancer.' No one had argued with Emmerich in a long time. 'What did you say?' he demanded. Jake almost expected a thunderbolt to come crashing into the dusk. . . . 'I said

I don't think it's carcinoma. I think it's a trichobezoar.' Then he told Emmerich about the hairs in the gastric juice, the trip to the Bronx, the visit to the furrier's back room and . . . [the patient's] nervous habit . . . [of licking his fingers]. . . . The surgeon, who never left his desk during a conference, stood up and walked to the window, deeply disturbed. After all, he was the Blickarzt, who was supposed to make the dramatic diagnosis at the very first glance. Instead there came to him a dispensary doctor with a theory that fitted the case like a glove and who had the audacity to throw the glove in his face. The diagnosis was preposterous. He turned around, looked at Jake broodingly and suddenly knew it was not preposterous at all. This man was no show-off, no sensation seeker. This was a good man and a very keen man. And of course the tumor had been completely movable. He returned to the desk, sat down and turned towards Jake. 'Whether you're right or wrong, it still is a brilliant diagnosis. I think you are right.'

The mass turns out to be a trichobezoar and the patient makes a full recovery.[201]

Consultations between equals

Occasional fictional passages capture the collegiate relationship between physicians as it exists in real life. In a partnership practice, a remark like 'Come and see old Phillimore, I don't like the look of him'[202] (which implies an admission of ignorance and a request for help) is much more likely than the ferocious infighting described in *The Practice*[71] or *A Wilderness of Monkeys*[131] (*see* pp. 72 and 81). Similarly, the telephone conversation between Dr Rieux and Dr Richard in Camus' *The Plague*[203] is more true to life than the 'war to the knife' in *My Brother Jonathan*[66] (*see* p. 72). Rieux has come across several patients with fever and lymph node enlargement and he is puzzled by this combination, which he has not previously encountered.

> On returning to his flat Rieux rang up his colleague Richard, one of the leading practitioners in the town. 'No', Richard said, 'I can't say I've noticed anything exceptional.' 'No cases of fever with local inflammation?' 'Wait a bit! I have two cases with inflamed glands.' 'Abnormally so?' 'Well,' Richard said, 'that depends on what you mean by normal.'[203]

The two physicians who look after Simenon's René Maugras,[204] a paralyzed and aphasic newspaper editor (*see* Volume 1, pp. 180–2), not only communicate but also cooperate with one another. Dr Pierre Besson d'Argoulet, the patient's usual physician and friend, transfers Maugras from a private facility to the care of Dr Audoire, a professor of neurology at a hospital for neurological disorders. Audoire, who is worried about Maugras' fatalistic attitude, contacts Besson, and the two doctors come to an understanding 'that they should each play their part.'[205] Audoire will treat Maugras' stroke on a strictly professional basis, while Besson d'Argoulet will provide friendly advice and admonition.

> This was how parents treated their children. When persuasion did not work, the mother would say to her husband: 'You try! You've got more

authority than I have. Perhaps if you shake him up a bit.' Besson was shaking him up.[204]

Slaughter provides several realistic descriptions of hospital consultations between different specialists. During a laparotomy for multiple abdominal bullet wounds, the hero of *No Greater Love*, [206] Dr Ted Bronson, a vascular and transplant surgeon, asks Dr Donald Taylor, a urologist who is assisting, what to do next. The right kidney has been torn apart.

> 'What do you think, Don?' he asked. 'No doubt about the fact that the right kidney is kaput', said the urologist. 'Should I explore the left one . . . too?'[206]

The question is inappropriate. Bronson is evidently not entirely familiar with the treatment of penetrating abdominal injuries, but the urologist's answer is neither patronizing nor sarcastic. He even shows Bronson the courtesy of pretending to consider an exploration of the left kidney but then rejecting the idea in favour of a 'better' (the correct) option. Taylor says:

> 'We can do that after you stop the haemorrhage by removing the right one. Or better still, unless there's a lot of blood in the urine from the left one . . . there's no need to add a second incision.'

Bronson manages to extricate himself without loss of face. 'My sentiments exactly', he concurs.[206]

There is also a bullet wound to the liver, and over the next few days the patient's liver functions deteriorate. Dr Bronson asks the chief of gastroenterology to see the patient, and the two physicians subsequently discuss the situation in the gastro-enterology office. After a few pleasantries the chief freely admits that he has no idea why the liver is failing, but that he considers it 'damn near . . . past redemption.'[207]

Slaughter also captures the pleasant casual encounters between medical colleagues that occur in places like hospital cafeterias and frequently end in serious, non-emotive 'shop talk'.[208] 'Dr Paul Fraser was ahead of [Dr Elizabeth MacGowan] in the cafeteria line but waited after paying his bill until she came through. "Sitting with anyone, Liz?" he asked.' The two sit down together and are subsequently joined by the transplant surgeon. The conversation ranges around amniocentesis, the survival rates of premature babies and, after the arrival of the surgeon, the progress of the hospital's star patient, the local political honcho with his multiple abdominal gunshot wounds.[208]

Social occasions: 'shop talk'

Relations between colleagues are generally harmonious at medical society banquets and similar functions. At the annual pre-Christmas dinner of the Australian College of Obstetricians and Gynecologists[209]

> beepers chirped from time to time, colleagues rose from their tables and hurried away to phones or to urgent deliveries, but there was a mood of generosity in the air, a camaraderie that no interruption could disturb, a willingness to laugh at anything [the guest speaker] said.[209]

On such agreeable occasions or at other times when hostilities are suspended, the participants discuss topics of mutual interest, such as their means of transportation.[27] They may also engage in medical 'shop talk', with its characteristic contents, expressions and attitudes. Topics are likely to include clinical problems and anecdotes, medical politics and gossip. The formal style of the early twentieth century has been replaced by medical shorthand and jargon, which some contemporary non-medical writers find offensive. The physicians' distinctive mixture of cynicism and compassion and the sardonic humour of clinical situations have only rarely been captured in works of fiction.

Sinclair Lewis's *Main Street*[210] contains one brief clinical conversation that sounds reasonably authentic. 'Say, doctor, what success have you had with thyroid for treatment of pain in the legs before childbirth?' However, the next question appears contrived: 'Doctor, what's been your experience with unilateral pyelonephritis? Buckburn of Baltimore advocates decapsulation and nephrotomy, but it seems to me . . .'.[210] A twenty-first-century reader will find it highly unlikely that doctors from Minnesota country towns would have lectured one another at a social encounter in 1920 about what 'Buckburn of Baltimore advocates' for unilateral pyelonephritis.[210]

By far the most convincing fictional account of contemporary medical shop talk is provided by Michael Crichton, who describes snatches of conversations overheard at a cocktail party.[211] The guests are academics, fellows and residents working at a Boston university hospital, the blood alcohol and noise levels are elevated, and the topics include clinical curiosities, lewd anecdotes and hospital gossip. The language is elitist medical jargon, superficially comprehensible to anyone familiar with medical terminology, but full of innuendoes and assumed background knowledge. Only sophisticated physicians with well-developed medical attitudes can join in.[211]

> 'They all get bacteremia sooner or later anyway . . .'
>
> 'And he was walking around – walking around, mind you – with a blood pH of seven point six and a potassium of one . . .'
>
> 'Well, what the hell do you expect of a Hopkins* man?'
>
> 'Sure you can correct the blood gases, but it doesn't help the vasculature . . .'
>
> 'Oliguric my ass. He was anuric for five days and he still survived . . .'
>
> '. . . in a 74-year-old man we just excised it locally and sent him home. It's slow growing anyhow . . .'
>
> '. . . liver reached down to his knees practically. But no hepatic failure . . .'
>
> 'She said she'd sign herself out if we didn't operate, so naturally we . . .'
>
> '. . . but the students are always bitching, it's a non-specific response . . .'
>
> 'Well, apparently this girl had bitten it off . . .'
>
> 'Really? Harry with that little nurse in Seven? The blonde?'
>
> '. . . don't believe it. He publishes more journal articles than most people can read in a lifetime . . .'
>
> '. . . metastases to the heart . . .'[211]

---

* *See* footnote on pp. 21–2.

The 'shorthand' language which doctors (especially hospital doctors) use among themselves ('he's gone down to be cathed'[212]) tends to irritate outsiders on account of both its form and its content. A remark like 'no fever, no rigors, normal bowel sounds'[212] would be considered perfectly reasonable in the context of a sit-down type of presentation, even though Kathryn Hunter considers such talk 'medicine's peculiar rhetoric of denial.' Hunter[212] also appears to resent remarks such as 'We sent the MI to the unit', which she believes dehumanizes the patient, while the residents argue that it does no such thing. They are aware that 'the MI' is a human being with a myocardial infarction, but for the moment the 'MI' or the need for a 'CABG' is more important than the patient's pain, his fears or the fact that he is a 62-year-old plumber.

As usual, the clearest fictional account of contemporary medical behaviour is to be found in one of Ravin's novels.[213] Clinicians, Ravin explains, do not use medical shorthand in order to confuse outsiders or to dehumanize their patients, but to indicate a system of priorities. When procedures have to be performed, investigations organized and various specialists notified, compassion and hand-holding must wait until the more urgent tasks have been completed. When Dr William Ryan, an intern at 'Manhattan Hospital', tells Arch, a young lawyer who shares his apartment, about one of his patients and inadvertently slips into hospital jargon[213]

> Arch was more appalled by Ryan's phrasing than his substance. 'What do you mean he's a melanoma? You mean he's a human being afflicted with melanoma?' . . . 'Arch, right now he's a melanoma. Monday, when I've got all the notes written, he might become Vince Cotti, human being with melanoma. But until then he's Vince Cotti, melanoma, pericardial effusion, lung mets, liver mets.'[213]

Summary

Writers of fiction exaggerate the prevalence and severity of fights between physicians and under-emphasize their collegiate relationships. They fail to appreciate the genuine respect that exists, especially in hospitals, between individuals who practise different branches of medicine or even the same specialty. The dearth of fictional descriptions of collegiality, compared with the plethora of colourful accounts of conflicts may be attributed to a 'preference for war over peace as a subject.'[1]

In the real world, humiliating encounters between colleagues have become particularly rare. Residents in university hospitals may amuse each other (and the senior staff) with anecdotes about the perceived ignorance or incompetence of physicians practising in centres of non-excellence, but such sentiments are rarely expressed in front of the offending physician, the patient or the patient's family. As residents mature, they learn not even to think along these lines.

Ritual case discussions during grand rounds and similar gatherings provide hospital physicians with mutual support and teaching exercises[214] rather than with opportunities for drawing attention to themselves. The doctor may not have many friends, but he has fine colleagues with whom he can share his anxieties and his job satisfaction. The 'surgical' behaviour described in Robin Cook's novels is recognizable, but it constitutes an aberration rather than the norm.

References

1 Petro JA (1992) Collegiality in history. *Bull N Y Acad Med.* **68**: 286–91.
2 James H (1884) Lady Barberina. In: *The New York Edition of Henry James. Volume 14.* Augustus Kelley, Fairfield, NJ, 1976, p. 18.
3 Gutheil TG and Gabbard GO (1993) The concept of boundaries in clinical practice: theoretical and risk management dimensions. *Am J Psychiatry.* **150**: 188–96.
4 Richardson S (1747–1748) The History of Clarissa Harlowe. In: Stephen L (ed.) *The Works of Samuel Richardson. Volume 8.* Henry Sotheran, London, 1883, p. 168.
5 Remarque EM (1945) *Arch of Triumph* (translated by Sorell W and Lindley D). Appleton Century, New York, pp. 261–2.
6 Auden WH (1972) Lines to Dr Walter Birk on his Retiring from General Practice. In: *Epistle to a Godson and Other Poems.* Faber and Faber, London, p. 16.
7 Norris CB (1969) *The Image of the Physician in Modern American Literature.* PhD Dissertation, University of Maryland, Baltimore, MD, p. 37.
8 Rinehart MR (1935) *The Doctor.* Farrar and Rinehart, New York, pp. 133–4.
8a O'Neill E (1928) Strange Interlude. In: *The Plays of Eugene O'Neill. Volume 3.* Random House, New York. 1955, p. 30.
9 Dawson WJ (1900) *The Doctor Speaks.* Grant Richards, London.
10 Mitchell SW (1901) *Circumstance.* The Century Company, New York, 1902, pp. 331–42.
11 Gaskell E (1864–1866) *Wives and Daughters.* Oxford University Press, Oxford, 1987.
12 Richardson HH (1917–1929) *The Fortunes of Richard Mahony.* Penguin, Harmondsworth, 1990.
13 Lewis S (1920) *Main Street.* Harcourt Brace and Company, New York, 1948.
14 Cozzens JG (1933) *The Last Adam.* Harcourt Brace and Company, New York, pp. 155–8.
15 Pritchett VS (1950) Passing the Ball. In: *The Complete Short Stories.* Chatto and Windus, London, 1990, pp. 332–45.
16 Faulkner W (1930) *As I Lay Dying.* Vintage Books, New York, 1985, p. 89.
17 Slaughter FG (1972) *Convention MD.* Hutchinson, London, 1973.
18 Cather W (1932) Neighbor Rosicky. In: *Five Stories.* Vintage Books, New York, 1956, pp. 72–111.
19 Caldwell T (1968) *Testimony of Two Men.* Collins, London, 1990, p. 225.
20 Hooker R (1968) *M.A.S.H.* William Morrow, New York, pp. 161–2.
21 Bernières L de (1994) *Captain Corelli's Mandolin.* Vintage, London, 1998.
22 Green G (1956) *The Last Angry Man.* Charles Scribner's Sons, New York.
23 Ibid., p. 188.
24 Ibid., p. 382.
25 Corris P (1999) *The Other Side of Sorrow.* Bantam Books, Sydney, pp. 107–23.
26 Hippocrates (attrib.) (fifth century BC) Precepts. In: *The Works of Hippocrates* (translated by Jones WHS). *Volume 1.* Loeb's Classical Library, Heinemann, London, 1972, p. 325.
27 Molière JBP (1665) Love's the Best Doctor. In: *The Plays of Molière* (translated by Waller AR). *Volume 4.* John Grant, Edinburgh, 1926, pp. 291–7.
28 Flaubert G (1857) *Madame Bovary* (translated by Steegmuller F). Modern Library, New York, 1982, pp. 68–9.
29 Dostoyevsky F (1880) *The Brothers Karamazov* (translated by Magarshack D). *Volume 2.* Penguin, Harmondsworth, 1977, p. 790.
30 Shaw GB (1906) The Doctor's Dilemma. In: *The Bodley Head Bernard Shaw: collected plays with their prefaces. Volume 3.* The Bodley Head, London, 1971, pp. 338–43.
31 Woolf V (1925) *Mrs Dalloway.* Zodiac Press, London, 1947, p. 106.

32 Mann T (1947) *Doctor Faustus* (translated by Lowe-Porter HT). Secker and Warburg, London, 1949, pp. 475–6.
33 Sanders L (1973) *The First Deadly Sin*. Berkley Books, New York, 1974, p. 91.
34 Palmer M (1998) *Miracle Cure*. Arrow Books, London, pp. 28–31.
35 Cao Xue Qin (also spelt Tsao Hsueh Chin) (1792) *The Story of the Stone* (also titled *The Dream of the Red Chamber)* (translated by Hawkes D). Penguin, Harmondsworth, 1973, p. 226.
36 Doctor X (Nourse AE) (1965) *Intern*. Harper and Row, New York, pp. 216–21.
37 Flaubert G, op. cit., pp. 144–5.
38 Ibid., pp. 204–5.
39 Ibid., p. 366.
40 Metalious G (1956) *Peyton Place*. Dell, New York, 1958, p. 64.
41 Bennett A (1923) *Riceyman Steps*. Cassell, London, 1947, pp. 264–5.
42 Green G, op. cit., pp. 2–9.
43 Gardner J (1963) *Nickel Mountain*. Alfred A Knopf, New York, 1973, p. 98.
44 Lewis S (1924) *Arrowsmith*. Signet Books, New York, 1961, p. 170.
45 Howells WD (1881) *Dr Breen's Practice*. James Osgood, Boston, MA, pp. 208–9.
46 Jewett SO (1884) *A Country Doctor*. Houghton Mifflin Company, Boston, MA.
47 Mauriac F (1927–1935) *Thérèse* (translated by Hopkins G). Penguin, Harmondsworth, 1959, p. 75.
48 Richardson HH, op. cit., p. 616.
49 Seifert E (1941) *Bright Scalpel*. Aeonian Press Inc., New York, 1973, p. 27.
50 Percy W (1987) *The Thanatos Syndrome*. Ivy Books, New York, 1991, p. 13.
51 Slaughter FG (1967) Doctors' Wives. In: *Four Complete Novels*. Avenel Books, New York, 1980, p. 8.
52 Roe F (1989) *Doctors and Doctors' Wives*. Constable, London, p. 241.
53 Sobel IP (1973) *The Hospital Makers*. Doubleday, Garden City, NY, pp. 349–58.
54 Palmer M (1998) *Miracle Cure*. Arrow, London, p. 51.
55 Ravin N (1989) *Mere Mortals*. Macdonald, London, 1990, p. 204.
56 Richardson S, op. cit., pp. 341–2.
57 Melville H (1850) *White Jacket*. LC Page, Boston, MA, 1892, pp. 232–49.
58 Cronin AJ (1937) *The Citadel*. Gollancz, London, p. 77.
59 Simenon G (1941). The Country Doctor. In: *The White Horse Inn and Other Novels* (translated by Ellenbogen E). Hamish Hamilton, London, 1980, pp. 203–27.
60 Van Der Meersch M (1943) *Bodies and Souls* (translated by Wilkins E). William Kimber, London, 1953, pp. 232–5.
61 Hemingway E (1929) *A Farewell to Arms*. Jonathan Cape, London, p. 105.
62 Posen S (2005) *The Doctor in Literature. Volume 1. Satisfaction or resentment?* Radcliffe Publishing, Oxford, p. 24.
63 Balzac H de (1836) *The Atheist's Mass* (translated by Bell C). Dent, London, 1929, pp. 1–20.
64 Martineau H (1839) *Deerbrook*. Virago Press, London, 1983, p. 518.
65 Young FB (1928) *My Brother Jonathan*. Heinemann, London, p. 127.
66 Ibid., p. 341.
67 Ibid., pp. 575–95.
68 Céline LF (1932) *Journey to the End of the Night* (translated by Manheim R). New Directions, New York, 1983, p. 259.
69 Cronin AJ, op. cit., pp. 164–73.
70 Slaughter FG (1969) Surgeon's Choice. In: *Four Complete Novels*. Avenel Books, New York, 1980, p. 273.
71 Nourse AE (1978) *The Practice*. Futura Publications, London, 1979, p. 27.
72 Ibid., p. 34.
73 Ibid., p. 108.

74 Percy W, op. cit., p. 104.

75 Richardson HH, op. cit., p. 408.

76 James MR (1919) Two Doctors. In: Byatt AS (ed.) *The Oxford Book of English Short Stories*. Oxford University Press, Oxford, 1998, pp. 97–104.

77 Braddon ME (1864) *The Doctor's Wife*. Oxford University Press, Oxford, 1998, pp. 308–11.

78 Ibid., p. 368.

79 Beauvoir S de (1964) *A Very Easy Death* (translated by O'Brian P). Andre Deutsch and Weidenfeld and Nicholson, London, 1966, pp. 10–12.

80 Goldsworthy P (1988) The Nice Chinese Doctor. In: *Bleak Rooms*. Wakefield Press, Adelaide, pp. 59–74.

81 Eliot G (1871–1872) *Middlemarch*. Penguin Books, Harmondsworth, 1988, p. 212.

82 Daudet LA (1894) *Les Morticoles*. Fasquelle, Paris, 1956, p. 47.

83 Ravin N (1985) *Seven North*. EP Dutton/Seymour Lawrence, New York.

84 Williams WC (1928) *Voyage to Pagany*. New Directions, New York, 1970, p. 148.

85 Bernhard T (1967) *Gargoyles* (translated by Winston R and Winston C). Alfred A Knopf, New York, 1970, p. 24.

86 Doyle AC (1894) His First Operation. In: *Round the Red Lamp*. John Murray, London, 1934, pp. 9–19.

87 Haggard HR (1898) *Doctor Therne*. Hodder and Stoughton, London, 1923, p. 72.

88 Ibid., pp. 86–8.

89 Maugham WS (1915) *Of Human Bondage*. Signet Classics, New York, 1991, pp. 646–9.

90 Ashton H (1930) *Doctor Serocold*. Penguin Books, London, 1936.

91 Cozzens JG, op. cit., 301 pp.

92 Ibid., p. 194.

93 Ibid., p. 203.

94 Ibid., pp. 173–4.

95 Ibid., p. 31.

96 Ibid., p. 161.

97 Ibid., p. 250.

98 Proust M (1913–1922) *Remembrance of Things Past* (translated by Scott-Moncrieff CK and Kilmartin T). *Volume 1*. Penguin, Harmondsworth, pp. 233–4.

99 Mitchell SW, op. cit., pp. 146–7.

100 Ibid., pp. 276–7.

101 Ibid., pp. 31–52.

102 Ibid., p. 453.

103 Jackson S (1954) *The Bird's Nest*. Farrar, Straus and Young, New York, pp. 32–5.

104 Green G, op. cit., p. 217.

105 Ibid., pp. 420–4.

106 Nourse AE, op. cit., pp. 22–3.

107 Ibid., p. 151.

107a Döblin A (1929) *Berlin Alexanderplatz* (translated by Jolas E). Continuum, New York, 2004, pp. 593–4.

108 Doctor X (Nourse AE), op. cit., p. 87.

109 Van Der Meersch M, op. cit., pp. 62–3.

110 Hailey A (1959) *The Final Diagnosis*. Bantam Books, New York, 1967, pp. 46–54.

111 Ibid., pp. 195–9.

112 Garcia Marquez G (1985) *Love in the Time of Cholera* (translated by Grossman E). Jonathan Cape, London, 1988, p. 112.

113 Ibid., pp. 11–13.

114 Nourse AE, op. cit., pp. 79–80.

115 Ibid., pp. 110–12.

116 Ibid., p. 573.

117 Caldwell T, op. cit., pp. 216–20.

118 Ibid., pp. 51–4.

119 Ibid., p. 73.

120 Ibid., pp. 132–8.

121 Ibid., pp. 87–8.

122 Ibid., pp. 157–67.

123 Ibid., p. 17.

124 Ibid., p. 347.

125 Ibid., p. 472.

126 Ibid., p. 468.

127 Ibid., pp. 75–8.

128 Ibid., p. 351.

129 Thompson M (1955) *Not as a Stranger*. Michael Joseph, London.

130 Thompson M (1951) *The Cry and the Covenant*. Pan Books, London, 1969.

131 Mitchell P (1965) *A Wilderness of Monkeys*. Arthur Barker, London.

132 Ibid., p. 275.

133 Ibid., pp. 171–7.

134 Ibid., pp. 78–9.

135 Ibid., p. 366.

136 Gerritsen T (1996) *Harvest*. Headline Publishing, London.

137 Ibid., pp. 10–14.

138 Fisher N (1994) *Side-Effects*. Hodder and Stoughton, London, pp. 41–4.

139 Palmer M (1996) *Critical Judgment*. Bantam Books, New York, pp. 7–14.

140 Sayers DL (1928) The Vindictive Story of the Footsteps that Ran. In: *Lord Peter Views the Body*. Gollancz, London, 1979, p. 167.

141 Bashford HH (1911) *The Corner of Harley Street: being some familiar correspondence of Peter Harding MD*. Constable, London, 1913, p. 14.

142 Williams WC (1934) Jean Beicke. In: *The Doctor Stories*. New Directions, New York, 1984, pp. 69–77.

142a Fontane T (1895) *Effi Briest* (translated by Parmée D). Penguin, London, 1967, p. 250.

143 Schnitzler A (1912) *Professor Bernhardi* (translated by Landstone H). Faber and Gwyer, London, 1927.

144 Ibid., p. 19.

145 Selzer R (1982) Imelda. In: *Letters to a Young Doctor*. Harcourt Brace, San Diego, CA, 1996, pp. 21–36.

146 Straub P (1988) *Koko*. Penguin, Harmondsworth, 1989.

147 Ibid., p. 93.

148 Kundera M (1984) *The Unbearable Lightness of Being* (translated by Heim MH). Faber and Faber, London, 1988, pp. 179–84.

149 Ibid., pp. 230–2.

150 Nourse AE, op. cit., 574 pp.

151 Ibid., p. 168.

152 Ibid., p. 298.

153 Ibid., pp. 124–6.

154 Irving J (2001) *The Fourth Hand*. Bloomsbury, London, pp. 26-44.

155 Ibid., p. 149.

156 Ibid., pp. 170–71.

157 Hecht B (1959) Miracle of the Fifteen Murderers. In: *A Treasury of Ben Hecht: collected stories and other writings*. Crown Publishers, New York, p. 191.

158 Glasser RJ (1973) *Ward 402*. Garnstone Press, London, 1974.

159 Ibid., pp. 55–6.

160 Doctor X (Nourse AE), op. cit., p. 247.

161 Ellis AE (1958) *The Rack*. Penguin, Harmondsworth, 1988.

162 Ibid., p. 33.
163 Ibid., p. 64.
164 Ibid., pp. 82–3.
165 Posen S, op. cit., p. 207.
166 Schneiderman LJ (1972) *Sea Nymphs by the Hour*. Authors' Guild Backinprint.Com, Lincoln, NE, 2000, pp. 55–8.
167 Frede R (1960) *The Interns*. Corgi, London, 1965.
168 Ibid., p. 23.
169 Cook R (1977) *Coma*. Pan Books, London, 1978, pp. 38–55.
170 Cook R (1981) *Brain*. Pan Books, London, pp. 42–53.
171 Douglas L (1935) *Green Light*. Angus and Robertson, Sydney, 1947, pp. 21–4.
172 Smollett T (1748) *The Adventures of Roderick Random*. Dent, London, 1964, pp. 92–3.
173 Sobel IP, op. cit., pp. 11–14.
174 Slaughter FG (1972) *Convention MD*. Hutchinson, London, 1973.
175 Ibid., p. 292.
176 Hailey A (1984) *Strong Medicine*. Dell, New York, 1986, pp. 137–41.
177 Mitchell P, op. cit., p. 13.
178 Reed B (1980) *The Verdict*. Simon and Schuster, New York.
179 Ibid., p. 69.
180 Deeping W (1925) *Sorrell and Son*. Cassell, London, 1927, pp. 299–306.
181 Posen S, op. cit., pp. 231–2.
182 Crichton M (Hudson J, pseudonym) (1968) *A Case of Need*. Signet, New York, 1969, pp. 308–11.
183 Bellaman H (1940) *King's Row*. Dymocks, Sydney, 1945, p. 451.
184 Osler W (1906) Unity, Peace and Concord. In: *Aequanimitas*. HK Lewis, London, 1920, pp. 447–65.
185 Havard J (1988) *Coming of Age*. Heinemann, London, pp. 121–2.
186 Wharton W (1981) *Dad*. Alfred A Knopf, New York.
187 Ibid., p. 130.
188 Stoker B (1897) *Dracula*. Penguin, Harmondsworth, 1993, p. 76.
189 Ibid., pp. 147–59.
190 Ibid., p. 428.
191 Ibid., pp. 353–7.
192 Dawson WJ (1900) A Surgical Operation. In: *The Doctor Speaks*. Grant Richards, London, pp. 3–28.
193 Martin du Gard R (1922–1940) *The Thibaults* (translated by Gilbert S). John Lane, The Bodley Head, London, 1939, pp. 532–40.
194 Ambler E (1974) *Doctor Frigo*. Fontana/Collins, Glasgow, 1976, pp. 130–1.
195 Reade C (1863) *Hard Cash*. Chatto and Windus, London, 1894.
196 Ibid., p. 180.
197 Ibid., p. 35.
198 Doyle AC (1894) The Curse of Eve. In: *Round the Red Lamp*. John Murray, London, 1934, pp. 89–108.
199 Proust M (1913–1922) *Remembrance of Things Past* (translated by Scott-Moncrieff CK and Kilmartin T). *Volume 2*. Penguin, Harmondsworth, pp. 354–5.
200 Bellaman H and Bellaman K (1948) *Parris Mitchell of King's Row*. Simon and Schuster, New York, p. 110.
201 Sobel IP, op. cit., pp. 63–71.
202 Percy E (1940) *Doctor Brent's Household*. English Theatre Guild, London, p. 24.
203 Camus A (1947) *The Plague* (translated by Gilbert S). Penguin, Harmondsworth, 1960, p. 20.
204 Simenon G (1963) *The Patient* (translated by Stewart J). Hamish Hamilton, London, 1963, p. 56.

205 Posen S, op. cit., pp. 180–82.
206 Slaughter FG (1985) *No Greater Love*. Hutchinson, London, pp. 37–8.
207 Ibid., pp. 137–8.
208 Ibid., pp. 43–4.
209 Goldsworthy P (1992) *Honk If You Are Jesus*. Angus and Robertson, Sydney, p. 5.
210 Lewis S (1920) *Main Street*. Harcourt Brace and Company, New York, 1948, pp. 302–3.
211 Crichton M (Hudson J, pseudonym), op. cit., pp. 215–16.
212 Hunter KM (1991) *Doctors' Stories*. Princeton University Press, Princeton, NJ.
213 Ravin N (1981) *MD*. Delacorte Press/Seymour Lawrence, New York, p. 70.
214 Bosk CL (1980) Occupational rituals in patient management. *NEJM*. **303:** 71–6.

CHAPTER 3

The doctor and religion

Hakims (= physicians) and priests are snake and tiger the world over.[1]

As a rule, we doctors don't believe in God.[2]

Historical background

In tribal cultures, medicine men use their communities' religious beliefs and practices to provide 'medical' treatment. These 'doctors' drive out evil spirits, control the weather and detect breakers of taboos[3] in addition to or as part of the process of healing the sick. In the Hippocratic tradition, medical (natural) and religious (supernatural) practices are generally regarded as separate disciplines, although even in contemporary Western societies many physicians consider themselves religious and participate in church activities. In a 1998 survey of more than 3000 US physicians, only 13% of respondents gave their religious affiliation as 'none', while 54% stated that they prayed at least once weekly.[4]

Fictional doctors, on the other hand, are rarely 'devout.' On the contrary, their indifference and hostility towards religion involve a great deal more than lax Sabbath observances[5] or irregular attendance at church.[6] There is an almost universal assumption that doctors who practise 'real' medicine would be unable to function if, during the course of their work, they retained the virtues of humility, resignation and a steadfast belief in whatever they had been taught. The perception of the physician as an irreligious individual is deeply entrenched in the non-medical literature, and extends from Old Testament times to the present day.

King Asa of Judah, whose 'heart was wholly true to the Lord',[7] is nevertheless censured for what is perceived as a regrettable lapse.

> In the thirty-ninth year of his reign, Asa was diseased in his feet and his disease became severe; yet even in his disease he did not seek the Lord but sought help from physicians [who, predictably, failed to cure him]. And Asa slept with his fathers, dying in the forty-first year of his reign.[8]

The author of the Book of Chronicles evidently finds it deplorable or at least incongruous that a reigning monarch of the Royal House of David should consult with medical doctors, an act perceived as incompatible with true faith. King Asa's physicians are not condemned (except by implication), but later Jewish scholars were obviously ambivalent towards doctors. The author of Ecclesiasticus admits that at times 'success lies in the hands of physicians',[9] but two verses later goes on to pray: 'He who sins before his Maker may he fall into the care of a physician.'[9] In a discussion of career choices, the compiler of the *Mishnah*[10] expresses strong disapproval of the medical profession and declares that '[Even] the best among physicians is destined for Gehenna.'[10] The text is ambiguous and may equally well be interpreted to mean 'The better the doctor the sooner he is likely to reach his destination below.'[10]

Early Christian writers discouraged the theory that diseases are due to natural causes, and most of them deprecate the intervention of physicians. Gregory of Tours contrasts the power of prayer and the intercession of saints with the painful and dangerous treatments administered by regular doctors. In his collection of miracles, Gregory narrates the story of a blind deacon who miraculously regained his sight after a night on his knees in the cell where St Martin had died some 200 years earlier.[11] He then goes on to denigrate medical treatment administered by secular physicians who rely on their medical skills rather than on the relics of St Martin:

> What [cure] such as this one, have doctors ever accomplished with their implements? Their efforts produce more pain than healing and . . . if caution is lacking . . . the doctor is providing eternal blindness for the wretched patient.[11]

By the late Middle Ages, the stereotype of the doctor with his fondness for gold and his lack of interest in religion seems to have become well developed. Chaucer's physician is familiar with the works of a variety of unbelievers, but 'his reading was but little of the Bible.'[12] The statement appears to be non-judgemental, implying that the doctor's lack of familiarity with the Scriptures is of little relevance to his professional skills. In the seventeenth century, Thomas Browne, in his treatise on what he did and did not believe,[13] began his work with the remark that in view of 'the general scandal of . . . [the medical] profession' it may come as a surprise to some that he practises any religion at all.

Ambroise Paré's statements, such as '[the surgeon who has achieved] some cure worthy of praise . . . is not to attribute it to himself but to God',[14] are widely cited but do not reflect the standard medical outlook, or even Paré's own way of thinking.[14] On the contrary, over the centuries, doctors and patients alike express the view that religion is relatively unimportant in a physician. Sterne's Corporal Trim, in the eighteenth century,[15] prefers to entrust his health and his savings to competent unbelievers rather than to religious zealots who lack 'moral honesty':

> I know the banker I deal with or the physician I usually call in . . . to be neither of them men of much religion. . . . Notwithstanding this I put my fortune into the hands of the one and . . . I trust my life to the honest skill of the other.[15]

The perception of the godless doctor in nineteenth- and twentieth-century fiction

Throughout the nineteenth and twentieth centuries, authors of fictional works take the doctor's indifference or hostility towards religion almost for granted. The theme transcends time, place and religious denomination. A typical early case is Balzac's Dr Denis Minoret, who trained during the Age of Enlightenment,[16] and who is described as a confirmed atheist.[17] Contemptuous of 'Church mummeries',[18] he has 'a horror of priests',[19] although he is fond of the local curé, a refined, well-educated man. 'Each hated the other's opinions but they esteemed each other's character.'[17]

Towards the end of his life the doctor, who is suspected of being 'in league with the devil',[20] becomes an active churchgoer, much to the chagrin of his relatives, who had hoped to inherit his money and who now face the prospect of having to 'share his estate with God.'[16]

Aggressive atheists like Dr Minoret[16–20] would not have been tolerated in the colony of Massachusetts in its early days, but even there the physician stood out for his lack of religious zeal.

> Skilful men of the medical and chirurgical profession . . . seldom, it would appear, partook of the religious zeal that brought other emigrants across the Atlantic. In their researches into the human frame . . . such men . . . lost the spiritual view of existence among the intricacies of that wondrous mechanism which seemed to . . . comprise all of life within itself.[21]

Bellamy's 'heathenish' Dr Gustav Heidenhoff,[22] another godless nineteenth-century physician, invents an electrical apparatus that removes feelings of guilt and depression. During a demonstration of the new gadget, Heidenhoff proclaims arrogantly and triumphantly that medical science is superior to religion:

> 'The ministers and moralists preach forgiveness and absolution on repentance, but the perennial fountain of the penitent's tears testifies how empty and vain such assurances are. I fulfil what they promise. They tell the penitent he is forgiven. I free him from sin' . . . and with an impressive gesture, the doctor touched the battery at his side.

Unfortunately, the 'Heidenhoff thought extirpator' fails to cure Madeline Brand's depressive illness.[22]

Dr Ledsmar in *The Damnation of Theron Ware*[23] has a medical degree but has not practised for many years. Instead, the doctor has become interested in other pursuits such as Assyriology and comparative religion[23] (*see also* p. 154). Despite his truancy from the medical profession, Ledsmar has not abandoned the traditional medical attitude towards religion. It is 'fully twenty years' since he 'last heard a sermon', and he views all creeds 'impartially from the outside.'[23] Naturally, Dr Ledsmar finds the scholarly Father Forbes more congenial than the Reverend Theron Ware, especially after Ware loses his innocence but retains his ignorance.[24]

The phenomenon of the ungodly physician is discussed in considerable detail in George Eliot's *Middlemarch*.[25] Mrs Harriet Bulstrode, a religious woman, tries to persuade her niece, Rosamond Vincy, not to get herself entangled with Dr Lydgate because, Mrs Bulstrode argues, physicians are, as a rule, lacking in faith. A devout doctor is almost a contradiction in terms.

> '[He] is very intellectual and clever. I like talking to such men myself, and your uncle finds him very useful. But . . . it is seldom a medical man has true religious views – there is too much pride of intellect.'[25]

(Rosamond takes no notice of her aunt's warnings and becomes the doctor's wife.)

George Eliot goes further. For a physician, an apparent lack of faith is almost obligatory, since his religious observances are liable to be regarded as a substitute for clinical competence.[26]

> Dr Sprague was more than suspected of having no religion, but somehow Middlemarch tolerated this deficiency in him. . . . Indeed, it is probable that his professional weight was the more believed in [because of] the world-old association of cleverness with the evil principle. If any medical man had come to Middlemarch with the reputation of . . . being given to prayer and of otherwise showing an active piety, there would have been a general presumption against his medical skill.[26]

Catholic counterparts of Dr Sprague appear in Willa Cather's *Shadows on the Rock*[27-29] and Robertson Davies' *What's Bred in the Bone*.[30] Cather's Euclide Auclair, an apothecary physician, although a practising Catholic, is highly sceptical of 'miracle cures' attributed to saints' relics,[28] and he is not at all intimidated by the Bishop of Quebec, whose notions of medical ethics differ from his own.[29]

Dr Joseph Ambrosius Jerome[30] is a more flamboyant character than Auclair,[27] and his medical activities are described in terms that would have been considered scatological in the nineteenth and early twentieth centuries. However, the central message is the same. The doctor's faith is questionable, but despite his unorthodox beliefs (or possibly because of them) his patients trust him.

> [Jerome] was locally believed to have powers of healing verging on the miraculous. He 'brought back' lumbermen who had chopped themselves in the foot with one of their terrible axes and were in danger of blood poisoning.

He also sews up knife wounds inflicted by bellicose Poles, and he manages to 'cure' patients with double pneumonia. Despite his religious affiliation

> he told women to have no more babies, and threatened their husbands with dreadful reprisals if this were not so. He blasted out the constipated and salved their angry haemorrhoids with ointments of opium. He could diagnose worms at a glance and drag a tapeworm from its lair with horrible potions. If not actually an atheist, the doctor was known to have dark beliefs nobody wanted to explore. He was rumoured to know more theology than Father Devlin and Father Beaudry clapped together. He read books that were on the Index, some of them in German. But he was trusted.[30]

Dr Benjamin Phillips, a Jewish physician,[31] believes in nothing. However, he practises mainly within his own community[32] and has to keep up appearances. He attends synagogue services,[33] and after his wife's death (brought about by an overdose of morphine administered by Dr Phillips) he observes the prescribed ritual mourning period.[34] However, in private he expresses his contempt for Jewish prayers and customs, 'exploded traditions invented by fools for fools',[35] and tells his mistress that 'immortality is a myth.'[36] After his ultimate rise to fame, Phillips abandons his religion and his people 'like a discarded garment; [and] he is scarcely known as an Israelite.'[33]

The Russian Orthodox version of the anti-religious doctor is represented by Dr Yefim Ragin, whose antagonism towards the Church blights his son's career. Young Andrew Yefimovich Ragin, the principal character of *Ward Number Six*,[37] might have turned into a good priest rather than an indifferent physician, if his overbearing medical father had not crushed the teenager's religious enthusiasm.

He was preparing for a church career, proposing to enter theological college after leaving school in 1863, but his father, a doctor of medicine and surgeon, supposedly uttered a scathing laugh and announced categorically that he would disown the boy if he became a cleric.[37]

Daudet's *Les Morticoles*[38] is a polemic anti-Utopian account of an island 'civilization' dominated by aggressively anti-religious physicians. Obviously in such a society there are no priests available to console the dying, and the Sisters of Charity have long since been dismissed from the hospitals[39] 'because their presence might bring back the old superstitions' (leur présence évaillait de vieilles superstitions). At school the children are taught that God does not exist,[40] and that men are descended from animals, animals from plants, and plants from rocks. All of this is an elaborate plot hatched by the physicians to make the rest of the population more tractable. 'People who believe they are descended from pebbles naturally let themselves get kicked about'[40] (celui qui se croit issu d'un caillou n'a plus qu'à se laisser rouler).

Hardly a role model for aspiring young physicians, Dr Ostermark in Strindberg's *The Father*[41] lacks the strength to resist becoming a participant in a marital dispute, and he makes decisions which are clearly not in the best interests of his patient.[42] However, Ostermark's attitude to religion is quite typical of a late-nineteenth-century European medical man. When the patient's brother-in-law, the local preacher, asserts that the Captain 'suffers from fixed ideas', the doctor retorts sarcastically 'I have a notion, Pastor, that *your* ideas are even more fixed.'[41]

Dr Edred Fitzpiers in Hardy's *The Woodlanders*[43] carries his agnosticism almost to extremes. He is quite prepared to provoke a minor scandal in a small English town (in the 1880s) by getting married in a registry office rather than a church. He subsequently relents (at his fiancée's insistence), but he believes that 'marriage is a civil contract' which is no more sacred than buying a home or making a will.[44]

This theme of the irreligious doctor persists in quite recent works of fiction. 'Doctor' Iannis in *Captain Corelli's Mandolin*[45] lacks formal medical training, but his attitude towards religion is very similar to that of 'proper' doctors. Father Arsenios, the local priest, regards the doctor as a 'notoriously godless man', and takes him to task for his non-attendance at church services. Iannis, although not a believer, regards the church with benevolent detachment rather than hostility. When the local Communist calls Arsenios 'a parasite', Iannis comes to the priest's defence.

> 'There are parasitic bacteria in the gut that aid digestion. . . . Priests are a kind of bacteria that enable people to find life digestible. Father Arsenios has done many useful things for those who seek consolation. He is a member of every family and he is the family for those who don't have one.'[46]

The two doctors who perform the autopsy on their late colleague in *Ingenious Pain*[47] display vestiges of superstition, but they express unconcealed contempt for the Reverend Lestrade, the friend and protector of the deceased. When Lestrade shows some reluctance to view their gruesome work at close quarters, one of them remarks 'The Reverend's interest is in the invisible tenant of the house, rather than the house itself. Heh?' When Lestrade reproaches the doctors for their lack of respect for the corpse, they jokingly advise him to take a purgative.[47]

Irma, Dr Nicholas Zajac's housekeeper in Irving's *The Fourth Hand*,[48] is relieved to find that her employer (and future husband) is not the praying type. Irma habitually prowls around the house stark naked in the hope that she might 'accidentally' come across the doctor and impress him with her well-developed body (*see* p. 41). One night, as she tiptoed

> past the doctor's closed bedroom door, Irma was halted by the baffling conviction that she'd overheard Dr Zajac praying. Prayer struck Irma, who was not religious, as a suspiciously unscientific activity for a hand surgeon. She listened at the door a little longer and was relieved to hear that Zajac wasn't praying [but reading out aloud from one of his son's books].[48]

Godless doctors and religious patients

The collective irreligious attitude of doctors may lead to communication problems with patients and antagonize religious relatives and friends. Authors who describe such antagonisms, such as Wilkie Collins in *The Moonstone*,[49] generally find themselves on the side of the 'atheistic' doctors. Miss Drusilla Clack,[50] whose name betrays Collins' bias, intends to elevate her dying aunt's mind by providing her with religious tracts, but to her bitter disappointment finds that

> the members of the notoriously infidel profession of medicine had stepped between me and my mission of mercy – on the quiet.[50]

Miss Clack is an intolerant fanatic, but the profession's reputation for 'ungodliness' may also cause problems with less aggressive individuals.

Maartens' *The Healers*[51] is a fanciful story involving telepathy and other forms of extrasensory perception, as well as a recently graduated medical hero who devises a new operation for the relief of mental retardation. However, some of Maartens' more serious remarks include accurate contemporary perceptions of medicine and medical men. When Kenneth Graye talks to Dr Edward Lisse about 'the God-given soul' of his idiot nephew,

> he looked anxiously askance at Edward, waiting for that horrible expression, the sort of hidden contemptuousness which comes so frequently when religion is mentioned, into the smileless eyes of the medical man.[52]

Patients who turn to their doctor for spiritual information and guidance are likely to be disappointed. Young Ben Gant in Wolfe's *Look Homeward Angel*,[53] who plans to enlist in the Canadian Army in 1914 and who fantasizes about his forthcoming martyrdom in France, is consulting Dr Coker, an earthy small-town physician. Ben is after a certificate of physical fitness, but he also wants answers to more fundamental questions: 'Where do we come from? Where do we go to? What are we here for?'. Coker gives the standard agnostic medical reply – he is a physician, not a priest.[54] As for life before or after death,

> 'I've seen them born and I've seen them die. What happens to them before or after I can't say.' 'Damn that!' said Ben. 'What happens to them in between?'

Coker refuses to be drawn into an argument about the purpose of life, and instead lists various enjoyable activities, much to the disappointment of Ben, who remarks, 'You're a great wit, Coker.'[54]

In Gerritsen's *Harvest*,[55] in a scenario very similar to that described by Wilkie Collins,[50] but taking place 130 years later, 84-year-old Mary Allen, who suffers from disseminated cancer[56] and whose treatment consists of continuous intravenous morphine,[57] expresses her wish 'to go to sleep and not to wake up.' Enter Mrs Allen's niece, Miss Brenda Hainey, who sincerely desires to make her aunt 'fully accept the Lord' before she dies.[58] Brenda objects to the morphine treatment not only because it may accelerate her aunt's death, but also because it makes the old lady drowsy and unable to pray. Here medical and religious values are in direct conflict. The doctors and nurses want to relieve the patient's physical pain and suffering, whereas the religious niece prefers her aunt to remain conscious (even if that means enduring pain) to prepare herself for the 'life to come.' The two attitudes are irreconcilable, and a violent confrontation ensues.[58] (The old lady subsequently dies from an overdose of morphine administered as part of a criminal conspiracy.)

The encounter between Sister John of the Cross, a cloistered Carmelite nun, and Dr Sheppard of the Los Angeles County Hospital[59] initially shapes up like any consultation between a deeply religious patient and an indifferent physician. Sister John, whose entire life, including her movements, her mode of speech and her thoughts, are all dedicated to pleasing God, regards her symptoms as an opportunity[60] – 'a means of achieving holiness.'[61] To the doctor, Sister John's ecstasies are typical features of temporal lobe epilepsy, and he recommends that the 'diseased' part of the nun's brain be excised. At the end of their first meeting, when Sister John says 'Peace be with you, Doctor,' he replies, 'Have a great day.'

Matters improve after Sister John's successful operation. She thinks of doctors as having dedicated their lives to others, and in her semi-delirious, post-operative state she draws a fanciful parallel between religious and medical establishments.[62]

> The spirit of obedience ruled in the hospital as it did in the cloister. Younger doctors yielded without hesitation to the will of their superiors, as if hoping to become perfect vessels for the greater will of medicine.[62]

Dr Sheppard draws parallels of his own. When the nun admits to him that she sometimes has doubts about everything, he talks about his own lack of confidence. During his first year of residency, he nearly left because he felt that he had entered a medical career 'for the wrong reasons.'[63] However, he stayed the course and became a successful and contented neurosurgeon. He explains to Sister John that he kept going because he discovered that 'everybody gets into medicine for the wrong reasons. It seems to come with the territory.'[63] On the day of her discharge from hospital, when the nun in her habit faces Dr Sheppard in his white coat, she feels 'like a frontier guard saying good-bye to her counterpart across the border,'[64] though the country she is leaving is neutral, not hostile.

Priestly and earthy physicians

In a masterful PhD dissertation, Carolyn Brimley Norris[65] classifies fictional physicians into two broad categories. The dividing line is not as sharp as that described by Norris, but the two groups are clearly distinguishable from each other. The 'Pan' doctor, epitomized by Dr George Bull in Cozzens' *The Last Adam*,[66] is an earthy, hardened sinner, coarse and cynical about everything except his own pleasures. The 'priestly' doctor, abstemious and usually celibate, is indifferent to material wealth and totally dedicated to the well-being of his patients. He cannot be bought, threatened or flattered, because he serves 'an invisible church'[65] with its own rituals, its own vestments and even its own 'desert tradition' (*see* p. 181). Dreiser's Dr Gridley, whose eyes peer 'all too kindly into the faces of dishonest men',[67] typifies this kind of physician. Neither Pan nor Priest is attracted to conventional religion. The Pan, who in biblical terminology would be described as 'a glutton and a drunkard', is too busy at the trough, while the Priest has his own set of values, which only partially coincide with those of the Church.

The physician's irreligious or anti-religious attitudes, which range from greater or lesser degrees of tolerance to total indifference to violent detestation, manifest themselves differently in the two classes of doctor. The 'Pan' doctor, vulgar in everything else, also tends to be coarse in his rejection of religious values. Tennyson's 'coarse and red' surgeon,[68] an aggressive unbeliever, sneers at Nurse Annie when she tells him that she prays for her poor crippled children:

> But he turned to me 'Ay, good woman can prayer set a broken bone?'
> Then he muttered half to himself but I know that I heard him say
> 'All very well – but the good Lord Jesus has had his day.'[68]

Dr Bull, the arch-Pan,[69] sloshes around in his bath singing 'with agile malice' about the 'Virgin's womb' in the second verse of 'O Come all ye Faithful', obviously trying to inject a lewd connotation into the carol.[69] Dr Matthew Swain in Grace Metalious' *Peyton Place*[70] is another earthy physician with a very simplistic attitude towards religion. Swain, who prefers playing poker to reading medical journals, uses foul language in public and drinks a great deal of alcohol. He 'hated . . . three things . . . in this world . . . death, venereal disease and organized religion . . . in that order.'[71]

Kathryn Hulme's Dr Fortunati in *The Nun's Story*[72] is yet another earthy character, despite his attachment to a hospital staffed by members of a religious order. Fortunati, 'an Italian with hot blood', does not practise poverty or chastity. He has a government salary and a mistress, and he goes off to weekend parties which leave him with 'bloodshot . . . eyes.' A confirmed agnostic, Fortunati amuses himself by making 'sardonic comments about the religious life', while the nuns refer to him as 'Beelzebub.'[73]

The priestly physician has neither need nor desire to express his opposition to religion through sarcastic or indecent remarks. Indeed, for most of the time he is sympathetic towards religious practices. He leads a blameless life even though his own concepts may not include God, sin, salvation or resurrection. Balzac's Dr Minoret[17] (*see* pp. 104–5 and pp. 231–2) is 'a Christian without knowing it.' He lives abstemiously and he secretly gives away large sums of money to the needy. Flaubert's Dr Larivière,[74] a very similar figure and described in almost identical terms,[75] is

> disdainful of decorations, titles and academies, hospitable, generous, a
> father to the poor, practising Christian virtues although an unbeliever. . . .

[He] might have been thought of as a saint if he hadn't been feared as a devil because of the keenness of his mind.[74]

Another priestly figure, Dr Thomas Thurnall in Kingsley's *Two Years Ago*,[76] is described as

> an ungodly man . . . [but] his morality was as high as that of the average; his sense of honour far higher. . . . He had seen men of all creeds and had found in all alike . . . the many rogues and the few honest men. [He did not believe] that any Being above cared for him, was helping him in the daily business of his life, that it was worthwhile asking that Being's advice, or that any advice would be given if asked for.[77]

In the last chapter of *Two Years Ago*, during an outrageously sentimental proposal of marriage,[78] Thurnall becomes a convert to Kingsley's version of Anglicanism, but throughout most of the book he is portrayed as a 'thoroughly genuine man, sincere and faithful to his own scheme of the universe', even though he has 'no creed at all.'[79]

Yet another priestly physician, 'Dr Colin', the hero of Graham Greene's *A Burnt-Out Case*,[80] has 'long ago lost faith in any god that a priest would have recognized.'[81] However, the doctor's lack of religious belief does not prevent him from spending his life in a remote leprosarium in the Belgian Congo, where he devotes all of his energies to the improvement of his patients. This atheistic, idealistic character is surrounded by 'true' believers and 'real' priests whose principles and accomplishments compare very unfavourably with those of the doctor. The 'rakish', bridge-playing bishop has 'the roving eye of an old-fashioned cavalier of the boulevards.'[82] Ryker, another member of the expatriate community, a colonial margarine manufacturer and a 'pious imbecile', spent six years in a seminary, where he presumably acquired his disgusting notions about 'Christian marriages' and a husband's 'conjugal rights.'[83] Father Thomas, a warped, intolerant man, has a genius for false judgements and wrong decisions.[84] Among these 'devout' fools, the doctor, with his lack of faith, stands out like a beacon of sanity and dedication. When asked 'Are you a happy man?', he replies 'I suppose I am. It's not a question that I've ever asked myself. Does a happy man ask it? I go on from day to day.'[85]

The chief medical character in Goldsworthy's *Honk If You Are Jesus*,[86] Dr Mara Fox, is a somewhat warped version of the priestly doctor. Mara, a preacher's daughter, who 'filled her quota of church-going during childhood many times over', might conceivably have become an ordained minister, but instead she turns into an atheistic zealot and trains as a gynaecologist. After getting 'into religion in a big way at fourteen . . . at fifteen I got out of religion in a big way.'[87] By the time we meet Dr Fox, a spinster in her mid-forties, she

> believes in nothing . . . beyond a few simple laws of nature . . . I liked also to occasionally renew my lack of faith. To attend church and confirm again all the worst memories of my childhood. To be, in a sense, Born Again as a non-believer.[87]

A fascinating description of a total transformation in a physician's religious convictions can be found in Tennessee Williams' *Summer and Smoke*.[88] Young Dr John Buchanan, who suddenly switches from Pan to Priest in the eighth scene of the play, simultaneously undergoes a reverse Pauline conversion. When his father, the old doctor, is fatally shot by one of John's criminal associates (*see* pp. 20–1), John changes from a dissolute playboy into a conscientious physician. With this metamorphosis comes a dramatic change in his attitude towards religious beliefs. John, who previously lived in symbiosis with the Reverend Winemiller and his family, suddenly feels constrained to fulminate against all faiths. He even tries to stop the preacher saying a prayer over his dying father.

> 'We don't want that worn-out magic. . . . You so right people, pious pompous mumblers, preacher and preacher's daughter all muffled up in a lot of worn-out . . . mumbo jumbo.'[88]

Doctor–priest encounters: harmless repartee and blazing hatred

Scenes describing friendly banter and verbal hostilities between priests and irreligious doctors abound in literature, especially nineteenth-century literature. The antagonism between the parties may become permanent and vicious, but more often the opponents develop a respect for each other and may even collaborate during a crisis. Dr Tom Thurnall in *Two Years Ago*[76] has, despite his agnosticism (*see* p. 111), established a very cordial relationship with Frank Headley, the Anglican curate, with whom he holds occasional religious disputations. Thurnall compares the curate's activities with those of a Yankee storekeeper. The curate protests: 'At least you will confess that I am not working for money.'

> 'No; you have your notions of reward and he has his. He wants to be paid by material dollars, payable next month; you by spiritual dollars, payable when you die. I don't see the great difference.'[79]

The two men nevertheless remain friends, and during a typhoid epidemic they work together to provide medical and social services for the helpless villagers, with the cleric clearly subordinate to the physician. 'The five real workers toiled on meanwhile in perfect harmony and implicit obedience to the all-knowing Tom.'[89]

A minor medico-clerical confrontation described by Bashford[90] involves 'a little cottage hospital . . . built, endowed, and kept lavishly up to date' by a middle-aged retired surgeon. This man, who went to sea at the age of fourteen, worked his way through medical school and practised among the highest as well as the lowest strata of society, is incensed when an 'ardent [and] sincere' young priest, newly arrived in the village, proposes to hold 'extra services' for the hospital patients. We do not hear by what compromise this little dispute is resolved, but Dr Peter Harding, who is not personally involved, considers the two protagonists to be 'very typical of all that is best (and possibly least reconcilable) on either side.'[91]

Dr Luke Serocold[92] regularly attends church, not because he believes in any religious doctrines, but because he enjoys the music and the ambience. Life after death, the resurrection of the dead and the notion of sin are not topics that he ponders over.[93] During a bout of depression he contemplates suicide,[94] but he rejects the idea, not because of a sense of wrongdoing but because he does not relish ending up as the subject of an inquest.[94] On St Luke's day (18 October 1929*),

---

* See footnote on p. 175.

while making house calls, he meets young Mr Carmichael, the Anglican vicar, in the street.[95] Carmichael, on his way to church, enquires:

> 'Aren't you going to worship your patron saint?' 'Only professionally, I'm afraid', said Doctor Serocold. 'I haven't time to do anything more for Saint Luke today.' 'I don't see how you could do anything better', the young man declared, and then a shade crossed his open and ingenuous countenance and he added: 'Yours is a more practical worship than mine, anyway. Sometimes I'm inclined to envy you.' [The doctor's response is quick and ironic.] 'Want to see your results quicker, do you?' 'Perhaps that's it', admitted the young man, with a wry face.[95]

Another doctor–priest encounter is described in Maurois' *Colonel Bramble*.[96] Dr O'Grady, who first appears as an Irish army doctor during the First World War, and resurfaces as a cynical 'Harley Street' psychiatrist after the Second World War (*see* p. 158), declares that he 'respect[s] the bitter wisdom of the Catholic faith',[97] and he never misses an opportunity to tease the Protestant army chaplain.[98] He professes admiration for the 'uncompromising attitude of the [Church] councils' and he asserts:

> so much [human] weakness and stupidity requires the firm support of an authority without the slightest tolerance. The curative value of a doctrine lies not in its logical truth but in its permanency.[99]

However, O'Grady's 'discourses' leave little doubt that despite his professed respect for the Catholic Church and his genuine contempt for its Protestant rivals, he is essentially an unbeliever. 'This universe of ours strikes me as completely non-moral. . . . The Gods have thrown up their job and handed it over to the Fates.'[97] The concept of an 'immortal soul' is quite foreign to him,[100] and he considers the behaviour of modern nations to be about as meaningful as fights between different colonies of ants.[101] O'Grady regales his friends with the story of one of his patients who suffers from bizarre nightmares due, he believes, to her inability to choose between her husband, at present on a business trip in Chile, and an old boyfriend, currently visiting from South Africa. The doctor offers the patient two treatment options, both of them guaranteed to relieve her symptoms: 'You either send your husband a telegram to say you are coming to join him and take the first boat, or you give way to temptation and become your friend's mistress.'[102]

According to O'Grady the two alternatives are equally efficacious from the medical point of view ('elles ont la même valeur médicale'), and he declines to recommend one or the other course of action. When the patient asks for his advice he comes out with the standard formula: 'I am a physician, not a priest.'[102] 'You're a miserable pagan', says the Reverend Jeffries when he hears this story. O'Grady does not reveal either to his fictional audience or to the reader whether or not his patient succumbs to her temptation.

The arguments between Dr Mouraille and the village priest in Chevallier's *Clochemerle*[103] represent a clownish sideshow rather than a serious discussion of important problems. Mouraille, an incompetent physician, meets the Curé Ponosse, a seasoned fornicator, in the street. Both men are heavy drinkers, although they are relatively sober on this occasion. Mouraille begins:

> 'Ah, there you are, you old grave-digger. Smelt a corpse, I take it!' 'Dear me, no, doctor' the Curé Ponosse modestly replies, . . . 'I have merely

come to finish off the job that you started so well. I give the whole credit to you.' Dr Mouraille is furious. 'You'll go through my hands one day yourself, you old dodderer.' 'I'm quite resigned to that, doctor. But you will also go through mine, without a word of protest.' . . . Dr Mouraille shows fight. 'Good God, Curé, you'll never get hold of me as long as I'm alive.'[104]

On the other hand, the dedication and single-mindedness of the 'clerical' and 'medical' protagonists in Bellaman's *King's Row*[105] make the conflict between them intense and vicious. The hero of the book, Dr Parris Mitchell, a psychiatrist at the state asylum, takes an instant dislike to Dr Cole, the new minister at the King's Row Presbyterian church, so that the conversation between the two becomes acrimonious almost as soon as they are introduced to one another. Cole talks about the 'nobility of medicine',[106] while Mitchell finds such sentiments pretentious.

'The physician doesn't think about nobility. Working with a case is just like mending anything else that's out of order. You find out what the trouble is, and then try to do something about it. It is in some respects no more romantic than plumbing.'[106]

Cole is not satisfied with this reply, and points out to Mitchell that as a physician he is doing 'God's work.' Mitchell interrupts:

'Excuse me, Dr Cole, I'm afraid that you are about to say that God in his wisdom has seen fit to afflict these his children.' Dr Cole stared and an ugly mottled flush darkened his face. 'I was indeed about to say something like that. Do you find fault with those words?' 'Has it occurred to you that if God in his wisdom has driven three thousand of our fellow citizens crazy for some secret purpose of his own, that it might be sacrilege for us to interfere and try to thwart his purpose?'[106]

The arguments are old and specious but the antagonism between the two men is real. At the funeral of a senior physician a week later, the Reverend Dr Cole preaches a sermon that obliquely criticizes Dr Mitchell for lacking 'sufficient humility of spirit and sufficient faith in the justice of Almighty God.'[106]

A more serious subsequent clash between this doctor and his clerical opponent occurs at the sitting of a commission of enquiry[107] that has been appointed to determine the 'guilt' of Benny Singer, the 'town idiot.' After years of torment inflicted by a gang of 'playful' adolescents, Benny has finally obtained a gun and shot two of his persecutors. Mitchell tries to convince the commission, which consists of three doctors and three lay people, that 'wilful murder' would not be an appropriate verdict and that Benny should be confined in a suitable institution.[107] The Reverend Cole expresses the majority view that 'it is our duty to hand this murderer over to the arm of the law and beyond that to trust to the mercy of the Lord Jesus Christ.' There is a predictable outburst from the Reverend Dr Cole when Dr Mitchell compares him to Pontius Pilate. Mitchell has the last word, but the half-witted Benny is executed.[107]

The doctor–priest interaction in Söderberg's *Doctor Glas*[108] also ends in bloodshed rather than harmless banter or a rancorous religious disputation. The two principal characters are a Lutheran pastor (Reverend Gregorius) and a family doctor (Dr Tyko Glas), who differ fundamentally in their outlook on life. Gregorius considers it:

self-evident his religion is the right one and . . . tends to regard those who reject it as . . . wicked people who are intentionally telling lies in order to bring others to perdition.[109]

The pastor lives by what he considers God's laws, which include a husband's 'conjugal rights.'[110] When his charming wife, Helga, finds her husband's sexual attentions repulsive and asks Dr Glas to relieve her of her loathsome obligations, he decides that the logical solution to her problem consists of the pastor's death. Glas has no moral scruples. Indeed, he uses the word 'moral' in its classical sense meaning 'according to custom.' 'I'm a traveller in this world; I look at mankind's customs and adopt those I find useful.'[111] Killing a parson may not be 'customary', but provided that it can be done without risk, it may be the 'correct' solution under the circumstances. Glas considers the physically hideous appearance of Gregorius[112] an additional argument in favour of ridding the world of this pest, and he uses his position of trust to poison the parson, hoping that this 'unusual' act will benefit Helga and her lover. The doctor is not apprehended, but none of the participants become happier as a result of this crime (*see also* p. 209).

The doctor hero in Remarque's *Arch of Triumph*[113] receives his lectures in piety from Eugénie, a nurse with limited intelligence but strong beliefs. 'You have no faith', Eugénie announces firmly, 'thank God I have my faith.' Dr Ravic admits his deficiency freely and then counters with the standard humanist argument: 'Faith can easily make one fanatical. That's why all religions have cost so much blood. . . . Tolerance is the daughter of doubt, Eugénie. That explains why you, with all your faith, are so much more aggressive toward me than I, lost infidel, am toward you.'[114]

One of the greatest fictional doctor–clergy encounters occurs in Somerset Maugham's short story, *Rain*.[115] A medical doctor (Alec Macphail) and a missionary (Mr Davidson), both stranded in Pago-Pago, find themselves in the same boarding house as Miss Sadie Thompson, a Californian prostitute, who proposes to set up a whorehouse in Samoa. Davidson is in no doubt concerning the course of action that should be used to deal with the evil Miss Thompson and her corrupting influence: 'If the tree is rotten it shall be cut down and cast into the flames.' He persuades the governor to send Miss Thompson back to San Francisco, where she will face a long jail sentence.[115] Dr Macphail, whose diffidence contrasts sharply with the missionary's sense of purpose, courage and eloquence, wants to protect Sadie from these moral policemen and tries (unsuccessfully) to make the governor change his mind. He then pleads with Davidson himself:

> 'Have you the heart to send her back to San Francisco?' said the doctor. 'Three years in an American prison. I should have thought you might have saved her from that.' 'Ah, but don't you see? It's necessary. Do you think my heart doesn't bleed for her? . . . You don't understand because you're blind. She's sinned and she must suffer . . . I want her to accept the punishment of man as a sacrifice to God.'[115]

Macphail, the unbeliever, who has no desire either to sniff out 'sin' or to eradicate it, is perceived to be a better Christian than Davidson, who is quite prepared to cast the first stone.[115] The story ends when Davidson succumbs to Sadie's physical charms and goes on to kill himself.

Are the two disciplines compatible?

A few authors regard medicine and religion as too far apart in their approaches to human suffering for the two disciplines even to coexist. Zola discusses the subject in detail in his priest–physician encounter, where, paradoxically, it is the doctor who defends the religious viewpoint. Pierre Froment, a priest who is hoping to regain his lost faith (and fails), meets Dr Chassaigne, an old family friend, now weak, white-haired and 'shaking with a slight tremor' during a pilgrimage to Lourdes.[116] The doctor, following a series of family disasters, has returned to religion after 40 years of indifference. However, in the process he has become disenchanted with medical science and has given up his practice, as if there were a contradiction between medicine and true faith. After prolonged discussions concerning the compatibility of medical practice and an honest belief in religion, Chassaigne and Froment decide (or at least Zola decides) that the two are incompatible.[117] The same sentiments are expressed on the return train journey by a distraught mother whose child dies during the pilgrimage: 'I should never have gone to Lourdes . . . perhaps the doctors would have saved her.'[118]

Dr Peter Harding in *The Corner of Harley* Street,[90] who describes his background as 'half-Protestant, half-scientific', makes a less complicated trip to Lourdes.[119] Quite by chance, he is offered an opportunity to accompany a group of British patients as their medical attendant, and he accepts the invitation, mainly out of curiosity.* Although respectful of the 'almost apostolic' faith of the pilgrims and full of admiration for the bishop leading the pilgrimage ('a statesman and a saint'), Harding dismisses the Lourdes miracles out of hand: 'I saw no instance, either then or later, of a Lourdes cure that could not be explained upon the observed and established lines of mental suggestion.' He feels a 'reverent' disdain for the 'stage-management of Lourdes',[120] but he also disparages other churches, which he considers irrelevant to his age: 'The various ecclesiastical bells . . . seem to contain almost less significance than the gramophone.'[121] Harding expresses some vague belief in his own version of muscular Christianity, 'The sun-browned Youth with His carpenter's wrists and His physical endurance',[121] but the doctor is essentially a worldly man whose main interest in religion consists of a deep anxiety that his teenage son may turn into an evangelical activist[122] (*see* p. 40).

In *The Healers*,[123] Dr Kevin Derry's son John, a school drop-out and drug addict, manages to rehabilitate himself by joining a commune where he and his companions 'live in the woods, farm, but mostly experience Jesus.' Kevin feels relieved rather than elated by the news: 'At least . . . his son was off drugs and busy at something not totally useless.' However, completely irreligious himself, he feels pessimistic about John's future: 'The boy would drift, seek new gods, all to no purpose.'[123]

The principal character in Cuthbert's *The Silent Cradle*, Dr Rae Duprey, loses her faith at the age of 13, when her mother bleeds to death in childbirth: 'How could . . . [God] be on her side if he let her mother die the way she did?' At the same time, Rae decides to 'become the world's greatest obstetrician so that no woman would have to go through what her mother did.'[124] Cuthbert implies that Rae exchanges her traditional Christian faith for another religion – a primitive belief in medicine.

---

* Sir Henry Bashford, the author of *The Corner of Harley Street*, actually accompanied a group of pilgrims to Lourdes (HJC Bashford, personal communication, 25 March 2003).

By the second half of the twentieth century, credulous folk have developed such a superstitious belief in the powers of 'Medical Miracles' that visits to the doctor are almost a substitute for attendance at church. Barbara Pym[125] describes this syndrome as observed in the waiting room of an English country doctor on a Monday morning.

> The patients had not on the whole been to church the previous day, but they atoned for this by a devout attendance at the place where they expected not so much to worship . . . as to receive advice and consolation. You might *talk* to the rector, some would admit doubtfully, but he couldn't give you a prescription. There was nothing in church-going to equal the triumphant moment when you came out of the surgery clutching the ritual scrap of paper.[125]

Writing from a Catholic point of view, Walker Percy[126] expresses his distaste for doctors who dabble in religious activities. His principal character asks:

> 'Are you a psychiatrist or a priest or a priest–psychiatrist? Frankly, you remind me of something in between, one of those failed priests who go into social work . . . or one of those doctors who suddenly decides to go to the seminary. Neither fish nor fowl.'[126]

Percy puts these sentiments into the mouth of a psychiatric patient, but they clearly reflect his own view that doctors and priests should not try to combine their separate roles.

Epidemics and other crises

Camus uses the setting of an epidemic[127] to describe an altercation between Dr Rieux and Father Paneloux, who meet in a makeshift hospital where a young boy dies despite the doctor's vaccine and the priest's prayers.[128] Paneloux is a highly intelligent, relatively tolerant man who tries in his own way to relieve suffering, but the contrast between the cleric and the physician remains. Camus' sympathies are clearly with the irreligious doctor who does not wish to concern himself with salvation: 'That's too big a word for me.'[128]

Similar crisis situations that bring physicians and priests into close proximity are described by Harriet Martineau,[129] Charles Kingsley,[76] Sinclair Lewis[130] and Graham Greene.[131] Dr Edward Hope in *Deerbrook*[129] and Dr Thomas Thurnall in *Two Years Ago*[76] collaborate with the local clergy during outbreaks of lethal contagious diseases. In both cases the cleric acts as a social worker, and is clearly subordinate to the physician.[89,132] Dr Hope[132] actually behaves more courageously (or more foolishly) than the Anglican rector, who sends his wife and children away, while Hope keeps his family in the epidemic-stricken area.[132]

The doctor–priest encounter between Dr Arrowsmith[130] and his old classmate the Reverend Dr Hinkley is less harmonious.[133] The two meet on a Caribbean island during a plague epidemic, but the doctor dislikes the preacher to such an extent that the two barely remain on speaking terms[133] (see p. 123).

In Greene's *The Honorary Consul*,[131] a doctor and a priest both become entangled with a group of insurgents. Father Leon Rivas joins the rebels, who he believes are acting in the interests of the poor. However, lacking ruthlessness, he is destroyed by his basic decency.[134] The physician, Dr Eduardo Plarr, is a more complex character. Plarr, who 'never went to mass except when he accompanied his mother on one of his rare visits to the capital',[135] declares himself uninterested in either the Bible or Marxism. He would have been willing, he says, to kill a child born without arms and legs if the parents had not been present.[134] He is 'able to fuck but unable to love', and he has made one of his patients pregnant. Nevertheless, although cynical about everything almost to the end, he retains a strong sense of duty, continues to work among slum-dwellers and finally sacrifices his life in an attempt to avert further bloodshed.[134]

A semi-historical account of the plague in seventeenth-century Milan[136] compares the behaviour of physicians and monks under crisis conditions, and reflects very unfavourably on the medical fraternity. In contrast to the conscientious and compassionate members of religious orders,[137] the doctors are not only callous but also incompetent and quite incapable of dealing with a medical catastrophe. The symptoms of the plague are well known to some of the older physicians, who have lived through a previous epidemic,[137] but the profession as a body goes through a massive ritual of denial.

> Many doctors . . . ridiculed the sinister prophesies and gloomy warnings of the minority. They had various names of ordinary diseases to describe all the instances of plague that they were called upon to treat.[137]

When the nature of the epidemic becomes appallingly clear, denial is no longer possible and some scapegoat has to be found to receive the blame for the disaster.[138] Many physicians, 'even those who had believed in the reality of the pestilence from the first', support the popular theory that the disease is being spread by malicious poisoners. Those doctors who are 'not very convinced of the truth of the stories about poisonous unguents' keep this opinion to themselves.[138] When it comes to helping the sick, the contrast between the doctors and the Capuchin monks becomes particularly sharp. At one stage 'the Lazaretto was left without any doctors',[139] and it is only with 'promises of great rewards and high honours' that 'some replacements were found, but not nearly as many as were needed.' By contrast, the Capuchins are willing to sacrifice their lives without receiving any material rewards. They 'arrived to serve as superintendents, confessors, administrators, nurses, cooks, distributors of clothing, washermen and in any capacity required.'[137] Old Dr Ludovico Settala is said to have been 'active and courageous' during the previous outbreak,[137] but if there are 'active and courageous' physicians during this epidemic, Manzoni does not mention them.

At the bedside of the dying patient

When it becomes obvious to the doctor that any further medical efforts are futile and that the time has come for the clergy to take over, he has a number of options. He may withdraw from the scene, indicating that his services are no longer required. He may elect to continue his therapeutic efforts even though these are now irrelevant, thereby delaying the activities of the non-medical professionals. Alternatively, he may join the clergy in their prayers for the dead and dying. Cable's *Dr Sevier*[140] compromises. He does not pray, but he agrees to read a few biblical verses to a dying patient.[141]

Schnitzler's *Professor Bernhardi*[142] does not compromise. He defies the clergy (in pre-First World War Vienna), and as a result he loses his job and ends up in jail.

Bernhardi, the chief of internal medicine in an institute of clinical research, has under his care Philomena Beier, an 18-year-old girl who is dying of what sounds like gram-negative septicaemia following an illegal abortion. The girl is unaware of her moribund condition, and Bernhardi, who wants her to have 'a happy death', perversely refuses admission to Father Reder, who has been summoned to give her the Last Sacrament.[143] The episode becomes charged with political and ethnic overtones (clerical versus liberal, Catholic versus Jew), and the differences between medical and clerical approaches towards euphoric terminal patients remain unresolved. (Philomena dies without the benefit of extreme unction.)

The clash between the protagonists of medical and religious attitudes in Ellen Glasgow's *Barren Ground*[144] produces less dramatic results, but as in Schnitzler's play,[142] the two points of view seem to be almost irreconcilable.[145] The doctor wants to relieve suffering in this world, while the patient's pious friend worries about what will happen to her soul (*see also* pp. 108–9). Dr Jason Greylock is hardly a 'typical' medical man. Not wanting to study medicine in the first place, he is forced into the profession by an overpowering father,[145] he never becomes fond of medical practice,[145] and eventually turns into the town drunkard.[146] Despite his isolation (*see* pp. 217–18) Greylock's attitude to the hereafter is very similar to that of mainstream doctors. Having reassured young Mrs Rose Emily Pedlar that she will recover from advanced tuberculosis, he informs Rose Emily's friend Dorinda Oakley that there is no hope. Both women belong to the local Presbyterian Church, and Dorinda is apprehensive about heaven and hell. She asks the doctor on the porch:

> 'Don't you think she ought to have time to prepare?' 'Prepare? You mean for her funeral?' 'No, I mean for eternity.' 'For eternity?' he repeated. 'Would you let her die, without time for repentance?' 'Repentance! Good Lord! What opportunity has she ever had to commit a pleasure?' Then, as if the discussion irritated him, he picked up his medicine case.[145]

Martin du Gard shows his physician-hero, Dr Antoine Thibault, engaged in religious debates on two occasions and with different priests.[147,148] The dispute with the Abbé Vécard takes place after the funeral of Thibault's father (whom the doctor had 'treated' with a large dose of morphine). The Abbé and the doctor employ the usual arguments and counter-arguments. 'Nothing I have observed', declares Thibault, 'warrants my believing that my childhood's God exists.' 'Can't you see', counters the Abbé, 'that your whole scheme of life, your conscientiousness, your sense of duty, your devotion to the service of your fellow men gives your materialism the lie? . . . Isn't [your conduct] a tacit admission that you are under orders from above?'[147] Dr Thibault counters that the concepts of 'prayer', 'sin', 'divine purpose' and 'natural religion' have become alien to him, and that he feels 'perfectly at home in . . . a godless world.' The Abbé fires his last salvo:

> 'Can you imagine what it's like . . . coming to the brink of life without discerning on the further shore an almighty merciful father stretching out his arms in welcome?' 'All that', Antoine put in briskly, 'I know as well as you do. . . . My profession, like yours, takes me to the bedside of the dying. I . . . have seen more unbelievers die than you have . . . and I wish I could give my patients in extremis an injection of belief.'

Thibault turns the Marxist concept of religion ('opium of the people') on its head. He has nothing against either opium or religion in circumstances where suffering has to be relieved. On the contrary, 'I dread a death without hope as much as a death-agony without morphia.'[147]

When, at the age of 37, Dr Thibault himself is on his deathbed (*see* pp. 236–8), the comforts of religion are not available to him.[148] He writes in his diary:

> Impossible to rid one[self] . . . wholly of the futile desire to find a 'meaning' in life. Even I, reviewing my career, often catch myself wondering: What was the point of it? It had no 'point.' None whatever. If we find it so hard to admit that obvious fact, the reason is simply that we have eighteen centuries of Christianity in our blood. But the more one thinks, the more one observes the outside world and one's own mind, the more apparent it becomes that life is pointless, 'signifying nothing.' Millions of beings take form on the earth's crust, live their little hour, procreate and pass away, making room for other millions, which like-wise in their turn will pass away. Their brief appearance has no significance . . . and nothing matters – except perhaps to get through this short lease of life with a minimum of suffering.[148]

A priest arrives and speaks about Antoine's 'Christian upbringing', but the dying doctor is not impressed: 'Not my fault if I was born with an itch for understanding and an incapacity for believing.' The doctor and the priest even argue about the Church's attitude to war. Thibault asks 'Why do your French and German bishops bless the flags and sing Te Deums to thank God for a bloody butchery?'[148] The priest gives the standard reply: 'A just war removes the Christian ban on murder.'[148] On his way out, he uses his final argument: 'Surely a man of your calibre can't admit that he will perish – like a dog!' Thibault replies 'What can I do about it if I'm an unbeliever – like a dog?' In his diary, the doctor describes the priest's departure.

> He stopped at the door and threw a curious look at me; a mixture of severity, surprise and sadness with (it seemed to me) a hint of affection. 'Why malign yourself, my son?' I don't think he'll come again.[148]

Doctors and pseudo-religions

Feminism, communism and other 'isms' hold no more appeal for physicians than old-fashioned religious movements. In *The Bostonians*,[149] Henry James introduces Dr Mary Prance to his readers at an assembly of feminists who are meeting in her landlady's apartment.[150] Mary is not enthusiastic about the sisterhood,[151] and she deprecates the eloquent speaker:

> 'I know more about women than she does . . . I know all she has got to say.' [The doctor] evidently didn't care for great movements.[151]

She withdraws from the meeting before anyone makes a speech.[152]

Steinbeck's encounter between a physician and a recent convert to Commun-ism[153] brilliantly illustrates the medical attitude towards the new ideology. Doc Burton, himself a left-wing sympathizer and 'fellow traveller', provides clinical help for a group of strikers, but does not share the dedication and wild-eyed fanaticism of militants like Jim Nolan, who recently joined the party. Jim, who has been shot in the shoulder by vigilantes, hopes to become a martyr to the cause of the proletariat, an ambition that he ultimately achieves.[153]

Jim stood beside the doctor. 'Better take good care of that shoulder', Burton advised, 'it might cause you some trouble later.' 'I don't care about it, Doc. It seems good to have it.' 'Yes, I thought it might be like that.' 'Like what?' 'I mean you've got something in your eyes, Jim, something religious. I've seen it in you boys before.' Jim flared: 'Well, it isn't religious. I've got no use for religion.' 'No, I guess you haven't. Don't let me confuse you with terms. You're living the good life, whatever you want to call it.' 'I'm happy', said Jim. 'And happy for the first time. I'm full up.' [The doctor responds]: 'I know. Don't let it die. It's the vision of Heaven.' 'I don't believe in Heaven', Jim said. 'I don't believe in religion.' 'All right, I won't argue any more. I don't envy you as much as I might, Jim, because sometimes I love men as much as you do, maybe not in just the same way.'[154]

Waltari's *The Egyptian*[155] is set in the fourteenth century BC, although the attitudes of the principal characters are clearly those of their mid-twentieth-century AD counterparts.[156] Sinuhe, spy, poisoner and 'physician' to Pharaoh, is an ordained priest, but he expresses a good deal of hostility towards 'real' priests whose priorities are different from his own. He loses his religious faith early in his career: 'As for the hope of immortality, I am as weary of that as I am of gods and kings.'[157] During the course of his life he meets priests of different persuasions, but he despises all of them. He is contemptuous of the hypocritical Theban priests of Ammon, their frenzy and their hocus pocus,[158] which he scrutinizes 'with the cold eye of a physician.'[159] However, so long as these clerics are left unmolested, they are essentially a tolerant bunch, and apart from enriching themselves by deceiving the poor and ignorant, they do little harm.

A Cretan priest is a more suspicious character: 'There was in his expressionless face something of sternness and cruelty.'[160] This evil creature turns out to be a murderer[161] who practises human sacrifice, but his misdeeds are confined to relatively few victims. In the opinion of Sinuhe, the worst kind of religion emanates from King Akhnaton, who introduces a new kind of worship and who preaches the universal brotherhood of man. The new religion, instead of bringing happiness to all, causes 'starvation, suffering, misery and crime.'[162] When the old order and the old religion are restored, Sinuhe, who has imbibed some of the new religion's unattainable ideals, is sent into exile because of his seditious views.[163]

Pasternak's Dr Yury Zhivago[164] believes in God, but he is sceptical about the orthodox view of heaven and contemptuous of all mass movements: 'People imagined that . . . they must all sing in chorus and live by . . . notions that were being crammed down everybody's throat.'[165] Zhivago has no time for catchphrases, whether tsarist or revolutionary, and it is not surprising that he is regarded as 'a mockery to that whole [Communist] world, an insult to it.'[165]

The doctor's concepts of 'good' and 'evil'

To a physician 'good,' 'evil,' 'sin' and 'divine punishment' are inappropriate concepts. Right and wrong refer to the correct way of arriving at a diagnosis or providing treatment, not to moral values. Physicians deal with notions like 'sick' and 'well', 'old' and 'young', 'risky' and 'safe', all of which are relative. Even the terms 'alive' and 'dead' take on different meanings in different contexts. 'Absolute' values are difficult to fit into this nebulous clinical scheme.

In *Elsie Venner*,[166] Oliver Wendell Holmes devotes an entire chapter to an after-dinner discussion between a doctor of divinity (Honeywood) and a doctor of medicine (Kittredge). 'We don't deal in absolutes', says the medical doctor.

> 'We know that food and physic act differently with different people; but you think the same kind of truth is going to suit, or ought to suit, all minds. We don't fight with a patient because he can't take magnesia or opium; but you are all the time quarreling over your beliefs as if belief did not depend . . . on early training.'[167]

Physicians, says Dr Kittredge, find it as difficult to blame the drunkard for his intemperate habits as to 'blame him for inheriting gout or asthma.' Finally, in a remarkable passage that antedates Freud by several decades, Holmes speaks of an old miser who 'has never got rid of that first year's teaching which led him to fill his stomach with all he could pump into it. . . . We are more lenient with human nature than theologians.'[167]

Dr Wilbur Larch in Irving's *Cider House Rules*[168] expresses similarly unorthodox views concerning good and evil. Larch, who provides an abortion service as well as a home for unwanted children, talks about the Lord's work (obstetrics) and the devil's work (abortions), but he evidently has his tongue in his cheek, and believes that both activities are necessary. The real devil's work gets done in the trenches in France, where 'the devil worked with shell and grenade fragments, with shrapnel and with the little dirty bits of clothing carried with a missile into a wound.'[168]

Solzhenitsyn[169] does not use this terminology, but he also concludes that 'good' and 'evil' in a medical setting assume different meanings from those that apply elsewhere: 'The doctor's voice bore no trace of bitterness . . . [towards an abusive patient] for she could see the fist-sized tumor under his jaw. Who could she feel bitter against? The tumor?'[169]

In a moving chapter in *Of Human Bondage*,[170] Somerset Maugham describes the experiences of a sensitive student (Philip Carey) during an afternoon at an outpatient clinic. The last paragraph sums up his thoughts on 'good and evil.'

> It was manifold and various; there were tears and laughter, happiness and woe; it was tedious and interesting and indifferent . . . it was sad and comic; it was trivial . . . death sighed in these rooms; and the beginning of life, filling some poor girl with terror and shame, was diagnosed there. There was neither good nor bad there. There were just facts. It was life.[170]

In a more flippant mood, Dr Salter, in John Mortimer's *Paradise Postponed*,[171] reaches the same conclusion and dismisses ethics, especially religious ethics, as irrelevant to medical practice. During a conversation between Salter and Fred Simcox, the son of the Reverend Simeon Simcox, Salter strongly disparages Fred's father and all that he stands for.

> 'Must be the religion that does it. . . . Secret sort of business, religion. All that whispering to God behind other people's backs.' [Fred feels protective of his father, who habitually takes up liberal causes] 'Do

you think he is wrong?' 'I don't deal in right and wrong. I deal in collywobbles and housemaid's knees.'[171]

Religious doctors

Although churchgoing doctors exist in literature, they are generally portrayed as clowns or hypocrites. The rare truly pious physician tends to be medically out of date or otherwise marginalized.

Religious clowns

Doctor Slop, the 'Man-Midwife' in *Tristram Shandy*, is a 'Papist',[172] which makes him an oddity in eighteenth-century England. Sterne uses Slop's curious religious beliefs and practices to illustrate the doctor's general clownishness.[172] While riding to see a patient, Slop, crossing himself at the wrong moment,

> let go of his whip and in attempting to save his whip . . . he lost the stirrup, on losing which he lost his seat and in the multitude of all these losses the unfortunate doctor lost his presence of mind. [He fell off his horse so that] the broadest part of him sunk about twelve inches deep in the mire.[172]

Another genuinely religious physician depicted as a poltroon is Sinclair Lewis's Ira Hinkley,[173] who holds both theological and medical qualifications (*see also* p. 117). Hinkley first meets Martin Arrowsmith, the irreligious hero of the story, in medical school. Martin, a future researcher, and Hinkley, who is preparing himself for a career as a medical missionary, are dissecting partners during the anatomy course. Hinkley is

> a graduate of Pottsburg Christian College and of the Sanctification Bible and Missions School. He had played football; he was as strong and nearly as large as a steer and no steer bellowed more enormously. He was a bright and happy Christian, a romping optimist who laughed away sin and doubt . . . [and] with annoying virility preached the doctrine of his tiny sect. Ira believed he could bring even medical students to bliss.[173]

Arrowsmith and Hinkley meet again[133] when both are working on a plague-stricken West Indian Island. Arrowsmith is trying out a new 'phage' system to treat the disease, while Hinkley is in charge of all the chapels of the Sanctification Brotherhood. Hinkley has lost some of his optimism but none of his bigotry.

> 'Oh Mart, if you only knew the wickedness of the natives and the way they lie and sing indecent songs . . . I've nursed the poor plague-stricken devils and I've told them how hellfire is roaring about them. . . . Oh Mart, after all these years you can't still be a scoffer.'

Arrowsmith is in no mood for arguments. He can only splutter (after Hinkley's departure) 'Now how do you suppose that maniac got here? This is going to be awful.'[133] (The two do not collaborate.)

Cronin[174] also provides a very unsympathetic picture of a doctor who displays 'active piety' but lacks medical skills.

> Dr Oxborrow, accompanied by his wife who played the portable har-
> monium, betook himself on Saturday afternoons to the nearby town of
> Fernely . . . and there, in the market, he would set up his little carpet-
> covered stand and hold an open-air religious meeting. . . . He wept
> unexpectedly and prayed even more disconcertingly. Once, when con-
> fronted by a difficult confinement, which defeated his own straining skill,
> he plumped suddenly upon his knees beside the bed and, blubbering,
> implored God to work a miracle upon the poor woman. [Dr] Urquhart,
> who detested Oxborrow, . . . had got upon the bed in his boots and
> successfully delivered the patient with high forceps.[174]

Yet another incompetent doctor prone to preaching and praying[175] comes from a
small Midwestern town, where in civilian life he conducts a general practice during
the week, and preaches in the Church of the Nazarene on Sunday. During the
Korean War, Dr Jonathan Hobson finds himself in the army doing 'a job for which
he was unprepared' and in the company of other medical officers who feel
uncomfortable with their devout tent-mate. The larrikin heroes in *M.A.S.H.*, who
despite their uncouth behaviour are competent surgeons, despise and ridicule this
simple soul with his limited medical and administrative skills. Hobson's military
career ends when his lengthy prayers irritate the Colonel, who has him sent back to
the USA 'to return to his general practice, his occasional excursions into minor
surgery and his church.'[175]

Hypocrites

Regular attendance at church was regarded as a prima facie sign of hypocrisy in a
medical man as early as the mid-eighteenth century. Launcelot Crab, a surgeon in
Smollett's *Roderick Random*,[176] and himself a depraved drunkard, bully and
womanizer, describes his rival, the apothecary, as 'a canting scoundrel who has
crept into business by hypocrisy and kissing the a-se of everybody.'[177] One of Crab's
drinking companions agrees: 'One might see with half an eye that the rascal has no
honesty in him by his going so regularly to church.'[177]

The two 'redneck' doctors in *Arrowsmith*[178] (*see also* p. 42) are quite blatant
about their religious observances. After criticizing Martin, who 'never goes to
church', one of them expresses the view that

> a priest or a preacher can send you an awful lot of business. . . . Great
> mistake for any doctor not to identify himself with some good solid
> religious denomination, whether he believes the stuff or not.[178]

Somerset Maugham's Dr Bob Nelson,[179] who practises in a small Michigan town,
expresses himself less crudely, but he is as insincere in his religious observances as his
'Leopolis' colleague.[178] Nelson, an agnostic, goes to church regularly 'because his
patients expected it of him', and he insists that his ward attend Sunday school 'for
the same reason.'[180]

Dreiser's Dr Glenn,[181] who refuses to perform an abortion on account of alleged
religious scruples, is a thoroughgoing fraud. He uses expressions like 'the sin of
destroying life' and 'my conscience will not permit me',[182] whereas in fact he has
only the vaguest notions of religion: He 'was inclined . . . to suspend judgment
between heaven and hell and leave it there, suspended and undisturbed.' With regard

to abortions, his main concern is not to get mixed up with cases that 'were illegal, dangerous and involved little or no pay', although he is willing, on occasions, to assist 'in extricating from the consequences of their folly several . . . heavily sponsored young girls of good family.' With Roberta, he assumes 'a firm and heartless attitude' and gives her medically incorrect advice: 'Even if anything were to be done, it wouldn't be advisable for you to do anything before . . . [you had waited] another two weeks.'[182]

The ship's doctor on the 'Vera' in Katherine Anne Porter's *Ship of Fools*[183] initially appears the only decent human being amongst a collection of freaks, clowns, sadists and criminals who are determined to lacerate one another, both figuratively and literally. Dr Schumann, a competent and conscientious physician,[184] curbs his tendency to gossip[185] and resists the sexual blandishments of 'La Condesa'[186,187] so that when he returns to Heidelberg he will be able to reassure his wife with a clear conscience that he has never been unfaithful.[187]

Schumann, a devout Catholic, takes his religion very seriously,

> believing in God, the Father, the Son and the Holy Ghost and the Blessed Virgin Mother of God . . . in a particularly forthright, Bavarian Catholic way.[188]

He accepts his Church's doctrines on Original Sin and Real Presence,[187] and confesses his transgressions to a particularly narrow-minded Spanish priest on board the ship.[189]

> Madness, he considered, having never separated the practice of his medical science from his theological beliefs, was the temporary triumph of Evil in the human soul.[188]

However, it gradually becomes apparent that the doctor's medical and religious facades conceal more sinister aspects of his personality. Schumann, who comes from 'the good old Junker class',[189] carries two duelling scars[190] – a relic, presumably, of his connection with an aristocratic fraternity during his university days. One of the scars looks recent rather than remote: 'Healed all these years . . . [it] still had a knotty surface.' Schumann controls his erotic desires for La Condesa and his jealousy of her other lovers by having her locked up in her cabin on narcotic drugs.[189,191] He contemplates with 'malicious satisfaction mixed with moral unction'[185] the physical injuries inflicted on one of the ship's lecherous inebriates by a female passenger. After a particularly exhausting evening

> he looked upon all . . . [patients] as his enemies. Without exception he rejected them all, every one of them, all human kinship with them, all professional duty except the barest tokens. He did not in the least care what became of any one of them. Let them live their dirty lives and die their dirty deaths . . . so much carrion to fill graves.[184]

These are not the sentiments of a person described by La Condesa as a 'preposterous, good, moral, dull, ridiculous . . . charming' man,[186] but those of a selfish individual concerned only with his own place in society and in heaven. Had Dr Schumann been alive ten years after the Vera's voyage, he would not have joined those of his colleagues who experimented on concentration-camp inmates. On the other hand, it would have been quite out of character for him to have lifted a finger to help a single holocaust victim.

The thin religious veneer of Doctor Walter ('Potsy') Luff in Green's *The Healers*[192] is also described with considerable distaste. Potsy, who no doubt considers himself a good Catholic, displays little interest in spiritual matters. However, he is fascinated by Vatican politics and the papal decorations of his father-in-law,

> a Knight of Malta and a Knight of St Gregory. You should see him in his uniform – plumed hat, sword, the works.[193]

Potsy, father of seven children[192] and husband of an alcoholic wife,[194] uses 'his father-in-law's leverage with the diocese' to obtain his first surgical appointment.[195] He is now the leading cardiac surgeon on Long Island, operating on the 'important' citizens of the area and earning over a million and a half dollars a year.[196] A prime example of the American conservative of the 1960s, Potsy supports the Vietnam War,[197] has 'a generalized contempt for anyone [with a skin] darker [than his own]',[195] and openly sneers at doctors who look after the poor and the disadvantaged.[195]

Sceptics who have not completely discarded their faith

Dr Wabanheim, the Jewish physician in *Les Morticoles*[198] who has, during his working days, been as cynical and unscrupulous as his 'gentile' colleagues (*see* Volume 1, pp. 79–80), interrupts his undignified deathbed ramblings (*see* p. 235) with superstitious Hebrew incantations, which provide him with little comfort. One of Mary Rinehart's doctors seems a little more sincere in his return to his childhood faith. He declares at the end of his life, 'It took four years of medical college to kill my belief in any sort of God, and forty years of practice to bring it back.'[199] Chris Arden, the medical hero of *The Doctor*,[199] does not know what to believe about life after death, but when he has to comfort his adopted teenage boy whose mother has just died, he gives it the benefit of the doubt:

> 'Death was either sleep – and sleep was a splendid thing, especially after pain – or . . . a new life . . . an open door, not a closed one.' . . . 'Which do you believe?' Chris hesitated. . . . What did he believe? 'I don't know, son', he said slowly. 'I think there must be a God and that if there is, he will take care of her.'[200]

Dr Richard Mahony's vague religious beliefs are criticized by two members of his family, for opposite reasons.[201] John Turnham, his brother-in-law, suspects that Richard is too religious for him,[202] while Polly, his wife, worries that he may not be religious enough.[203]

Turnham, devastated by the death of his wife, has locked himself into his room with a loaded revolver, and becomes abusive when Richard tries to visit him. As soon as he opens the door, he snarls 'Have you too come to preach and sermonize? If so, you can go back where you came from. I'll have none of that cant here.' Mahony replies 'I'm here as your doctor', he avoids any 'reference to the mystery of God's ways',[202] and by listening quietly to Turnham's outbursts against his family and the Almighty, he finally manages to calm him down.

On the other hand, Polly Mahony[203] worries about the laxity of her husband's beliefs. Mahony, who is 'kind to the poor and the sick and hadn't missed a single Sunday at church since their marriage', has his doubts about certain passages in the book of Genesis, and believes 'that God might be worshipped according to any creed.' Polly is afraid that 'if once he got the reputation of being an infidel . . . nobody would want him as a doctor at all.'[203] Polly need not have worried. Dr Mahony's numerous practice troubles do not stem from his religious beliefs or from a lack of them. During his prosperous days, he takes good care not to discuss his religious convictions and doubts with his patients. He subsequently deteriorates mentally and physically, takes up a naive form of spiritualism and announces his beliefs at a public gathering, much to the amusement of the townspeople and the disgust of the Bishop, 'who held spiritualism to be of the devil.'[204]

In his love–hate relationship with the Catholic Church, Dr Jonathan Ferrier,[205] who has not 'been to Mass for years',[206] goes out of his way to insult the local priest, Father Thomas McNulty, even though the two men maintain a professional relationship.[207] Like other irreligious physicians, Ferrier continues to practise Christian virtues (other than humility; *see* pp. 80–1), although he never refers to his activities in these terms. When a young seminarian asks to see Father McNulty about a suicide attempt, the doctor gives the priest some medical advice:

> 'Don't quote platitudes at him. Don't express any horror at what he's tried. Don't for God's sake talk about sin. . . . Keep your mouth shut as much as possible and just listen if he talks, and if he doesn't, don't talk either.'[208]

Ferrier's attitude towards God and the Church is rebellious rather than indifferent. When Father McNulty comes to see him late one night, Ferrier, who has been drinking, asks the priest 'What's up? . . . Someone died, thank God?' 'Yes.' [The deceased is a ten-year-old girl.] 'Congratulations. She's well out of it. What does anyone have to live for?' After several similar outbursts of defiance, Ferrier relents, reveals his genuine anguish and sends a message of sympathy to the grieving parents.[207] The doctor continues to brandish his fist at heaven, but he remains a believer, albeit a rebellious one. After assisting at a salpingectomy for an ectopic pregnancy, Ferrier baptizes the fetal tissue, unconcerned by the 'indulgent smiles of the interns.'[209] At the end of the story we find Dr Ferrier on his knees in St Leo's Church, confessing his sins to Father McNulty.[210]

Unlike Dr Ferrier,[205–210] Walker Percy's Dr Thomas More[211] neither loves nor hates the Catholic Church. Educated in a parochial school[212] where the nuns 'did a . . . good . . . job on us',[213] More is no longer sure what he believes,[214] and regards himself as a Catholic 'only in the remotest sense of the word.'[215] His children, although baptized Catholics, are attending a Pentecostal school,[216] and he is too indifferent to protest. He also happens to be an alcoholic who has served a two-year jail sentence for illegally selling prescriptions for sedatives and stimulant drugs to interstate truck drivers[217] (*see* p. 218).

Despite his multiple flaws, this marginalized doctor, whose nostalgia for his childhood religion enables him to triumph over his evil opponents,[211] is portrayed as a sane member of the medical profession, fighting against 'successful' and fanatical social engineers. Moreover, the impaired doctor strikes up a friendship with Father Simon Rinaldo Smith, an alcoholic and somewhat addled priest who has spent some time in a home 'for impaired priests, mostly drunks.'[218] Father Smith models himself on St Simeon Stylites, and establishes his home in a six-foot-square fire tower,[218] where he ruminates and rambles but comes out with some profound truths.

Dr Thomas More, like his historical namesake, sacrifices the prospect of a pleasant and lucrative second career ('divorce facilitation with . . . aging yuppies, crisis intervention with their stoned-out teenage children'[219]) for the sake of a principle. He has retained his 'psychiatric faith', and believes that deeply buried within each person is a soul like the biblical treasure buried in a field.[220] As an 'old-fashioned shrink' who wants to heal the psyche, he is suspicious of psychotrophic drugs and persists in trying to help patients by making them talk. He continues to befriend Father Smith, the eccentric old priest who plays the role of a garrulous, demented patient combined with that of an inspired and inspiring teacher. Although the doctor refuses to serve Mass routinely, he sometimes helps in emergencies, especially during a disorganized and somewhat farcical consecration ceremony.[219]

The devout doctor

An eighteenth-century Anglican priest[6] finds it noteworthy that two doctors who live and practise in his parish, while displaying different attitudes towards theological questions, are both faithful members of his church. He remarks:

> It is not to be supposed . . . that a physician should be a regular attendant at morning and evening prayers . . . but within the measure of their ability . . . both these persons fulfilled their obligations as loyal members of the Church of England. [Dr Quinn was] . . . a plain honest believer, not enquiring over closely into points of belief. [Dr Abell] interested himself in questions to which Providence . . . designs no answers to be given us.[6]

Dawson's Dr John Selkirk,[221–225] another loyal (and complacent) member of the Anglican Church, holds traditional beliefs that include 'sin' and 'divine punishment', and would no doubt have joined those of his colleagues who condemned and ridiculed cures for syphilis, on the grounds that the threat of sexually transmitted diseases was necessary for the maintenance of moral discipline.[226] Selkirk persuades a woman whose husband had deserted her many years earlier not to enter into a relationship with another man, because such a union would dishonour her daughter.

> She loves and trusts you and will no doubt grow up to honour you. But if you do this wrong, the day will come when you will stand ashamed before the questioning eyes of your child.[222]

One of Dawson's stories is a fanciful 'temperance tale' dressed up as a clinical anecdote and containing the usual message that drinkers have to pay a high price for their insobriety. The patient is an alcoholic woman whose only daughter lies on her deathbed, and 'we stood . . . in that awful silence which is our tribute to the majesty of death.' The drunken mother chooses this particular moment to flounce into the sickroom and attempts to cheer up the assembled company by singing 'Charlie is my Darling.'[223] The singing is forcibly and abruptly terminated, the daughter dies and the mother 'loses her mind' at that instant: 'She was a child again, a simple, ignorant, loving, beautiful child, and if she lived to old age she would be nothing else.'[223]

When Dr Selkirk discovers that 'James Farquharson' has led a somewhat licentious life, he appoints himself God's detective and informs the father of

Farqhuarson's betrothed of the moral turpitude of his prospective son-in-law.[224] It comes as no surprise that this judgemental and moralistic doctor (who would have been atypical even in 1900) is firm in his religious faith. When a patient requests some prayers just before her operation, her husband, 'a doubter', refuses on the grounds that the recitation of prayers would make him feel hypocritical.[225] The doctor has no such scruples.

> So I bowed my head and repeated the immortal prayer in which all the sorrow and pain of the world seems to be summed up. 'Finally we commend to Thy fatherly goodness all those who are anyways afflicted or distressed in mind, body or estate. . . . That it may please Thee to comfort and relieve them . . . giving them patience under their sufferings and a happy issue out of all their afflictions.'[227]

The patient recovers her health, and the husband, no doubt inspired by the doctor, recovers his faith.[225]

Unlike the self-righteous Dr Selkirk,[221-225] who practises among the London rich, Dr Herzenstube, in Dostoyevsky's *The Brothers Karamazov*,[228] works as a family physician in a small Russian town. He is a member of one of the German evangelical sects, and the locals regard him as 'an excellent and pious man.' Despite his stubbornness, his ridiculous mannerisms and his 'heavy . . . self-satisfied German wit',[228] Herzenstube gives the impression of a conscientious and compassionate doctor who is not ashamed to confess his ignorance when baffled by a difficult medical problem.[229] At the murder trial of Dmitry Karamazov, Dr Herzenstube is one of the witnesses who have to testify whether or not the accused is insane. In his rambling evidence he tells the court how he first met Dmitry:

> 'when he was a little chap so high, abandoned by his father in the backyard where he used to run about in the dirt without boots and his little breeches hanging by one button.'[228]

Herzenstube buys the neglected little boy a bag of nuts and tries to teach him some rudimentary Christian doctrine.[228] Many years later Karamazov returns to thank the doctor – no one else had ever bought him any nuts. The doctor's evidence continues:

> 'And then I remembered the happy days of my youth and the poor boy without boots . . . and I embraced him and blessed him. And I wept. He laughed but he also cried – for a Russian often laughs when he should be crying. But he cried, I saw it. And now, alas . . .'[228]

At this point there is an emotional outburst from the dock. 'I'm crying now, too, you dear old man', the prisoner calls out.[228] Herzenstube may be a 'dear old man', but there is reason to believe that his knowledge of medicine is thoroughly out of date.[228]

Another genuinely religious physician is described by Garcia Marquez in *Love in the Time of Cholera*.[230] Dr Juvenal Urbino, the principal character in the book, 'a physician and a believer',[231] is a devout traditional Catholic who has no difficulty in reconciling his faith (and his occasional lapses) with his medical practice. He attends mass regularly,[232] does not visit his patients on days of obligation,[233] kneels in the street when the archbishop's carriage drives past,[234] and during a bout of marital disharmony he suggests to his wife that they go to the archbishop for arbitration.[235]

When his patients died, 'he ushered them out of this world with a final sign of the cross and some words for the salvation of their souls.'[236] Urbino's piety is rewarded with a papal decoration; he is awarded a Knighthood of the Order of the Holy Sepulchre.[234]

In his younger days, Urbino may have been the leading physician of his home town, but by the time we meet him he has become far removed from mainstream medicine and may no longer understand the concept. Openly suspicious of advances in medical theory and practice, he has turned into an anachronistic Don Quixote whose clinical skills are obsolete,[232] and who spends his time playing chess and training his parrot to recite passages from St Matthew's gospel – in Latin.[237]

Yet another profoundly religious physician, Dr Sagiura in Paige Mitchell's *A Wilderness of Monkeys*,[238] believes that medicine is 'the purpose for which . . . [he] was created.' He has now received a 'call' to set up a first-rate diagnostic clinic, and he informs his colleagues at a business meeting that 'God willing' he will fulfil his 'destiny' with or without their assistance. The other partners in the practice are opposed to this divinely inspired scheme, and a nasty legal fight ensues (*see* p. 81).

The atypical, pious doctor, although rare, persists in contemporary novels. Hannah Alexander's *Solemn Oath*[239] relates the adventures of Dr Lukas Bower in the Emergency Department of the 'Knolls, Missouri' Community Hospital. Despite his licence to practise medicine, Dr Bower does some strange things. Soon after his arrival in Knolls, he behaves like a first-year medical student, studying the illustrations in his anatomy textbook during a meal at the local restaurant, with the predictable result that he is mistaken for a pervert.[240] He has a degree in osteopathy and performs spinal manipulations.[241] However, he functions credibly enough as an emergency-room physician, feeling pulses, listening to hearts,[242] delivering babies,[243] suturing lacerations,[244] rushing in and out of examination areas and briskly ordering emergency medications.[242] He achieves one miraculous cure, diagnosing and relieving a cardiac tamponade in his arch-enemy, who is trapped in a partially destroyed building that is about to collapse.[245]

Lukas is no ordinary TV doctor – he is a latter-day Kildare with a stethoscope in one hand and a Good News Bible in the other. He makes the local drunk 'give it all to Christ',[246] and then pays pastoral visits to check whether the new convert is coping.[247] He prays for guidance and help when confronted with difficult clinical problems,[245,248] and to give thanks when his patients recover.[249] He feels attracted to a somewhat brittle female medical colleague (Dr Mercy Richmond), who reciprocates his emotions,[250] but he then reluctantly decides to terminate the relationship because she does not 'allow God to take control.'[251] The book ends on a happy note. Mercy becomes a believer[252] so that all impediments to a union with Lukas are swept away.

This edifying tale is quoted at length because Lukas, a Christian who happens to be a doctor, is a totally uncharacteristic product of a Western medical school (if indeed he graduated from a regular medical school). In a university hospital, Lukas's powerful religious convictions would have marginalized him from mainstream medical life with its scepticism, its black humour, its 'sympathetic detachment' from human suffering and its ambiguous code of ethics. Indeed there are allegations that Lukas 'was dismissed from his residency program' and that he landed in Knolls 'because he couldn't make it in the city.'[249] In the Knolls Emergency Room, working with a team of nurses, radiographers and ambulance officers, Lukas is well qualified to combine the roles of a 'fisher of men' and a biblical 'beloved physician.' However, as a twenty-first-century Western doctor he would be regarded as a failure by more distinguished members of the medical profession.

Frank Huyler[253] tells the story of a deeply religious black woman who trusts the Lord to cure her recurrent venous thrombi and pulmonary emboli so long as she believes in him with sufficient faith. Her attending physician, a lay Baptist minister, quotes scripture to convince her that she ought to be taking anticoagulants, but the patient counters by quoting contradictory scriptural material. She refuses to take her medication and, as expected, she dies from a pulmonary embolus. At autopsy the pathologist displays the fatal clot. 'Would any of you mind if I said a prayer?', asks the physician/minister, and when there is no overt objection, he goes on to recite the Lord's Prayer.[253]

> We all said Amen and . . . there was a silence until the pathologist, an uneasy witness, cleared his throat. 'Well,' he said, 'I should really be getting back to it.'

The pathologist, who feels ill at ease when prayers are recited over a blood clot, is a typical doctor. The lay preacher is not.

Dr Chris Arden, Mary Roberts Rinehart's hero, is not a firm believer in any faith[200] (*see* p. 126). However, he is granted – on a very transient basis – a genuine religious experience familiar to most doctors who have worked with obstetric patients. After the birth of a healthy infant, Chris, holding the child in his arms,

> had for a moment that old feeling . . . of knowing what God had felt when He looked on His work and found it good.[199]

The nostalgic non-believer

Occasional fictional physicians express regret and nostalgia concerning their lost faith. Balzac's Dr Desplein,[254] a distinguished surgeon and an aggressive atheist, declares 'I swear to you I would give my whole fortune if faith such as [this simple water carrier's] could enter my brain.' Herman Wouk's Dr Keith,[255] who is dying of malignant melanoma, has this to say in his last letter to his only son, who is currently serving on a minesweeper in the South Pacific:

> I'm afraid we haven't given you much [religion], not having had much ourselves. But I think, after all, I will mail you a Bible before I go into the hospital. . . . There is a lot of everyday wisdom in it . . . I came to the Bible, as I did to everything in life, too late.[255]

Summary

Fiction writers seem almost unanimous in the view that physicians, during the course of their training and their work, acquire sets of values that are notably different from those of the Church. They may have a strong sense of duty and they may practise Christian virtues, but their ideas of 'good' and 'evil' are conditioned by their experiences of human suffering and by their attempts to relieve it.[256] They do not believe in heaven or hell but, in the end, they may get to the right place.[257]

References

1   Kipling R (1901) *Kim*. Pan Books, London, 1978, p. 235.
2   Čapek K (1929) Giddiness (translated by Selver P). In: *Tales From Two Pockets*. Allen and Unwin, London, 1967, pp. 177–83.
3   Grim JA (1983) *The Shaman*. University of Oklahoma Press, Norman, OK.
4   Meier DE, Emmons CA, Wallenstein S, Quill T, Morrison RS and Cassel CK (1998) A national survey of physician-assisted suicide and euthanasia in the United States. *NEJM*. 338: 1193–202.
5   Bennett A (1923) *Riceyman Steps*. Cassell, London, 1947, pp. 51–2.
6   James MR (1919) Two Doctors. In: Byatt AS (ed.) *The Oxford Book of English Short Stories*. Oxford University Press, Oxford, 1998, pp. 97–104.
7   The Bible, Revised Standard Version. Oxford University Press, New York, 1977, I Kings, 15: 14.
8   The Bible, Revised Standard Version. Oxford University Press, New York, 1977, II Chronicles, 16: 12–13.
9   The Bible, Revised Standard Version. Oxford University Press, New York, 1977, Ecclesiasticus, 38: 13–15.
10 *Mishnah* (*c.* 180 AD) (translated by Danby H). Oxford University Press, London, 1933, p. 329.
11 Gregory of Tours (*c.* 580 AD) The Miracles of the Bishop Saint Martin. In: *Saints and their Miracles in Late Antique Gaul* (translated by Van Dam R). Princeton University Press, Princeton, NJ, 1993, p. 238.
12 Chaucer G (*c.* 1390) The Canterbury Tales. In: Fisher JH (ed.) *The Complete Poetry and Prose of Geoffrey Chaucer*. Holt, Rinehart and Winston, New York, 1977, pp. 17–18.
13 Browne T (1642) Religio Medici. In: Keynes G (ed.) *The Works of Sir Thomas Browne. Volume 1*. Faber and Faber, London, 1964, p. 11.
14 Paré A (1564) *Ten Books of Surgery* (translated by Linker RW and Womack N). University of Georgia Press, Athens, GA, 1969, p. 153.
15 Sterne L (1759–1767) *The Life and Opinions of Tristram Shandy, Gentleman*. Odyssey Press, New York, 1940, p. 136.
16 Balzac H de (1841) *Ursule Mirouët* (translated by Bell C). Dent, London, 1925, p. 13–19.
17 Ibid., pp. 26–9.
18 Ibid., p. 53.
19 Ibid., p. 9.
20 Ibid., p. 39.
21 Hawthorne N (1850) *The Scarlet Letter*. Ohio State University Press, Columbus, OH, 1971, p. 119.
22 Bellamy E (1880) *Dr Heidenhoff's Process*. AMS Press, New York, 1969, p. 105.
23 Frederic H (1896) *The Damnation of Theron Ware*. Harvard University Press, Cambridge, MA, 1960, pp. 69–78.
24 Ibid., p. 233.
25 Eliot G (1871–1872) *Middlemarch*. Penguin Books, Harmondsworth, 1988, p. 330.
26 Ibid., p. 211.
27 Cather W (1931) *Shadows on the Rock*. Virago, London.
28 Ibid., p. 124.
29 Ibid., p. 253.
30 Davies R (1985) *What's Bred in the Bone*. Penguin, Harmondsworth, 1988, pp. 49–50.
31 Danby F (Frankau J) (1887) *Dr Phillips: a Maida Vale idyll*. Garland Publishing, New York, 1984.
32 Ibid., p. 187.

33 Ibid., pp. 335–40.
34 Ibid., p. 287.
35 Ibid., p. 27.
36 Ibid., p. 47.
37 Chekhov AP (1892) Ward Number Six. In: *The Oxford Chekhov* (translated by Hingley R). *Volume 6.* Oxford University Press, London, 1971, p. 129.
38 Daudet LA (1894) *Les Morticoles.* Fasquelle, Paris, 1956.
39 Ibid., pp. 30–4.
40 Ibid., p. 42.
41 Strindberg A (1887) The Father. In: *Twelve Plays* (translated by Sprigge E). Constable, London, 1962, p. 47.
42 Posen S (2005) *The Doctor in Literature. Satisfaction or resentment?* Radcliffe Publishing, Oxford, pp. 175–6.
43 Hardy T (1886–1887) *The Woodlanders.* Oxford University Press, Oxford, 1988.
44 Ibid., pp. 125–9.
45 Bernières L de (1994) *Captain Corelli's Mandolin.* Vintage, London, 1998.
46 Ibid., p. 53.
47 Miller A (1997) *Ingenious Pain.* Harcourt Brace, New York, pp. 5–8.
48 Irving J (2001) *The Fourth Hand.* Bloomsbury, London, p. 42.
49 Collins W (1868) *The Moonstone.* Perennial Classics, Harper and Row, New York, 1965.
50 Ibid., p. 222.
51 Maartens M (1906) *The Healers.* Constable, London.
52 Ibid., p. 79.
53 Wolfe T (1929) *Look Homeward Angel.* Charles Scribner's Sons, New York, 1936.
54 Ibid., p. 353.
55 Gerritsen T (1996) *Harvest.* Headline Publishing, London.
56 Ibid., pp. 31–3.
57 Ibid., pp. 66–7.
58 Ibid., pp. 124–34.
59 Salzman M (2000) *Lying Awake.* Knopf, New York.
60 Ibid., p. 47.
61 Ibid., p. 121.
62 Ibid., p. 152.
63 Ibid., p. 159.
64 Ibid., p. 165.
65 Norris CB (1969) *The Image of the Physician in Modern American Literature.* PhD Dissertation, University of Maryland, Baltimore, MD.
66 Cozzens JG (1933) *The Last Adam.* Harcourt Brace and Company, New York.
67 Dreiser T (1919) The Country Doctor. In: *Twelve Men.* Constable, London, 1930, pp. 102–22.
68 Tennyson A (1880) In the Children's Hospital. In: Ricks C (ed.) *The Poems of Tennyson.* Longmans, London, 1969, pp. 1261–3.
69 Cozzens JG, op. cit., p. 279.
70 Metalious G (1956) *Peyton Place.* Dell, New York, 1958.
71 Ibid., p. 9.
72 Hulme K (1956) *The Nun's Story.* Pan Books, London, 1959.
73 Ibid., pp. 116–22.
74 Flaubert G (1857) *Madame Bovary* (translated by Steegmuller F). Modern Library, New York, 1982, p. 364.
75 Rothfield L (1992) *Vital Signs: medical realism in nineteenth-century fiction.* Princeton University Press, Princeton, NJ, p. 46.
76 Kingsley C (1857) Two Years Ago. In: *The Works of Charles Kingsley. Volume 8.* Reprinted by Georg Olms, Hildesheim, Germany, 1969.

77 Ibid., p. 36.
78 Ibid., p. 494.
79 Ibid., p. 165.
80 Greene G (1961) *A Burnt-Out Case*. Heinemann and The Bodley Head, London, 1974.
81 Ibid., p. 15.
82 Ibid., p. 68.
83 Ibid., pp. 38–42.
84 Ibid., pp. 100–5.
85 Ibid., pp. 144–5.
86 Goldsworthy P (1992) *Honk If You Are Jesus*. Angus and Robertson, Sydney.
87 Ibid., pp. 94–6.
88 Williams T (1948) Summer and Smoke. In: *The Theatre of Tennessee Williams. Volume 2*. New Directions, New York, 1971, pp. 218–19.
89 Kingsley C, op. cit., p. 303.
90 Bashford HH (1911) *The Corner of Harley Street: being some familiar correspondence of Peter Harding MD*. Constable, London, 1913.
91 Ibid., pp. 204–10.
92 Ashton H (1930) *Doctor Serocold*. Penguin, London, 1936.
93 Ibid., p. 14.
94 Ibid., pp. 30–1.
95 Ibid., p. 72.
96 Maurois A (1919–1921) *Colonel Bramble* (translated by Wake T). Jonathan Cape, London, 1937.
97 Ibid., pp. 180–1.
98 Ibid., pp. 53–7.
99 Ibid., p. 215.
100 Maurois A (1919–1950) *Les Silences du Colonel Bramble: les discours et nouveaux discours du Dr O'Grady*. Grasset, Paris, 1950, pp. 378–86.
101 Ibid., p. 403.
102 Ibid., pp. 244–57.
103 Chevallier G (1936) *Clochemerle* (translated by Godefroi J). Secker and Warburg, London, 1952.
104 Ibid., pp. 182–3.
105 Bellaman H (1940) *King's Row*. Dymocks, Sydney, 1945.
106 Ibid., pp. 376–80.
107 Ibid., pp. 430–40.
108 Söderberg H (1905) *Doctor Glas* (translated by Austin PB). Chatto and Windus, London, 1963.
109 Ibid., p. 40.
110 Ibid., p. 23.
111 Ibid., p. 95.
112 Ibid., pp. 13–14.
113 Remarque EM (1945) *Arch of Triumph* (translated by Sorell W and Lindley D). Appleton Century, New York.
114 Ibid., p. 39.
115 Maugham WS (1920) Rain. In: *Collected Short Stories. Volume 1*. Pan Books, London, 1975, pp. 9–48.
116 Zola E (1894) *Lourdes* (translated by Vizetelly EA). Chatto and Windus, London, 1896.
117 Ibid., pp. 142–3.
118 Ibid., p. 450.
119 Bashford HH, op. cit., pp. 130–9.
120 Ibid., p. 147.
121 Ibid., pp. 214–16.

122 Ibid., pp. 40–1.
123 Green G (1979) *The Healers*. Melbourne House, London, pp. 491–2.
124 Cuthbert M (1998) *The Silent Cradle*. Simon and Schuster, London, p. 7.
125 Pym B (1980) *A Few Green Leaves*. EP Dutton, New York, p. 13.
126 Percy W (1977) *Lancelot*. Farrar Straus and Giroux, New York, pp. 4–5.
127 Camus A (1947) *The Plague* (translated by Gilbert S). Penguin, Harmondsworth, 1960.
128 Ibid., pp. 173–9.
129 Martineau H (1839) *Deerbrook*. Virago Press, London, 1983.
130 Lewis S (1924) *Arrowsmith*. Signet Books, New York, 1961.
131 Greene G (1973) *The Honorary Consul*. Simon and Schuster, New York.
132 Martineau H, op. cit., pp. 472–509.
133 Lewis S, op. cit., pp. 351–2.
134 Greene G, op. cit., pp. 255–67.
135 Ibid., p. 36.
136 Manzoni A (1827) *The Betrothed* (translated by Penman B). Penguin, Harmondsworth, 1983.
137 Ibid., pp. 566–76.
138 Ibid., p. 603.
139 Ibid., p. 594.
140 Cable GW (1885) *Dr Sevier*. James R Osgood and Company, Boston, MA.
141 Ibid., p. 62.
142 Schnitzler A (1912) *Professor Bernhardi* (translated by Landstone H). Faber and Gwyer, London, 1927.
143 Ibid., pp. 32–3.
144 Glasgow E (1925) *Barren Ground*. Virago, London, 1986.
145 Ibid., pp. 64–71.
146 Ibid., pp. 360–2.
147 Martin du Gard R (1922–1929) *The Thibaults* (translated by Gilbert S). John Lane, The Bodley Head, London, 1939, pp. 870–89.
148 Martin du Gard R (1936–1940) *Summer 1914* (translated by Gilbert S). John Lane, The Bodley Head, London, 1940, pp. 1057–75.
149 James H (1886) *The Bostonians*. Penguin, Harmondsworth, 1984.
150 Ibid., p. 58.
151 Ibid., pp. 67–8.
152 Ibid., p. 73.
153 Steinbeck J (1936) *In Dubious Battle*. Heinemann, London, 1970.
154 Ibid., p. 161.
155 Waltari M (1945) *The Egyptian* (translated by Walford N). Panther Books, London, 1960.
156 Ibid., pp. 51–2.
157 Ibid., p. 5.
158 Ibid., pp. 31–3.
159 Ibid., p. 240.
160 Ibid., p. 151.
161 Ibid., p. 167.
162 Ibid., p. 255.
163 Ibid., pp. 348–50.
164 Pasternak B (1957) *Doctor Zhivago* (translated by Hayward M and Harari M). Pantheon, New York, 1958.
165 Ibid., pp. 404–21.
166 Holmes OW (1861) Elsie Venner. In: *The Works of Oliver Wendell Holmes. Volume 5*. Houghton Mifflin, Boston, MA, 1892.
167 Ibid., pp. 313–28.

168 Irving J (1985) *Cider House Rules*. Bantam Books, New York, 1986, p. 68.
169 Solzhenitsyn A (1968) *Cancer Ward* (translated by Bethell N and Burg D). The Bodley Head, London, 1971, pp. 55–7.
170 Maugham WS (1915) *Of Human Bondage*. Signet Classics, New York, 1991, pp. 445–6.
171 Mortimer J (1985) *Paradise Postponed*. Penguin, Harmondsworth, 1986, p. 105.
172 Sterne L, op. cit., p. 106.
173 Lewis S, op. cit., pp. 16–17.
174 Cronin AJ (1937) *The Citadel*. Gollancz, London, pp. 163–4.
175 Hooker R (1968) *M.A.S.H.* William Morrow and Company, New York, pp. 19–27.
176 Smollett T (1748) *The Adventures of Roderick Random*. Dent, London, 1964.
177 Ibid., pp. 33–7.
178 Lewis S, op. cit., p. 171.
179 Maugham WS (1944) *The Razor's Edge*. Penguin, Harmondsworth, 1963.
180 Ibid., pp. 258–9.
181 Dreiser T (1925) *An American Tragedy*. Signet Classics, New York, 1964.
182 Ibid., pp. 397–407.
183 Porter KA (1945–1962) *Ship of Fools*. Little Brown, Boston, MA, 1962.
184 Ibid., pp. 468–9.
185 Ibid., p. 492.
186 Ibid., pp. 117–21.
187 Ibid., pp. 196–205.
188 Ibid., pp. 113–15.
189 Ibid., pp. 346–50.
190 Ibid., pp. 16–17.
191 Ibid., p. 316.
192 Green G, op. cit., pp. 236–7.
193 Ibid., pp. 178–9.
194 Ibid., pp. 143–4.
195 Ibid., p. 159.
196 Ibid., p. 356.
197 Ibid., p. 311.
198 Daudet LA, op. cit., pp. 267–74.
199 Rinehart MR (1935) *The Doctor*. Farrar and Rinehart, New York, p. 95.
200 Ibid., p. 495.
201 Richardson HH (1917–1929) *The Fortunes of Richard Mahony*. Penguin, Harmondsworth, 1990.
202 Ibid., p. 120.
203 Ibid., pp. 160–4.
204 Ibid., p. 725.
205 Caldwell T (1968) *Testimony of Two Men*. Collins, London, 1990.
206 Ibid., p. 16.
207 Ibid., pp. 61–3.
208 Ibid., p. 129.
209 Ibid., p. 330.
210 Ibid., pp. 447–8.
211 Percy W (1987) *The Thanatos Syndrome*. Ivy Books, New York, 1988.
212 Ibid., p. 130.
213 Ibid., p. 137.
214 Ibid., p. 395.
215 Ibid., p. 48.
216 Ibid., pp. 384–6.
217 Ibid., pp. 27–9.
218 Ibid., p. 125.

219 Ibid., pp. 394–9.
220 The Bible, Revised Standard Version. Oxford University Press, New York, 1977, Matthew, 13: 44.
221 Dawson WJ (1900) *The Doctor Speaks*. Grant Richards, London.
222 Ibid., p. 220.
223 Ibid., pp. 92–7.
224 Ibid., pp. 169–204.
225 Ibid., pp. 20–8.
226 Donzelot J (1977) *The Policing of Families* (translated by Hurley R). Hutchinson, London, 1980, p. 172.
227 *Book of Common Prayer According to the Use of the Church of England*. Cambridge University Press, Cambridge, 1968, p. 42.
228 Dostoyevsky F (1880) *The Brothers Karamazov* (translated by Magarshack D). *Volume 2*. Penguin, Harmondsworth, 1977, pp. 789–95.
229 Dostoyevsky F (1880) *The Brothers Karamazov* (translated by Magarshack D). *Volume 1*. Penguin, Harmondsworth, 1977, pp. 211–12.
230 Garcia Marquez G (1985) *Love in the Time of Cholera* (translated by Grossman E). Jonathan Cape, London, 1988.
231 Ibid., p. 35.
232 Ibid., pp. 11–13.
233 Ibid., p. 15.
234 Ibid., pp. 47–8.
235 Ibid., p. 32.
236 Ibid., p. 242.
237 Ibid., p. 24.
238 Mitchell P (1965) *A Wilderness of Monkeys*. Arthur Barker, London, p. 275.
239 Alexander H (2000) *Solemn Oath*. Bethany House Publishers, Minneapolis, MN.
240 Ibid., p. 244.
241 Ibid., p. 63.
242 Ibid., pp. 26–35.
243 Ibid., p. 169.
244 Ibid., pp. 283–9.
245 Ibid., pp. 334–5.
246 Ibid., p. 161.
247 Ibid., pp. 235–7.
248 Ibid., p. 178.
249 Ibid., pp. 224–6.
250 Ibid., p. 217.
251 Ibid., p. 262.
252 Ibid., p. 351.
253 Huyler F (1999) Faith. In: *The Blood of Strangers*. University of California Press, Berkeley, CA, pp. 19–22.
254 Balzac H de (1836) *The Atheist's Mass* (translated by Bell C). Dent, London, 1929, pp. 1–20.
255 Wouk H (1951) *The Caine Mutiny*. Cape, London, 1954, p. 63.
256 Rushmore S (1934) The care of the patient as the religion of the physician. *NEJM*. **211**: 1081–7.
257 Benét SV (1938) Doc Mellhorn and the Pearly Gates. In: *Tales Before Midnight*. Heinemann, London, 1940, pp. 102–24.

CHAPTER 4

Versatile scholars or ignorant boors?

Conflicting perceptions of what there is and what there should be

> Like many doctors . . . [Jean Doutreval] was . . . very artistic and interested in everything.[1]

> Doctors, as a rule, are the least curious of men.[2]

These contradictory statements concerning the physician's extra-curricular interests, both published in 1943,* reflect two perceptions which go back to classical times. The Apollo–Aesculapius tradition portrays medicine as part of general and priestly knowledge, and doctors as men of arts, letters and magic.[3] By contrast, Hippocrates' aphorism 'the art is long and life is short',[4] which has become generally accepted as a behavioural guide for the medical profession, obliges physicians to spend most of their time studying matters pertaining to their trade. It follows that doctors raised in the Hippocratic tradition lack the opportunity to acquaint themselves with non-medical subjects, and that many of them develop into one-sided individuals.

Medical teachers to this day debate the relative merits of these conflicting approaches. Some deplore the predominance of the 'Hippocratic' attitude in medical education, and endeavour to rectify this state of affairs.[5,6] Others express scepticism about curricula that attempt to 'teach' humanistic values to medical students.[7] Oliver Wendell Holmes, one of the most famous nineteenth-century medical educators, saw it as part of his duty to emphasize the essentially specialized nature of the doctor's knowledge and to caution young medical graduates against taking even shallow draughts from the spring of non-medical learning.[8] Despite his own wide interests, Holmes warned the members of the Bellevue Graduating Class of 1871

> against all ambitions and aspirations outside of [their] profession. . . . Medicine is the most difficult of sciences and the most laborious of the arts. It will task all your powers of body and mind if you are faithful to it. Do not . . . linger by the enchanted stream of literature. . . . The great

---

* The extracts come from different geographical settings. The 'cultivated, artistic' Dr Doutreval in *Bodies and Souls*[1] is a junior physician on the staff of the Angers University Hospital in western France, whereas Raymond Chandler's doctor who lacks curiosity[2] is in private practice in Los Angeles.

practitioners are generally those who concentrate all their powers on their business.[8]

In *Elsie Venner*,[9] Holmes goes further. Dr Kittredge, the idealized small-town physician, appears to deprecate even the reading of medical journals and books. He expresses the view that

> practical experience [is more important than] all the science in the world. When a man . . . lives among sick folks for five and thirty years . . . if he hasn't got a library of five and thirty volumes bound up in his head at the end of that time he'd better . . . sell his horse and sulky.

Holmes would have been well aware that in the absence of books and journals 'thirty-five years' experience' may well become 'one year's experience thirty-five times', but he evidently considered personal observations more important for busy practising doctors than any form of book learning.

William Osler, although not quite as negative about extramural pursuits as Holmes, nonetheless accepts the restricted outlook of doctors as virtually inevitable,[10] regardless of their degree of dedication to medicine.

> On the one hand are the intense ardent natures, absorbed in their studies and quickly losing interest in everything but their profession. . . . On the other hand are the bovine brethren who think of nothing but the treadmill and the corn.[10]

In her exceptional PhD dissertation, Carolyn Norris[11] makes the same distinction, using a different terminology. Osler's 'intense, ardent natures' are equivalent to Norris's 'priestly' physicians, who are abstemious, idealistic and totally dedicated to their patients. The 'bovine brethren' are Norris's earthy 'Pan'-type doctors who, although capable of hard work, are devoted largely to their own pleasures. Neither kind is likely to display a great deal of scholarly versatility. The priest is completely absorbed in his profession, while the Pan, who lacks the mental capacity and/or the inclination to take an intelligent interest in his chosen subject, can hardly be expected to tackle another discipline.

Authors of fiction portray both versatile and unidimensional doctors, contrasting the surprising erudition of some members of the profession with a total ignorance of non-medical topics among others. The scholarly physician predominates in the nineteenth century, the ignoramus in the twentieth. Some one-sided individuals, such as Proust's Dr Cottard,[12] succeed professionally, but a great many, including Charles Bovary[13] and Chekhov's doctors,[14–16] are no more than medical drudges. A few successful doctors attempt to acquire 'culture' but generally succeed only in making themselves ridiculous. Achievements in fields of endeavour outside medicine do not necessarily add to a physician's diagnostic or therapeutic abilities, or to his stature within the medical and lay communities.

The ignorant boor

Dickens' uncouth and impoverished medical students, who fail to pay their rent,[17] hold drunken parties and engage in various tricks to attract patients after setting up in practice,[18] are highly unlikely to develop an interest in 'cultural' pursuits. The cynical and superficial attitudes of these embryonic doctors towards the sufferings of a hospital patient are illustrated in this widely quoted conversation:

> 'You're late, Jack', said Mr Benjamin Allen.' 'Been detained at Bartholomew's', replied Hopkins. 'Anything new?' 'No, nothing particular. Rather a good accident brought into the casualty ward.' 'What was that, sir?' inquired Mr Pickwick. 'Only a man fallen out of a four pair of stairs window – but it's a very fair case – very fair case indeed.' 'Do you mean the patient is in a fair way to recovering?' inquired Mr Pickwick. 'No', replied Hopkins carelessly. 'No. I should rather say he wouldn't. There must be a splendid operation, though, tomorrow – magnificent sight if Slasher does it.'[17]

Admittedly, Hopkins and Allen are only students, assuming an attitude of flippancy for the benefit of Samuel Pickwick. However, neither their way of thinking nor the level of their conversation suggests the slightest awareness of humanistic values.

Charles Bovary's lack of clinical competence[13] is not counterbalanced by non-medical skills. Drama, music and painting mean nothing to him.[19]

> When he had lived in Rouen, . . . he had never had any interest in going to the theatre. . . . He couldn't swim or fence or fire a pistol. . . . This man could teach you nothing, he knew nothing, he wished for nothing.[19]

Chekhov presents an entire gallery of intellectually impoverished physicians,[14–16] most of them misfits and malcontents (*see* pp. 185–8) who derive little satisfaction from either their clinical or their spare time activities. Dr Kirilov, the unhappy country physician in *The Enemies*,[14] loathes the 'idle rich' who (to him) smell of 'scent and prostitutes.' He despises their 'noble act of money-grabbing', their insincere 'humanitarian ideas' and especially their cultural pursuits, for which he has neither time nor inclination. Kirilov regards the musical activities of Aboghin, a member of this wealthy set, as trivial and frivolous. It is not clear from the text whether Kirilov does not know or affects not to know the difference between a trombone and a cello. What is clear is his hatred and contempt for Aboghin's cultured way of life, which he twice compares to the endeavours of a castrated rooster.[14]

Dr Dimitry Startsev,[15] financially more successful and politically less radical than Kirilov, suffers from the same cultural impairment and is considered a boor even in his own unsophisticated environment. Startsev becomes briefly infatuated with Catherine Turkin, the daughter of typical Chekhovian provincials. Her father is full of clichés and stale jokes: 'Why did the cowslip? Because she saw the bullrush.' Mrs Turkin is a tedious, middle-aged flirt: 'You can be my new boyfriend. My husband is jealous – oh! He's quite the Othello! – But we'll try to behave so he won't notice anything.' Catherine, who is called 'Pussy' by her parents, 'is considered a musical genius . . . in the town of S . . . but her piano playing is noisy and she lacks talent.' She refuses Startsev's proposal of marriage in order to 'dedicate her life to music', but after four years at the Moscow Conservatorium she acknowledges and accepts her limitations. She returns home and attempts to rekindle the extinguished fire, but by now Startsev has lost interest in her. He has becomes fat, self-centred and rich.

> He has a vast practice in the town and scarcely time to draw breath. Already he owns an estate and two town houses. . . . He has grown ill-humoured and irritable. When taking surgery he usually loses his temper

and bangs his stick impatiently on the floor. 'Pray confine yourself to answering my questions!' he shouts unpleasantly. . . . He lives alone. It is a dreary life, he has no interests.[15]

The Turkins may be provincial in their outlook, but they maintain some interest in music and literature and they remain jolly and cheerful despite Catherine's gradual transformation into an old maid. Dr Startsev, on the other hand, lacks even the most elementary cultural accomplishments, and his symbolic stick comes to represent the tyranny of an irascible old man rather than the staff of Aesculapius.[15]

Dr Ivan Chebutykin in *Three Sisters*[16] is largely untroubled by his laziness and his ignorance, which he discusses without inhibitions: 'Since I left the university I haven't lifted a finger. I've never even read a book. I've read nothing but newspapers.'[16]

Indeed, whenever he appears on stage, Chebutykin is either combing his beard or reading tabloids, which seem to provide him with his postgraduate education. He has forgotten whatever medical facts he had managed to cram into his brain, presumably at the last minute before his examinations. When Andrew Prozorov, who has put on a great deal of weight, develops shortness of breath and asks his friend Chebutykin for informal advice, he obtains the response 'Why ask me? I don't know, dear boy. Don't remember.' The doctor blames himself[16] for the death of a patient because he lacks the insight to realize that in all probability this woman would have died regardless of whether she had been given the 'right' or the 'wrong' treatment (in 1901). During bouts of alcoholic remorse Chebutykin regrets his general ignorance, which is almost as vast as his lack of medical information: 'A couple of days ago, at the club, they were talking about Shakespeare and Voltaire. I've never read them, never read a word of them, but I managed to look as if I had.'[20]

For most of the time Chebutykin seems unconcerned about his lack of general and medical knowledge, and oblivious to his clownishness.

Chevallier's Dr Mouraille[21] is another incompetent and ignorant individual who did not attain his narrow outlook through excessive study in the medical library. He

> was a heavy drinker with a taste . . . for appetizers before meals, a habit acquired in his student days. That period had been very prolonged and devoted impartially to racing, poker, drinking at cafés, visits to houses of pleasure, country excursions and parties at the university.[21]

'The exception that proves the rule'

Several authors take the doctor's ignorance for granted and express surprise when the odd medical character turns out to have read more than his textbooks. Henry James in *The Middle Years*[22] comments that it is rare 'to find a bristling young doctor . . . enamored of literary form', but then goes on to present young Dr Hugh, a connoisseur of serious writing, as an exception.* Somerset Maugham uses the same device. 'Medical men aren't much interested in literature', remarks Dr Philip Carey in *Of Human Bondage*[23] when he finds, to his surprise, that old Dr South has read Smollett's *Peregrine Pickle*. Sarah Orne Jewett's Dr Leslie,[24] himself 'a scholar in other than medical philosophies', is very conscious of the cultural limitations of his

---

* Dr Hugh's love of books and writing makes him neglect his patient who revenges herself by cutting him out of her will.

colleagues.[25] Family practitioners, says the doctor, rarely make good local historians, despite their knowledge of the district.

> 'We haven't time to do any writing. . . . That's why our books amount to so little for the most part. The active men who are really to be depended upon as practitioners are kept so busy that they are too tired to use the separate gift for writing even if they possess it, which many do not.'[25]

The editor of an 'arty' magazine in Segal's *Doctors*[26] expresses the view that the notion of a 'literary doctor' is almost a contradiction in terms, 'like benign cancer', although he manages to find one exception to this rule (a psychiatrist). Hank, the old country doctor in Busch's *A History of Small Ideas*,[27] owns many good books, 'not the sort you'd expect a country doctor – any doctor – to be reading.'

Medicine: 'A'; other pursuits: 'D'

It is hardly surprising that medical fools and drunkards, who have forgotten whatever they were taught during their university years, display few signs of proficiency in non-medical subjects. Dr Allen and Dr Hopkins,[17] who practise under the name of 'Sawyer, late Nockemorf'[18] (*see* pp. 140–1) and will never amount to anything more distinguished than medical mediocrities, are unlikely to make any contributions to either medical or non-medical knowledge. More interesting is the paradox of those doctors who possess finely honed medical skills, but whose understanding of other branches of learning is almost non-existent. Balzac's Dr Desplein,[28] a serious and highly successful surgeon, obviously ranks far above Dickens' clowns in the medical hierarchy. Nevertheless, he lacks the breadth of knowledge that would have made him 'the great figure of his age.'[28] Desplein's educational limitations preclude the publication of scientific papers, so he 'made no original contributions to medical science' and has to content himself with the role of a performer: 'The glory of a surgeon is like that of an actor . . . their talent leaves no trace when they are gone.'[28]

Chekhov's hard-working and idealistic Dr Osip Dymov,[29] whose academic career is terminated by his early death, is not interested in art, drama or literature, in sharp contrast to his brainless wife, who dabbles in various artistic activities but performs indifferently at all of them (*see also* pp. 17–18 and 32). HG Wells' recent Montpellier graduate who 'looks after' Edward Ponderevo,[30] and prolongs his life by a few hours, evidently lacks the experience necessary to decide when to give and when to withhold treatment. No conversational details are provided, but the doctor is simply dismissed as 'one of those half-educated young men.'

The arch-prototype of the professionally successful but otherwise ignorant physician is represented by Proust's 'illiterate' Dr Cottard,[12,31] who practises in Paris during the days when diagnostic acumen was considered to be a 'mysterious gift' bestowed on a few chosen individuals (*see* Volume 1, pp. 112–13). Cottard is believed to have developed this flair to a high degree,[31] but his medical ability provides him with no 'superiority in the other departments of the intellect.' Medical skills, declares Proust, may be present in 'a person of the utmost vulgarity',[31] and he goes on to show that Cottard is a social climber with the general knowledge and the manners of a not particularly intelligent high-school student.[32] He is devoid of any artistic or literary training, but always ready to tell a bad joke or use an inappropriate pun.[12] When his loyal wife organizes musical soirées for his colleagues 'in the hope that [they] might one day make him Dean of the Faculty', Cottard, whose 'unsparing endeavours to cultivate the wilderness of his ignorance'[12] do not include classical music, removes himself to another room where he plays cards with a few like-minded friends.[33]

Unlike Cottard,[12,31–33] Sinclair Lewis's famous medical hero, *Martin Arrowsmith*,[34] at least has enough insight to recognize and acknowledge his educational deficiencies. Arrowsmith realizes early in his career that

> he was half educated. He was supposed to be a college graduate but he knew nothing of economics, nothing of history, nothing of music or painting. Except for hasty bolting for examinations he had read no poetry . . . and the only prose besides medical journalism at which he looked nowadays was the baseball and murder news in the Minneapolis papers.[34]

Martin, who goes on to become a clinical researcher, makes valiant efforts to improve his general knowledge. He announces to his wife, Leora, that they are 'going to get educated, if it kills us',[34] and proceeds to carry out his threat by reading European history aloud to Leora, 'who looked interested or at least forgiving.' He also 'took up' literature, but 'it cannot be said that he became immediately and conspicuously articulate.'[34] Remarkably and paradoxically, Martin's classmate and negative role model, the 'bloodless and acquisitive' Angus Duer, whose sole aim in life is to become a 'successful' surgeon, is familiar with the works of Bach and Beethoven.[35]

Other successful physicians whose ignorance gives rise to comment include Sir William Bradshaw, Virginia Woolf's prominent psychiatrist.[36] Fictional psychiatrists are usually portrayed as being well versed in non-medical subjects[26,37–40] and exempt from censures of boorishness, but not Bradshaw, who is of 'low birth' and 'the son of a shopkeeper.' He has jostled his way up to the top of the London social ladder and now charges outrageous fees, but he continues to resent patients who show any signs of being well educated.[36] Sir William is a snob with

> a natural respect for breeding and clothing. . . . There was in Sir William, who had never had time for reading, a grudge, deeply buried, against cultivated people who came into his room and intimated that doctors, whose profession is a constant strain upon all the highest faculties, are not educated men.[36]

On the other hand, Graham Greene's unnamed 'Herr Professor'[41] accepts his own ignorance as a fact of life and displays no hint of resentment. The professor, whose background is not revealed,

> had never been seen reading anything other than medical books. . . . Once questioned on Madame Bovary's poisoning, he had professed complete ignorance of the book, and another time he had shown himself to be equally ignorant of Ibsen's treatment of syphilis in 'Ghosts.'[41]

Joyce Carol Oates provides yet another example of a medical 'high-tech cave man.' The hero of *Wonderland*,[42–46] Dr Jesse Vogel, is a brilliant neurosurgeon whose perception of literature, if it ever existed, has completely atrophied. After an exceptionally traumatic childhood, Jesse works his way through medical school and, despite his financial problems, he graduates at the top of his class.[42] During his residency he makes such a favourable impression on Dr Roderick Perrault, the leading neurosurgeon of the town, that within a few years he is taken into partnership at the Perrault Clinic,[43] and when Perrault's health deteriorates, Vogel takes over the entire establishment.[44] This gifted, competent and ambitious man with his prodigious memory[46] is 'tone-deaf' when confronted with serious literature.[42]

> He was unable to follow a plot. He was unable to see the careful evolution of a story. The necessary pattern, the rhythm that demanded completion . . . what did all these things mean? He had not understood, though he had tried.[42]

Jesse's appreciation of the visual arts is even worse.

> What the hell did she see in these paintings? All this mess was a mockery of life, of the natural forms of life. Deterioration of vision. . . . 'All this is useless' he said. 'There is no value to it.'[45]

Even the names of the Impressionist painters are foreign to him. When, during the search for his runaway daughter (*see* pp. 46–7), Jesse finds himself in a painters' colony,[46] he meets an energetic old artist who has produced multiple pictures of a barn – 'different angles and lighting.' A young member of the group tries to explain:

> 'You know – Monet – The Haystacks – that sort of thing.' 'What?' 'Monet.' Jesse smiled in confusion. Money? 'Like The Haystacks and Water Lilies, playing around with different light' . . . Jesse could not pay any attention to all this.[46]

Andrew Miller's James Dyer, another brilliant surgeon,[47] has similar problems with literary appreciation: 'He reads no novels and the few plays he has seen . . . have made precious little sense to him.'

In general, contemporary authors of medical fiction imply that doctors lack culture, regardless of their background and their 'refined' or 'uncouth' behaviour (*see also* p. 147). Robin Cook's Dr Curt Mannerheim,[48] like Jesse Vogel[42–46] a prominent neurosurgeon, is portrayed as the foul-mouthed dictator of the operating room[48] who makes no pretence to gentility. Cook does not discuss Mannerheim's leisure pursuits, but the reader is left to assume that chamber music and literature are not among them.

Ignorance of non-medical subjects is not confined to leaders of the profession. Theodore Dreiser's hypocritical Dr Glenn 'was able to consider himself at least fairly learned . . . because of the ignorance and stupidity of so many of those around him.'[49] Dr Raste in *Riceyman Steps*, a general practitioner in a decaying London suburb[50] and 'a simpleton in regard to books',[51] behaves like an oaf when trying to buy 'a Shakspere.' When the bookseller asks whether he wants an illustrated version, the doctor responds 'I suppose it would be nice to have pictures to look at',[51] but finally settles for a non-illustrated edition, declaring that 'After all, Shakspere is for reading, isn't it?'[51] The book is a considerable success with the doctor's precocious daughter,[52] whereas the doctor himself seems to lack the time or the inclination to read even a single play in detail. He remarks during a subsequent visit to the bookshop: 'By the way, I've been reading that Shakspere. Very fine, very fine. I shall read it all one of these days.'[53]

Another functionally illiterate general practitioner, Francis Brett Young's Dr John Hammond,[54] represents a 'sad spectacle' at the age of 72.

> Apart from his work the old man had no interests. The sports of his youth had vanished along with it. There remained not one diversion from which he could extract even a vicarious pleasure. He could not read; for reading is a habit and habits are not to be acquired in the twilight of life.[54]

Other philistine physicians include Dr Milton Haggett in Howard's *The Late Christopher Bean*.[55] Haggett may be a competent and compassionate general practitioner but his 'notions of art belong to the lower animals.' This assessment of the doctor's art appreciation is originally formulated by Christopher Bean, the artist, who is also Haggett's patient. When, after Bean's death (of tuberculosis and alcoholism), the doctor finds himself in possession of one of the artist's paintings, he uses it to fix a leak in the roof of his hen house.

> I was looking round for something watertight and I found that picture. Fine thick oil paint . . . and there wasn't no reason to set much store by it.[55]

At the time of this artistic outrage, Bean's work is virtually unknown, but as Bean becomes famous over the next few years, the doctor's appreciation of art does not improve.[55]

Yet another physician who lacks creative ability and artistic imagination is Susan Cheever's oncologist, Dr Macklin Riley (*see* Volume 1, pp. 66–7 and 183). Riley does not possess any works of art he can vandalize, but he has visited the Frick Gallery where the Holbein paintings 'give him the creeps.'[56] Dr Chris Arden, Mary Roberts Rinehart's hero,[57] does not destroy or openly reject works of art, but his interest in the cultural activities of Vienna appears no greater than that of his wife, the unspeakable Catherine (*see* p. 14), who is bored by them and cannot wait to return to the USA.[58]

Updike's Dr Pennypacker[59] may be 'county-famous in his trade in a county where doctors were as high as the intellectual scale went', but he clearly demonstrates his inadequacies in both the professional and intellectual departments. His medical treatment of Clive Behn is manifestly inappropriate (*see* Volume 1, p. 156), while his achievements in the 'cultural' sphere also leave a great deal to be desired. 'The enlarged tinted photograph of a lake in the Canadian wilderness . . . which . . . covered one whole wall' of the waiting room denotes poor taste, the doctor does not seem to understand his patient's allusion to 'cobwebs in a Durer print', and the most important part of his annual fishing holiday evidently consists of the various freeways he navigates on his way from Pennsylvania to upstate New York.

> 'Once a year I pass through your territory', . . . Pennypacker droned on . . . 'Down the turnpike, up the New Jersey Pike, over the George Washington Bridge, up the Merritt, then up Route 7, all the way to Lake Champlain. To hunt the big bass. There's an experience for you.'[59]

In some hospital novels, the entire medical staff appears devoid of even the remotest sign of any 'civilized' pursuits. In Fearing's *The Hospital*,[60] the priestly Dr Gavin, now on his deathbed, can recall nothing other than his pioneering days in surgery and the instruments, now obsolete, that he has designed. Dr Thomas Kane[61] uses his spare time to go fishing and to dabble in share speculations (with catastrophic results). Significantly, the only well-read character in *The Hospital* is the laundry attendant, who draws a salary of 40 dollars a month.[62]

Shem's *The House of God*[63] contains a long list of medical boors. The 'Fat Man', a weird but competent physician, celebrates his free evenings by watching *The Wizard of Oz*, stuffing himself with 'blintzes' and salami, and indulging in perverted sexual fantasies about Dorothy and the Tin Man.[63] Dr Roy Basch, who appears to have derived no civilizing benefits from his Rhodes Scholarship, can think about only two topics – sex and his dislike of patients. Basch walks out of a performance of Handel's *Messiah* because the soprano sounds 'menstrual.'[64] Jo, a graduate of Radcliffe[65] and the Harvard Medical School,* the most ruthlessly competitive resident in 'The House of God', has

> dedicated her whole life to [medicine] and had little energy for anything else. . . . She's been in her apartment over a year and she still hasn't unpacked her stereo.[65]

Wayne Potts, a depressed and incompetent gentleman from South Carolina who goes on to kill himself, appears devoid of any non-medical skills even prior to his disintegration.[66] Only Chuck, the black intern who made it into medical school on the basis of affirmative action quotas,[67] excels at any extra-curricular activity. He is a talented basketball player.

Alfred Boone, Lucas Marsh's rich and cynical room-mate,[68] seems almost proud of his animosity towards 'artistic' pursuits, and openly flaunts his anti-intellectualism. He is particularly contemptuous of two 'arty' pathology technicians who have hung prints by Van Gogh, Pisarro and Sisley in their apartment, and whose paperback collection includes works by Sterne and Swift.[68,69]

> 'They're nice, nice people, couple of middle-aged girls trying desperately to substitute art and culture . . . for a home in the suburbs and . . . [intending] to take a trip to Europe once before they die like they always planned . . . when they were at Smith or Radcliffe or South Scrotum or wherever. . . . Since when did a doctor need culture?' 'Are you kidding?' 'I don't mean the wealthy ones, that suddenly go in for culture . . . I mean the run-of-the-mill doctor. The guy who probably hasn't read six books in his life . . . and music makes him nervous'. . . . 'I don't say what you say is true. But even if it is . . . what chance do [doctors] get to read? Or go to the opera? Or an art gallery?' 'They don't. And they haven't any natural bent toward those things. Their cultural background is zero. And you might as well face it, son. They know their trade – we hope – and without their medical knowledge, stripped of it, they're about where they were when they left high school. If there.'[69]

El Saadawi,[70] writing from an entirely different background, expresses almost identical sentiments.

> Why should medical students be interested in an art exhibition? What good was a painting or a story or a piece of music to them?

Medical students are not even interested in current affairs. Bahia Shaheen, the main character in *Two Women in One*, is quite unaware that there will be a transport

---

* *See* footnote on pp. 21–2.

strike in Cairo on a particular day, and she has no idea why the tram and bus drivers would want to stop work. 'Don't you live on this planet?' asks a student from another faculty. One of his friends comments: 'Medical students don't care about anything other than studying and memorizing their lectures. It's the law and arts students who know something about strikes.'[71] The old-fashioned medical education system is partly to blame: 'The dissecting room and the lectures, learnt by rote, parroted back in examinations and then forgotten for ever – nothing else mattered.'[70]

Ignorant medical husbands and their well-read wives

The cultural discrepancies involving ignorant doctors and their well-read wives, such as the educational gap between Dr and Mrs Kennicott[72] are discussed in Chapter 1 (pp. 31–2). Carol Kennicott tries desperately and unsuccessfully to interest her husband in drama and poetry. Dr Will Kennicott, whose hobbies include property speculation and hunting, remains completely impervious to his wife's cultural blandishments and declares: 'Gosh, I wish I could appreciate that highbrow art stuff . . . I guess I'm too old a dog to learn new tricks.'[72] Carol, a librarian, regards her husband, who is basically a decent character and a competent practitioner, as 'a dollar-chasing roughneck.'[73]

Cronin's Dr Andrew Manson (see p. 32),[74] one of the major medical heroes of twentieth-century fiction, is a meticulous and considerate physician. Until his temptation and fall, he pursues a constant fight against entrenched, self-satisfied bureaucrats wherever he finds them, and he longs for a position where he can practise 'scientific medicine.' This shining example of a medical graduate has never heard of Anthony Trollope until Christine, his schoolteacher wife, enlightens him.[75] At a dinner party attended by the Mansons and Professor Challis, a medical academic,

> the conversation . . . turned to music, to the qualities of Bach and then . . . to Russian literature. [Andrew] heard mentioned the names of Tolstoy, Tchekov (sic), Turgenev, Pushkin with his teeth on edge. Tripe, he raged to himself, all unimportant tripe. Who does this old beaver think he is? I'd like to see him tackle a tracheotomy. . . . He won't get far with his Pushkin there. Christine, however, was enjoying herself thoroughly. Andrew saw her smiling at Challis, heard her take part in the discussion. . . . And later, as Challis approvingly patted Christine on the hand, . . . [Andrew became jealous.] Can't old bird's-nest keep his paws to himself?[75]

Similarly, Dr Kevin Redden, a Belfast surgeon in Moore's *The Doctor's Wife* (see p. 33), suffers from cultural dwarfism when compared with his wife Sheila, who 'was fond of reading and the theatre. Redden . . . never opened a book.'[76] After Mrs Redden has run off with a postdoctoral fellow, Dr Redden wanders aimlessly around his empty house and briefly lingers in her room.

> This was . . . her sewing room, the room in which she paid household bills, read sometimes and did God knows what else he knew nothing

about. Floor to ceiling two walls of the room were books. . . . He went . . . to the shelves staring at book spines as though he might find hidden in them some proclamation of who she really was. Those large volumes on the bottom shelves had been her father's; sets of Shakespeare, Milton, Dryden, Pope; green and gold volumes of the works of George Bernard Shaw. There were some French books – Gide and Valéry and Anatole France and small books of poetry, mostly in French. And Hemingway and Saki and Joyce's *Ulysses*, which he remembered dipping into years ago as a dirty book. . . . Always stuck into books; poetry, plays and novels. A lot of rot. He remembered her chatting with Brian Boland about 'modern writers.' Rubbish. As if reading some bloody novels makes her better than me.[77]

Dr Redden's hate-filled musings continue in this vein for some time. He particularly resents his wife's lover's PhD in literature 'in James Joyce's laundry lists' or some such rubbish. 'Nattering away about Camus and Yeats and what have you, and she's so happy that she's not with me.'[77] (Sheila Redden leaves her literary lover within days, but she can no longer tolerate her anti-intellectual husband and does not return to him.)

Who is the better doctor?

When the medical performance of a versatile doctor is compared with that of an uncultured colleague, the verdict is generally in favour of the 'refined' individual, although at times neither of them is able to help the patient. Obviously, in an emergency, when a particular technique is called for, 'culture' is as irrelevant to the participating personnel as it is to a basketball player on the court. The difference becomes important when the doctor has to provide a long-term plan, explanations and reassurance.

Proust contrasts the 'illiterate' Dr Cottard (*see* p. 32 and pp. 143–4) with Dr du Boulbon, 'a superior man with a profound and inventive intellect',[78] who has the common sense to adjust treatment modalities to individual patients and a talent for coining felicitous expressions. It is Dr du Boulbon who is made to formulate the aphorism: 'If [non-organic illness] . . . is capable of deceiving the doctor, how should it fail to deceive the patient?'[78] Du Boulbon's talent for formulating medical observations and his appreciation of great literary works do not assist him in his medical practice. On the contrary, he is quite capable of keeping 'all his patients waiting until he had finished Bergotte's latest volume.'[79] In the end, neither the boorish Cottard nor the erudite du Boulbon are able to diagnose Marcel's grandmother, who dies within a few weeks of having been informed that she suffers from 'nervous weakness.'[78]

Hemingway[80] contrasts two seriously flawed emergency-room doctors – Doc Fischer, a Jewish abortionist and gambler with a veneer of 'culture', and Dr Wilcox, a stupid and aggressive 'gentile' who is ignorant and proud of it. Fischer affects 'a certain extravagance of speech' which impresses the storyteller as being 'of the utmost elegance.' He asks about 'news along the Rialto', and he refers to his fellow residents as 'confrères'. Despite the artificiality and superficiality of Fischer's conversational tricks, he shows at least some understanding of the 16-year-old boy who comes into the emergency room complaining of 'awful lust' and asking to be castrated. Fischer's colleague, Dr Wilcox, the classic and unrepentant boor, talks in expletives and tries to throw the young lad out. When the inevitable happens and the boy mutilates himself with a razor, Wilcox does not know how to deal with this emergency, which is not listed in 'The Young Doctor's Friend and Guide'[80] (*see also* Volume 1, pp. 155–6).

Wolfe, who presents a scenario of four medical men breakfasting together,[81] seems to regard literary sophistication as a distinct shortcoming in a doctor. The four doctors belong to different social and educational strata. Dr Hugh McGuire, a drunkard, and Dr Coker, the funeral director's friend, clearly regard themselves as tradesmen in the tradition of barbers and horse-gelders, who also act as blood-letters and surgeons. No boundary of professionalism or cultural attainments divides them from the local townspeople (*see also* Chapter 2, p. 63). Dr Jefferson Spaugh, originally from an Allegheny mountain town and 'brought up on salt pork and cornbread', has become gentrified with 'country club and University of Pennsylvania glossings.' Despite his foppishness, his social pretensions and his professional success ('he gets drunk with the best families'), Spaugh is as 'low and coarse' as the two older physicians.[81] By contrast, Dr Dick Ravenel, who comes from 'old money' and trained at Johns Hopkins,* looks and acts like a professional man. He has 'silver aristocratic hair', he owns the 'Ravenel Hospital' and he presents papers at surgical meetings. Dr McGuire, who calls Ravenel a 'literary sawbones', does not perceive his colleague's cultural achievements as an advantage.

> McGuire belched into the silence loudly . . . 'Literature, literature, Dick', he returned portentously, 'it's been the ruin of many a good surgeon. You read too much, Dick . . . you know too much. The letter killeth the spirit, you know. . . . I'm no scholar, Dick. I've never had your advantage. I'm a self-made butcher. I'm a carpenter, Dick. . . . I'm a diamond in the rough. . . . I'm a practical man.'

Ravenel, despite his Johns Hopkins background, his wide reading and his own sobriety, declines to operate on a woman with a large ovarian cyst, and tacitly admits that even in his inebriated state the unscholarly McGuire is the better surgeon of the two.[81]

Bellow's *Seize the Day*[82] contrasts the behaviour of two doctors towards an unfortunate young man, Tommy Wilhelm, who comes to them for help with his social and financial problems. One of the doctors (Dr Adler), Tommy's father (*see* p. 48), is a 'real' retired internist who has had a standard medical school education. The other ('Doctor' Tamkin) is a bogus physician whose 'training' is the result of a vivid imagination, eclectic reading and an ability to insinuate himself into the confidence of unsuspecting victims. Dr Adler, who now resides at a hotel on a permanent basis, is regarded by his fellow guests as a man with wide interests: 'You can discuss any subject with him.'[83] In fact, the doctor displays no such conversational powers. He talks about himself and about his children (as an extension of himself), he uses a few medical phrases such as 'respiratory center',[84] and he informs Tommy that one of his neighbours suffers from 'a bone condition, which is gradually breaking him up.'[85] He has become obsessed with his own health,[85] and spends his time being massaged and undergoing hydrotherapy. His conversation is cool, precise, laconic and uninteresting.[82–85] On the other hand, the bogus 'Doctor'

---

* *See* footnote on pp. 21–2.

Tamkin displays a wide range of interests. He is full of sensational case histories, he boasts about his inventions and his linguistic skills ('A friend of mine taught me [Greek] when I was in Cairo'[86]), and he analyzes the gyrations of the stock market using mathematical and psychological terminologies. Tamkin may not be a scholar, but he is certainly versatile.

Neither 'doctor' is capable of helping Tommy Wilhelm, the chronic loser. His father rejects him, while the 'versatile' Tamkin swindles him out of his last few dollars.

The three doctors in *Augustin, ou, Le maître est là*[87] represent a hierarchy of educational accomplishments. At the bottom is a general practitioner from Cantal who combines competence with vulgarity whenever he appears. During his first meeting with Professor Augustin Méridier, he discusses what he considers to be a suitable academic subject – the duration of university courses in different faculties.[88] Asked for some treatment to relieve the agony of a dying infant, he replies in pompous and meaningless medical-school jargon 'It's all in the physiological areas.'[89] The consultant physician from Clermont at least shows some insight. After ordering absolute rest for Augustin's mother, he declares 'Absolute statements are never true, but in this instance I want you to behave as if they were' ('Les opinions absolues ne sont jamais vrais, mais faites comme si elles l'étaient').[90] He apologizes for the pointlessness of his trip (which costs the Méridiers 1000 francs), but explains that in desperate cases an out-of-town consultant finds it hard to refuse to make the journey.[90] The third of Malègue's physicians, a Paris lung specialist, is a true scholar, despite some undesirable personality traits.[91] He has a vast knowledge of extra-curricular subjects, and although his literary talents have had to take second place in recent years, they are still discernible in his scientific articles, which are masterpieces of clarity. None of the three doctors make any impact on the sufferings of the Méridiers, who lose three out of four family members in the course of a year.[87]

Simenon[92] also presents two doctors who differ from each other not only in their approaches to the patient (*see* Volume 1, pp. 180–2), but also in their educational achievements. Professor Pierre Besson d'Argoulet,[93] a prominent Paris physician, is being

> considered as a candidate . . . for the Académie Francaise . . . on the strength of his three books on Flaubert, Zola and Maupassant. He was already a member of the Academy of Medicine.

His colleague, Professor Audoire, who in the Métro would have been indistinguishable from a minor clerk, is well versed in the literature of neurology but not in the writings of Zola and Flaubert. The patient recovers following the joint efforts of the two doctors, both of whom arouse considerable resentment. Besson's literary accomplishments are notable mainly for the year of Simenon's publication. By 1963, the species of professor of medicine who could write significant books on literary topics would have been almost extinct in English-speaking countries.

In Lilian Ross's story,[94] the versatile psychiatrist is also the better doctor. Unlike the thin-lipped, intense, dissatisfied and incompetent Dr Al Blauberman, his intelligent colleague Doctor Ben 'Sailboat' Selzer combines a successful practice with multiple hobbies. Selzer 'always looked relaxed and happy.' His name appears regularly 'in the indexes of leading psychiatric journals', he is a keen sailor, he knows 'a lot of sailing songs, which he sang in a near professional baritone voice' and he is 'a tremendous rumba dancer.' Al Blauberman's name never appears in the journals, and he is not invited to parties.

Scott Fitzgerald's well-known Dr Richard Diver,[95] educated at Yale, Johns Hopkins* and Vienna, Rhodes scholar and writer (or at least planner) of psychiatric texts,[96] is obviously an erudite and gracious person. Through his marriage into a stupendously wealthy family he is introduced to the multilingual atmosphere of the French Riviera of the 1920s and becomes a leading member of that world. However, despite or possibly because of his multiple interests (he is, among other things, a good carpenter[97] and, until his physical decline, an accomplished water skier[98]), he functions poorly as a clinician. Unlike his stodgy partner, Franz Gregorovious, with his burgeoning practice, Richard drifts away from psychiatry and towards alcoholism. At the end of the book, we find him incapable of functioning even in general practice.[99]

'Culture' as a disadvantage

Some authors display no ambivalence towards 'literary' physicians. Far from being objects of admiration, these 'versatile scholars' are treated as misfits, with colleagues and patients concluding (rightly or wrongly) that a fascination with literature or music or archaeology denotes a lack of involvement in clinical activities. A range of 'artsy-fartsy' pursuits may represent a sign or even a cause of marginalization, followed by a 'descent' into one of the subcultures, while a strong attachment to a particular non-medical field of endeavour may cause a doctor to relocate in another profession.[100]

Dr Long Ghost, the ship's surgeon aboard the 'Julia' in Melville's *Omoo*,[101] represents the typical marginalized doctor. He 'quotes Virgil and talks of Hobbs of Malmsbury, besides repeating poetry by the canto, especially Hudibras.'[115] The 'Long Doctor' may be intimate with literary works, but he has obviously been excreted from mainstream medicine, he has divested himself of whatever dignity he once possessed, and he now acts the part of a prankster more frequently than that of the physician.[101]

Dr Matthew O'Connor in *Nightwood* (see p. 221),[102] another brilliant talker, can lecture for hours on abstruse subjects such as the biblical text 'Watchman What of the Night?' O'Connor's interests include history and anthropology as well as religion, but his alcoholism and his gynaecological activities have cost him his licence to practise, and he has sufficient insight to appreciate that despite his erudition (or possibly because of it) he is now classified with 'the scorned and the ridiculous.'[103]

Richardson's Dr Richard Mahony[104] holds regular medical qualifications and is not quite as marginalized as Dr Long Ghost[101] and Dr Matthew O'Connor.[102–103] Mahony tries his hand at a number of hobbies, such as collecting butterflies, annotating the book of Genesis and practising spiritualism. He travels widely and he appreciates music and literature, but he lacks any kind of originality, and his ability to practise medicine declines even before he becomes mentally and physically ill.[104]

Similarly, Zola's Dr Pascal Rougon[106] is a man of wide-ranging interests, including marine biology, embryology, morbid anatomy, new forms of therapy

---

* *See* footnote on pp. 21–2.

and, above all, human genetics. Paradoxically his obsession with the idea of 'racial degeneration',[107] particularly as applied to his own family, does not prevent him from impregnating his niece.[108,109] Unfortunately, Doctor Pascal's acquaintances regard him as an eccentric, so when his banker absconds with his savings, leaving him destitute, his reputation as a 'half-cracked genius'[110] makes it impossible for him to resume the practice of medicine.

Weir Mitchell, who regards Dr Archer's wide interests[111] as a source of strength (*see* p. 157), uses a different scale of values for Dr Ezra Wendell, the chief medical character in *In War Time*,[112] whose multiple pastimes include 'poetry and nature.'[113] Far from regarding the doctor's non-medical activities as commendable, Weir Mitchell treats them as a failing (*see also* p. 212). Wendell, an effeminate medical failure, who

> should never have been a doctor[112] . . . did many things well [but none of his endeavors was pursued] with sufficient intensity of purpose or with such steadiness of effort as to win high success in any of them.[114]

His 'sensible' sister reprimands him: 'You will have to love your books and microscope and botany a little less and study human beings more.'[114]

Mitchell speculates that if Wendell could have found an academic post 'in some quiet college nook'[114] his multiple interests might have been advantageous. However, to a practising physician they are a positive hindrance: 'He was known among doctors as having contributed nothing to their journals save barren reports of cases.' Naturalists regard him 'as a clever amateur.'[115]

Dr Yury Zhivago[116] is more than a man with many talents. He writes outstanding poetry[117] and philosophical commentaries, though his unorthodox religious and political views land him in trouble with the communist authorities. Early in his career

> his interest in the physiology of sight was in keeping with other sides of his character – his creative gifts and his preoccupation with imagery in art and the logical structure of ideas.[118]

Had there been no war and no revolution, Zhivago might have become a competent or even great ophthalmologist, combining his literary and professional skills. Had he been a common medical hack, he might have been able to accommodate to the new regime. Instead, he spends several years of his life roaming about the ruins of the Russian empire and, after his return to Moscow, 'losing his skill as a doctor and writer.'[119]

Schnitzler's Dr Oskar Bernhardi,[120] an assistant physician at the Vienna Medical Institute headed by his father, has presumably been appointed on merit rather than on nepotistic grounds. The younger Bernhardi, a rather colourless figure, is a musician of sorts and has composed a new waltz ('Quick Pulses') for the hospital ball.[121] However, neither Bernhardi Junior with his Strauss imitations, nor the other characters in the play with their propensity to quote Latin tags,[122] seem as dedicated or as competent as the redneck Dr Kennicott[72,73] (*see* pp. 32 and 148).

Against the background of Seifert's McCord medical dynasty,[123] literary aspirations may become a veritable threat. The 'eminent McCords', who are pillars of society in a Midwestern city, live in the *Saturday Evening Post* opulence of the 1950s. The children address the older men in the family as 'sir', the new hospital addition is going to be called the 'McCord Tower' and the family is terrified of a newspaper scandal which might inform the public that all is not well in this genteel clan.[124] In such a setting, a rebellious young family member with a medical degree and an acquaintance with the writings of Nietzsche and Marx becomes a menace to the established order and an object of suspicion.

The doctor father in Bernhard's *Gargoyles*,[125] a country general practitioner in Austria after the Second World War, feels estranged from his medical colleagues, who constantly discuss their properties and their cars. Deprived of professional contacts (*see* p. 75), the doctor uses his free time to study Kant, Marx, Diderot and Nietzsche, borrowing the relevant books not from a colleague or a public library, but from another marginalized individual, a Jewish property developer.[126]

Saramago's unnamed ophthalmologist,[127] a kindly, somewhat mediocre doctor, is 'a man with a taste for literature and . . . a flair for coming up with the right quotation.'[128] He remembers scraps of the *Iliad*, especially the esteem that Homer expresses for physicians,[128] although in his own case such esteem is hardly justified. When the epidemic strikes and the ophthalmologist loses his sight, he is no more resourceful than the other blind patients who have not had the benefit of a classical or a medical education (*see* pp. 44 and 205).

Dr Whistler's literary erudition[129] fails to hide his sinister personality. Whistler, the surgeon in charge of a burns unit, 'had a degree in philosophy from Harvard and he made sure we knew it. On rounds he would decorate his remarks with literary quotations: Li Po or Shakespeare.'[129] Whistler is also familiar with Golding's *Lord of the Flies*, with the *Bhgavad Gita* and with many details pertaining to poisonous snakes of various habitats. Underneath his kindly, intelligent and well-educated exterior, Whistler is a freak. He actually enjoys cutting dead skin away from patients with third-degree burns.

> He loved the razor in his hand, the heat, the faint coppery smell of blood.
> . . . 'It's like slaughtering a hog', Dr Whistler said happily.[129]

Goethe's Doctor Faust, the epitome of a Renaissance scholar, initially functions quite successfully as a physician. His patients worship him, but he finds the theory and practice of medicine intellectually stifling,[130] and gives up his clinical work to devote himself to the 'pursuit of happiness' (*see also* pp. 190–1). Weir Mitchell's Dr Owen North[131] attends unending dinner parties where he and his scholarly friends discuss painters, poets, religious topics, military tactics and Arabian folk tales. Dr North occasionally mentions the fact that he is a member of the medical profession, but throughout most of the book he might as well have been a retired history professor.[131]

Moynihan[100] provides details of numerous historical physicians who leave the profession in pursuit of excellence in other occupations, some of them far removed from medicine. These 'truants' are an extraordinarily well-educated group, but at least one of them, Dr Thomas Young, is a little too versatile. Young, a linguist, a musician, a mathematician, an artist and an archaeologist, as well as a physician,[132] is regarded by his medical contemporaries as 'too engrossed in other pursuits.' Most of Moynihan's truants, by definition, feel cramped within the profession and therefore differ from their colleagues who continue to labour in the medical vineyard. During the nineteenth and early twentieth centuries, these versatile scholars provided an inspiration to writers of fictional works. In more recent times, a physician who is also an Egyptologist or an astronomer is likely to be regarded by his peers and his patients as an eccentric, and is unlikely to be portrayed favourably.

The doctor who 'goes in for culture'

Occasional medical characters try, with varying degrees of success, to overcome their educational deficiencies. They become literary name droppers or ritualistic attendees at symphony concerts, but in the process they make themselves faintly ridiculous. Bernard Shaw's Sir Ralph Bloomfield Bonnington[133] considers himself a literatus, and quotes various poetical works at appropriate and inappropriate moments. However, his knowledge of English literature is as superficial as his grasp of modern therapeutics, and after the death of Louis Dubedat in *The Doctor's Dilemma* he recites a grotesque Shakespearean fruit salad.[133]

Margaret Sargent in Mary McCarthy's *The Company She Keeps*[134] evaluates her psychiatrist's cultural activities with gentle malice. The doctor's visits to the theatre are seen as part of a facade and of no more significance than his annual pilgrimage to the seaside, or his wife's elegant clothes.

> You see about six plays a year. Your wife makes a list of the things that are really worthwhile, and you check them off one by one. You get the tickets well in advance and you generally take another couple with you. You never go on the spur of the moment; you never take standing room. Sometimes somebody in your party knows the girl who is playing the ingénue, and then you go backstage afterwards. You meet some of the actors and think it's a lot of fun. . . . You like the movies and you never miss one that the *New Yorker* recommends. . . . In the summer you commute to your mother-in-law's place at Larchmont or Riverside. There's a nice crowd of young doctors there and you kid each other about who is going into the water first. . . . Your wife has a three-quarter-length silver fox coat.[134]

Green's inventory of the extramural pursuits of Dr Harry Hemitz is less gentle.[135] Hemitz, the competent but deceitful surgeon in *The Last Angry Man*,[135] has managed to claw his way up from a Brooklyn tenement to a lucrative surgical practice. After publicly announcing his 'arrival' by purchasing an ostentatious mansion, Hemitz decides that he needs to 'improve himself.'[136] He hires an instructor to teach him painting, he learns to play the violin, he sets up a laboratory in his basement to study 'the effects of anesthetics on different generations of rats', he buys classical books by the set 'in tooled leather bindings' and he takes boxing lessons. Harry is a talented pupil, at least as far as boxing is concerned, but despite all his 'cultural', 'physical' and 'research' activities, he remains an ignorant dilettante who is considerably less conversant with humanistic values than his former mentor and subsequent victim, Dr Samuel Abelman, whose hobbies include gardening and the works of Henry David Thoreau. Hemitz's frenetic endeavours cause his premature demise.[137] He 'had to have the fastest, biggest . . . speedboat, . . . he smashed into a dock and the boat went up in flames.'

Likewise, the 'versatility' of Dr Kreck in Schneiderman's *Sea Nymphs by the Hour*[138] is that of a rich child amusing himself and becoming bored by a variety of expensive toys.

> Watson Kreck was Associate Clinical Professor of Neurology, a title granted him in exchange for three hours per week of neurological pyrotechnics on the wards of the Paradiso Veterans Administration

Hospital. Time was precious to Dr Kreck, and the three hours drove him to exhaustion, piled as they were on top of his bustling practice . . . and the supervision of his ranch, his schooner, his vineyards, his subdivisions, his ex-wives, his trips abroad, his soaring fortune in drug company securities and his collapsing golf game.[138]

The practising doctor as a civilized gentleman

In contrast to this negative image, several nineteenth-century works contain accounts of physicians whose outlook and behaviour have obviously been shaped by the humanist tradition and who are able to combine a liberal education and a variety of interests with the practice of good medicine. The saintly Dr Benassis in Balzac's *The Country Doctor*[139] is the very antithesis of the unidimensional specialist in the more recent literature. Benassis serves as the mayor of his village, he helps to reorganize agriculture and industry in the district, and he advises the local people on legal matters. His wide range of interests enables him to discuss religion, politics and economics in the light of facts and theories available at the time.

Kingsley's Dr Edward Thurnall,[140] the idealized and romanticized nineteenth-century physician, combines clinical ability with compassion for his patients and a familiarity with non-medical subjects.

> A purer or gentler soul never entered a sick room with patient wisdom in his brain and patient tenderness in his heart. [He was] beloved and trusted by rich and poor . . .

Despite his large and lucrative practice, Thurnall is also 'something of a geologist . . . a botanist and an antiquarian',[140] who uses a microscope to perform 'research' activities during his spare time.

Another 'civilized' medical man is described by Elizabeth Gaskell in *Wives and Daughters*.[141] Dr Robert Gibson has 'an unusually good library . . . for his station in life.'[141] Despite his busy country practice, he reads widely and is able to converse with or at least listen to 'the leaders of the scientific world . . . [who] valued his appreciation. . . . By and by he began to send contributions of his own to the more scientific of the medical journals.'[141] Unfortunately for Dr Gibson, apart from the occasional scientific guest at the Castle, his contact with 'intelligent and cultivated society' is limited, so that his intellectual activities are reduced to religious disputations with the local vicar, a kindly man with a very restricted intellect.

Professor Abraham Van Helsing[142] is another example of a nineteenth-century versatile medical scholar. Apart from his multiple clinical accomplishments (*see* p. 89) and his familiarity with obscure disorders,[143] he is a repository of knowledge about priestcraft and witchcraft. His powers of deduction equal those of Sherlock Holmes.

> He is a seemingly arbitrary man, but this is because he knows what he is talking about better than anyone else. He is a philosopher and a metaphysician and one of the most advanced scientists of his day; and he has, I believe, an absolutely open mind. This, with an iron nerve, a

temper of the ice-brook, an indomitable resolution . . . and the kindliest
and truest heart that beats . . . [143]

One major difference between the 'cultured' nineteenth-century doctor and his
contemporary 'boorish' counterpart is the social relationship between the medical
man and the community. The urbane physician of 1880 is frequently a family friend
who has seen the children grow up, who dines at his patients' homes on a regular
basis (*see* p. 62) and who takes a considerable interest in the non-medical affairs of
his charges. Such doctors, who see no conflict of interest between their roles as
friends and as medical advisers, have to display at least some flexibility in their
interests and topics of conversation.

The medical hero in Weir Mitchell's *Circumstance*, Dr Sydney Archer, clearly
belongs to the versatile category. His medical interests range from bullet wounds of
the chest[144] to the treatment of Parkinsonism.[145] His non-medical activities include
music and art, although he no longer has the time to draw and paint.

> If anyone now knew of his skill . . . with brush and pencil . . . it was when
> he lectured and the ready hand on the blackboard made clear to the eye
> what he was striving to teach.[146]

Archer watches helplessly as a devious adventuress, appropriately named Lucretia
Hunter, insinuates herself into the household of his friend and patient, John
Fairthorne. Mrs Hunter makes the old man turn his back on his family, and induces
him to leave her a large sum of money in his will. As part of the scheme, a more
tractable medical attendant is recruited to displace the straight-shooting but
troublesome Dr Archer.[147] Despite his dismissal, the doctor continues to discharge
his responsibilities as a family friend. He takes it upon himself to warn the deceitful
Mrs Hunter that if she goes too far, she will get nothing at all: 'If you are to have too
much, enough to injure others, I can easily show that Mr Fairthorne is now unfit to
mend or make a will.'[148] It is difficult to envisage a twentieth-century medical
technocrat voluntarily engaging in such a fight except as a reluctant witness in court.
Archer's personal involvement, on the other hand, is portrayed as a positive
characteristic.

Dr Peter Harding of 'Harley Street, London', a prosperous middle-aged English
physician of the Edwardian period[149] (*see also* pp. 40, 82, 112, and 174), may not
qualify as a scholar, but there can be no doubt about his versatility. At the outset,
Harding seems to belong to the boorish category, despite his gentlemanly veneer. He
is obviously a snob who, when visiting his teaching hospital on the eastern side of
London, holds his nose to block out 'the inexorable smell of . . . human
unwashedness.'[150] He compares railway stations on the fancy side of town, where
the 'sun-tanned country squire . . . [whose] luggage is of well-ripened leather . . . is
lavish with his tips',[151] with those on the unfashionable side, where passengers
smoke 'cheap cigarettes', where 'baggage [is tied] up with string . . . and dribbly
children' embark for trips to squalid seaside resorts. Harding leaves no doubt as to
the side with which he identifies. His recreations are those of the English upper class
of 1910, such as 'rugger' football,[152] golf[153] and trout-fishing,[154] while his circle of
friends (some of whom are also his patients) consists of titled ladies, professional
men, army colonels and members of the upper hierarchy of the Anglican church.[155]

Within these 'blimpish' limitations, Dr Harding displays considerable erudition
and a great deal of intellectual curiosity. Although his opinions on modern trends in

art and music are predictably reactionary, he is at least aware of what is happening. He refers to Impressionism as 'the Bedlamite echoes of Van Gogh . . . that . . . soil our walls in the name of progress.'[156] He detests the music and the librettos of Richard Strauss's operas, which he describes in terms such as 'obscene', 'decadent' and 'pathological', but he knows enough (or believes that he knows enough) about the subject to be critical.[156] He reads voraciously,[157] although he may miss essential parts of a novel's plot.[158] His views on sex education, while a little naive, are remarkably modern.[158]

Dr Stirling in Arnold Bennett's *The Old Wives' Tale*[159] also has a broad general knowledge. Stirling, a 35-year-old Scot practising in Stoke-on-Trent, is a man

> of broad sympathies who could discuss with equal ability the flavour of whisky or of a sermon, and he had more than sufficient tact never to discuss either whiskies or sermons in the wrong place. He had made a speech (responding for the learned professions) at the annual dinner of the Society for the Prosecution of Felons, and this speech (in which praise of red wine was rendered innocuous by the praise of books – his fine library was notorious) had classed him as a wit with the American Consul.[159]

Yet another versatile scholar is the medical dinner guest in Wells' *The Time Machine*,[160] a talented botanist who immediately recognizes that the time traveller has brought back with him an unknown species of 'gynaeceum.' This man also has sufficient awareness of mechanical engineering to appreciate the workmanship of the time-machine prototype,[160] and he obviously has a good grasp of history.

André Maurois' Dr O'Grady, a psychiatrist by profession, is able to function both as an army surgeon[161] and as an obstetrician.[162] O'Grady, a man of 'real artistic culture',[163] psychoanalyses historical personages such as Talleyrand[164] and displays a great deal of interest in sociological and economic problems[165] (*see* p. 113). O'Grady's opinions may not be original, and his psychiatric success stories seem somewhat superficial,[165] but he is undoubtedly familiar with non-medical scholarly works and he has an aversion to single-minded doctors such as Proust's Professor Cottard,[12] whom he mentions by name.[166]

Despite his *King's Row* background, Bellaman's Dr Parris Mitchell[167] turns into a genuine cosmopolitan character. He speaks several languages, he appreciates music and his interests include French cathedrals. The 'idlers around the courthouse' who constitute a kind of Greek chorus in *King's Row* (*see* p. 228) regard Mitchell, who studied in Vienna, as 'one of the finest doctors for crazy people there is in this part of the country.' A little doubt is expressed about the doctor's sanity.

> 'Some says you have to be a little crazy to understand the lunatics.' . . .
> 'Well, I've heard that a lot of them highly educated doctors is a little off.'
> 'Yes, I guess studying so hard does that.'[167]

However, the consensus emerges that Dr Mitchell, who in addition to his medical accomplishments has also made a great deal of money, is a 'smart fellow.'[167]

The species of multifaceted physician is still to be found towards the end of the twentieth century, although works describing such characters tend to be set in earlier time periods. Shreve's *Fortune's Rocks*,[168] published in 1999 but set at the turn of the nineteenth century, tells the story of Dr John Haskell who, despite his age, his devoted wife and his teenage children,[169] succumbs to the physical and intellectual charms of a 15-year-old girl. Dr Haskell is no common paedophile. He makes up for his deviant behaviour by his constancy towards the young girl, the two marry after his divorce from his first wife, and the marriage turns out a remarkably happy one.[168] Haskell possesses numerous talents in addition to his medical skills. He is a gifted writer[169] and a keen amateur photographer.[170] Most importantly, this Boston patrician has a well-developed social conscience. Together with some colleagues he documents the appalling state of health of the mill workers,[170] he actively campaigns to improve their 'living and working conditions',[169] and he ends up practising among the poor and the marginalized.

'Doctor' Iannis in *Captain Corelli's Mandolin* has received his medical education (if one can call it that) 'in the wardrooms of ships and from a popular medical encyclopedia.'[171] On the island of Cephalonia, where the patients pay their doctor with chickens, crayfish and aubergines, Iannis practises a primitive kind of medicine, extracting teeth, administering enemas and removing foreign bodies from ears.[172] Despite his lack of a formal education, Dr Iannis writes skilfully about local history,[171] and he becomes the natural leader when a crisis erupts.[173] His familiarity with island wildlife and veterinary medicine[171] enables him to treat a variety of animals, and he knows enough about politics to engage in debates with the local Communist (*see* p. 107).[174] Iannis, whose knowledge is not profound and who displays no evidence of originality in any of his multiple activities, may not be a scholar, but his versatility strikes the reader as more 'genuine' than the contrived activities of Dr Hemitz at the easel or on the violin[136] (*see* p. 155). Obviously, if a patient who required abdominal surgery was to be given a choice between Hemitz and Iannis, he would be safer in the hands of the half-educated but technically skilful Hemitz. However, if an operation were to prove unsuccessful, Iannis with his multiple skills would be more likely to provide comfort and consolation.

Patrick O'Brian's Dr Stephen Maturin,[175] another refined physician from the past, is a ship's doctor who has written a textbook on 'Diseases of Seamen.'[176] He is also a philosopher, an intelligence agent, an accomplished cellist[177] and a classical scholar.[178] He speaks fluent French.[179] Maturin knows all about the 'left-wing' political doctrines of the times ('equality, the perfectibility of human nature and the essential goodness of mankind'[180]) but, despite his Catholic background and his attitude towards 'empires and colonies',[179] he supports King George, whom he considers a lesser evil than Napoleon and the democratic Americans.[180]

Dr Juvenal Urbino in *Love in the Time of Cholera*,[181] whose very name suggests antiquity and urbanity, is another example of a well-educated cultured physician of the nineteenth century, even though at the time of his death (at the age of 81) the first three decades of the twentieth century have passed, and by the time the story is published his type has become virtually extinct. Urbino, who graduated in medicine from the University of Paris in the 1870s, is multilingual, an avid reader of 'novels and works of history',[182] a devotee of classical music[183] and an excellent chess player.[182] He is the founder and lifetime president of the local medical society. 'He organized the construction of the first aqueduct, the first sewer system, and the covered public market.'[184] His other achievements include the foundation of the School of Fine Arts and the restoration of the Drama Theatre. Urbino's frenetic cultural and civic activities are remarkable for their breadth rather than for their depth ('He does so many things . . . so that he will not have to think'[185]), but without doubt his achievements are legion.[184] Clinically the doctor is trapped in the time warp of his medical education and the even greater time warp of the decayed colonial South American city[186] where he was born, and where he practises for more than half a century (*see also* pp. 43–4, 80, 129–30).

Historically, the publication of *The Story of San Michele*[187] constitutes something of a watershed, bringing to an end the stereotype of the scholarly medical hero of nineteenth- and early twentieth-century literature. The type persists a little longer in Continental and South American literature,[93,118,163,182] and is still to be found among fictional psychiatrists,[26,37,40,188] but mainly in nostalgic accounts of physicians who practised in the past or who are relics of the past. Contemporary physicians, whether uncouth[48] or genteel,[123] alcoholic[21] or abstemious,[42] acquisitive[82] or generous,[189] share one common characteristic – they received their education in medical schools, and 'medical training does not make for conversational sweetness.'[190] Even the atypically thoughtful and tolerant Henry Perowne,[191] a contemporary neurosurgeon who takes an interest in architecture, ethics and music, has a blind spot when it comes to literature. When Henry's daughter and his father-in-law, both of them literary people, try to explain to him how a piece of poetry 'scans', all he can think about are MRI scans.[192]

'Culture' as a form of doctor–patient communication

Very occasionally, cultural experiences shared between doctor and patient provide a means for an exchange of ideas that might not otherwise have taken place. Proust's Professor E, who has fitted Marcel's grandmother into his busy schedule at short notice,[78] uses his familiarity with literature to put the patient at ease: 'Since he knew that my grandmother was a great reader and was himself one, he devoted the first few minutes to quoting various favourite passages of poetry appropriate to the glorious summer weather.' However, he then went on to perform a very thorough examination, repeated some of his quotations, and finally, when the patient was out of the room, pronounced sentence: 'Your grandmother is doomed.'[78]

William Carlos Williams' Mrs Yates,[193] a classics major from Cornell, is married to a man whose education is considerably inferior to her own. The marriage is remarkably happy, but Mrs Yates evidently requires intellectual stimulation from time to time. She and her physician have both read Plato, and she seems pleased when, while discussing religious rites for the dying, he mentions Socrates, who 'took the cup quietly without religion.'[193] Similarly, a crucial conversation between Walker Percy's Donna Stubbs and her psychiatrist, Dr Thomas More,[194] would not have been possible if both had not been conversant with Harper Lee's *To Kill A Mockingbird*.[195] Donna, who had been sexually abused by her father, declared to Dr More during one session

> 'You look . . . like . . . Atticus Finch who messed with Scout.* Wouldn't Scout love that?' 'Would she?' I asked her. She told me.[194]

Obviously, both doctor and patient have to be familiar with a particular work if it is to be employed as a means of communication. The technique fails when Bennet's Dr Stirling[159] mentions Zola's *Downfall* to Sophia Baines, one of his patients, and

---

* Apart from the fact that a motherless girl sits on her father's lap at the age of eight, there is no hint in Harper Lee's book[195] that 'Atticus messed with Scout.'[194]

obtains no response. Stirling is familiar with the history of France, the siege of Paris, the Commune and Zola's works. Sophia, who lived in Paris during the relevant period and speaks fluent French, has never read the book.[159] Communications based on literary works fail even more miserably when an educated patient finds that the doctor is not familiar with a crucial piece. Helen Ayling,[196] suffering from postnatal depression, is beside herself when she discovers that her supposedly well-read psychiatrist, Dr Dougald Argyle, has never even heard of *Finnegan's Wake*. She fears that all her literary allusions have fallen on deaf ears, she angrily accuses the doctor of deceiving her, and she asks him derisively in one of her lengthy letters whether he has heard of the author: 'Have you ever heard of a person called James Joyce? Or were you away the day he was in fashion, fighting a war to make the world safe for charlatans?'[197]

Summary

Authors of fiction, like medical educators, are divided about the extent to which doctors are or should be the recipients of a broad humanistic education. It is generally assumed that the doctor's extra-curricular pursuits, although not necessarily improving his medical skills, tend to make him a more interesting man. However, in developed countries the scholarly physician has been largely replaced by the competent technologist who may not be interested in poetry, history or music, but who is able to diagnose and treat his patients' diseases. Contemporary doctors who engage seriously in non-medical pursuits are likely to be marginalized from mainstream medicine.

References

1 Van Der Meersch M (1943) *Bodies and Souls* (translated by Wilkins E). William Kimber, London, 1953, p. 120.
2 Chandler R (1943) *The Lady in the Lake*. Vintage Books, New York, 1976, p. 21.
3 Green JP (1993) Physicians practicing other occupations, especially literature. *Mt Sinai J Med.* 60: 132–55.
4 Hippocrates (*c.* 400 BC) Aphorisms. In: *The Works of Hippocrates* (translated by Jones WHS). *Volume 4.* Loeb's Classical Library, Heinemann, London, 1943, p. 99.
5 Charon R, Banks JT, Connelly JE *et al.* (1995) Literature and medicine: contributions to clinical practice. *Ann Intern Med.* 122: 599–606.
6 Snow CP (1973) Human care. *JAMA.* 225: 617–21.
7 Little M (2001) Does reading poetry make you a better clinician? *Int Med J.* 31: 60–1.
8 Holmes OW (1871) The young practitioner. In: *The Works of Oliver Wendell Holmes. Volume 9. Medical essays 1842–1882.* Houghton Mifflin, Boston, MA, 1892, p. 384.
9 Holmes OW (1861) Elsie Venner. In: *The Works of Oliver Wendell Holmes. Volume 5.* Houghton Mifflin, Boston, MA, 1892, pp. 210–11.
10 Osler W (1903) The master-word in medicine. In: *Aequanimitas.* HK Lewis, London, 1920, pp. 365–88.
11 Norris CB (1969) *The Image of the Physician in Modern American Literature.* PhD Dissertation, University of Maryland, Baltimore, MD.
12 Proust M (1913–1922) *Remembrance of Things Past* (translated by Moncrieff CKS and Kilmartin T). *Volume 1.* Penguin, Harmondsworth, 1985, pp. 217–25.
13 Flaubert G (1857) *Madame Bovary* (translated by Steegmuller F). Modern Library, New York, 1982.

14 Chekhov AP (1887) The Enemies (also titled Two Tragedies, or Antagonists) (translated by Fen E). In: *Short Stories*. Folio Society, London, 1974, pp. 58–72.

15 Chekhov AP (1898) Doctor Startsev. In: *The Oxford Chekhov* (translated by Hingley R). *Volume 9*. Oxford University Press, London, 1975, pp. 51–66.

16 Chekhov AP (1900–1901) Three Sisters. In: *The Oxford Chekhov* (translated by Hingley R). *Volume 3*. Oxford University Press, London, 1964, pp. 74–7.

17 Dickens C (1837) *The Pickwick Papers*. Signet Classics, New American Library, New York, 1964, pp. 479–84.

18 Ibid., p. 583.

19 Flaubert G, op. cit., pp. 46–7.

20 Chekhov AP (1900–1901) Three Sisters. In: *The Oxford Chekhov* (translated by Hingley R). *Volume 3*. Oxford University Press, London, 1964, p. 113.

21 Chevallier G (1936) *Clochemerle* (translated by Godefroi J). Secker and Warburg, London, 1952, p. 58.

22 James H (1893) The Middle Years. In: *The New York Edition of Henry James. Volume 16*. Charles Scribner's Sons, New York, 1937, p. 87.

23 Maugham WS (1915) *Of Human Bondage*. Signet Classics, New York, 1991, p. 645.

24 Jewett SO (1884) *A Country Doctor*. Houghton Mifflin Company, Boston, MA, p. 94.

25 Ibid., p. 141.

26 Segal E (1988) *Doctors*. Bantam Books, New York, 1989, p. 387.

27 Busch F (1984) A History of Small Ideas. In: *Too Late American Boyhood Blues*. David R Godine, Boston, MA, pp. 150–70.

28 Balzac H de (1836) *The Atheist's Mass* (translated by Bell C). Dent, London, 1929, pp. 1–20.

29 Chekhov AP (1892) The Butterfly. In: *The Oxford Chekhov* (translated by Hingley R). *Volume 6*. Oxford University Press, London, 1971, pp. 61–82.

30 Wells HG (1909) *Tono Bungay*. Ernest Benn, London, 1926, p. 414.

31 Proust M, op. cit., p. 536.

32 Ibid., pp. 275–7.

33 Ibid., p. 467.

34 Lewis S (1924) *Arrowsmith*. Signet Books, New York, 1961, pp. 163–4.

35 Ibid., pp. 25–6.

36 Woolf V (1925) *Mrs Dalloway*. Zodiac Press, London, 1947, p. 108.

37 Barker P (1996) *The Ghost Road*. Viking, London.

38 Fitzgerald FS (1934) *Tender is the Night*. Penguin, Harmondsworth, 1998.

39 Bellaman H (1940) *King's Row*. Dymocks, Sydney, 1945.

40 Percy W (1987) *The Thanatos Syndrome*. Ivy Books, New York, 1988.

41 Greene G (1963) Dream of a Strange Land. In: *Collected Stories*. The Bodley Head and William Heinemann, London, 1972, pp. 281–97.

42 Oates JC (1971) *Wonderland*. Vanguard Press, New York, pp. 246–50.

43 Ibid., pp. 371–9.

44 Ibid., p. 432.

45 Ibid., pp. 327–8.

46 Ibid., p. 395.

47 Miller A (1997) *Ingenious Pain*. Harcourt Brace, New York, p. 175.

48 Cook R (1981) *Brain*. Pan Books, London, pp. 42–3.

49 Dreiser T (1925) *An American Tragedy*. Signet Classics, New York, 1964, p. 398.

50 Bennett A (1923) *Riceyman Steps*. Cassell, London, 1947.

51 Ibid., pp. 12–15.

52 Ibid., p. 185.

53 Ibid., p. 52.

54 Young FB (1928) *My Brother Jonathan*. Heinemann, London, p. 309.

55 Howard S (1932) The Late Christopher Bean. In: Warnock R (ed.) *Representative Modern Plays*. Scott Foresman and Company, Chicago, 1952, pp. 136–59.
56 Cheever S (1987) *Doctors and Women*. Methuen, London, 1988, p. 197.
57 Rinehart MR (1935) *The Doctor*. Farrar and Rinehart, New York.
58 Ibid., p. 277.
59 Updike J (1963) The Persistence of Desire. In: *Pigeon Feathers and Other Stories*. Andre Deutsch, London, pp. 12–26.
60 Fearing K (1939) *The Hospital*. Ballantine Books, New York, pp. 90–91.
61 Ibid., pp. 52–3.
62 Ibid., pp. 55–8.
63 Shem S (1978) *The House of God*. Richard Marek, New York, pp. 74–81.
64 Ibid., p. 209.
65 Ibid., pp. 91–8.
66 Ibid., p. 277.
67 Ibid., pp. 29–30.
68 Thompson M (1955) *Not as a Stranger*. Michael Joseph, London, pp. 141–2.
69 Ibid., pp. 189–92.
70 El Saadawi N (1975) *Two Women in One* (translated by Nusairi O and Gough J). El Saqi Books, London, 1985, p. 39.
71 Ibid., p. 80.
72 Lewis S (1920) *Main Street*. Harcourt, Brace and Company, New York, 1948, p. 120.
73 Ibid., p. 175.
74 Cronin AJ (1937) *The Citadel*. Gollancz, London.
75 Ibid., pp. 156–9.
76 Moore B (1976) *The Doctor's Wife*. Jonathan Cape, London, p. 145.
77 Ibid., p. 207.
78 Proust M (1913–1922) *Remembrance of Things Past* (translated by Moncrieff CKS and Kilmartin T). *Volume 2*. Penguin, Harmondsworth, 1985, pp. 311–28.
79 Proust M (1913–1922) *Remembrance of Things Past* (translated by Moncrieff CKS and Kilmartin T). *Volume 1*. Penguin, Harmondsworth, 1985, p. 102.
80 Hemingway E (1933) God Rest You Merry, Gentlemen. In: *The Complete Short Stories of Ernest Hemingway*. Scribner Paperback Edition, Simon and Schuster, New York, 1998, pp. 298–301.
81 Wolfe T (1929) *Look Homeward Angel*. Charles Scribner's Sons, New York, 1936, pp. 170–80.
82 Bellow S (1956) *Seize the Day*. Penguin, New York, 1998.
83 Ibid., p. 12.
84 Ibid., p. 34.
85 Ibid., pp. 42–4.
86 Ibid., pp. 61–9.
87 Malègue J (1932) *Augustin, ou, Le maître est là*. Volume 2. Spes, Paris, 1935.
88 Ibid., p. 120.
89 Ibid., p. 328.
90 Ibid., pp. 277–83.
91 Ibid., pp. 415–16.
92 Simenon G (1963) *The Patient* (translated by Stewart J). Hamish Hamilton, London.
93 Ibid., p. 45.
94 Ross L (1961) The ordeal of Dr Blauberman. *The New Yorker*. 13 May, p. 13.
95 Fitzgerald FS (1934) *Tender is the Night*. Penguin, Harmondsworth, 1998.
96 Ibid., pp. 129–30.
97 Ibid., p. 200.
98 Ibid., pp. 303–6.
99 Ibid., p. 338.

100 Moynihan BGA (Lord Moynihan) (1936) *Truants: the story of those who deserted medicine yet triumphed*. Cambridge University Press, Cambridge.
101 Melville H (1847) *Omoo*. Dent, London, 1907, pp. 9–10.
102 Barnes D (1936) *Nightwood*. Faber and Faber, London, 1985, pp. 115–55.
103 Ibid., pp. 223–32.
104 Richardson HH (1917–1929) *The Fortunes of Richard Mahony*. Penguin, Harmondsworth, 1990.
105 Ibid., pp. 160–64.
106 Zola E (1893) *Doctor Pascal* (translated by Kean V). Elek Books, London, 1957, pp. 30–31.
107 Ibid., p. 102.
108 Ibid., p. 144.
109 Ibid., p. 257.
110 Ibid., p. 198.
111 Mitchell SW (1901) *Circumstance*. Century Company, New York, 1902.
112 Mitchell SW (1885) *In War Time*. Century Company, New York, 1913, p. 63.
113 Ibid., p. 103.
114 Ibid., pp. 20–29.
115 Ibid., p. 198.
116 Pasternak B (1958) *Doctor Zhivago* (translated by Hayward M and Harari M). Pantheon, New York.
117 Ibid., pp. 523–58.
118 Ibid., p. 79.
119 Ibid., p. 465.
120 Schnitzler A (1912) *Professor Bernhardi* (translated by Landstone H). Faber and Gwyer, London, 1927.
121 Ibid., p. 23.
122 Ibid., p. 59.
123 Seifert E (1969) *Bachelor Doctor*. Collins, London, 1971.
124 Ibid., p. 17.
125 Bernhard T (1967) *Gargoyles* (translated by Winston R and Winston C). Alfred A Knopf, New York, 1970.
126 Ibid., pp. 21–2.
127 Saramago J (1995) *Blindness* (translated by Pontiero G). Harvill Press, London, 1997.
128 Ibid., pp. 21–8.
129 Huyler F (1999) Burn. In: *The Blood of Strangers*. University of California Press, Berkeley, CA, pp. 93–8.
130 Goethe JW (1808) *Faust. Part 1* (translated by Latham AG). Dent, London, 1928, p. 31.
131 Mitchell SW (1900) *Dr North and His Friends*. Century Company, New York.
132 Moynihan BGA (Lord Moynihan), op. cit., pp. 32–7.
133 Shaw GB (1906) The Doctor's Dilemma. In: *The Bodley Head Bernard Shaw: collected plays with their prefaces. Volume 3*. The Bodley Head, London, 1971, p. 423.
134 McCarthy M (1942) *The Company She Keeps*. Penguin, Harmondsworth, 1975, pp. 185–6.
135 Green G (1956) *The Last Angry Man*. Charles Scribner's Sons, New York.
136 Ibid., pp. 325–33.
137 Ibid., p. 344.
138 Schneiderman LJ (1972) *Sea Nymphs by the Hour*. Authors' Guild Backinprint.Com, Lincoln, NE, 2000, p. 55.
139 Balzac H de (1833) *The Country Doctor* (translated by Marriage E). Dent, London, 1923.
140 Kingsley C (1857) Two Years Ago. In: *The Works of Charles Kingsley. Volume 8*. Reprinted by Georg Olms, Hildesheim, Germany, 1969, pp. 18–19.

141 Gaskell EC (1864–1866) *Wives and Daughters*. Oxford University Press, Oxford, 1987, pp. 32–8.

142 Stoker B (1897) *Dracula*. Penguin, Harmondsworth, 1993.

143 Ibid., p. 147.

144 Mitchell SW (1901) *Circumstance*. Century Company, New York, 1902, pp. 278–93.

145 Ibid., p. 143.

146 Ibid., p. 53.

147 Ibid., p. 231.

148 Ibid., pp. 331–42.

149 Bashford HH (1911) *The Corner of Harley Street: being some familiar correspondence of Peter Harding MD*. Constable, London, 1913.

150 Ibid., p. 13.

151 Ibid., p. 18.

152 Ibid., p. 38.

153 Ibid., p. 57.

154 Ibid., p. 102.

155 Ibid., p. 217.

156 Ibid., pp. 49–51.

157 Ibid., pp. 219–23.

158 Ibid., p. 84.

159 Bennett A (1908) *The Old Wives' Tale*. Hodder and Stoughton, London, 1964, pp. 461–3.

160 Wells HG (1894–1895) The Time Machine. In: *Selected Short Stories*. Penguin, Harmondsworth, 1958, pp. 7–83.

161 Maurois A (1919–1921) *Colonel Bramble* (translated by Wake T). Jonathan Cape, London, 1937, p. 88.

162 Ibid., p. 213.

163 Ibid., p. 154.

164 Maurois A (1919–1950) *Les Silences du Colonel Bramble. Les discours et nouveaux discours du Docteur O'Grady*. Grasset, Paris, 1950, pp. 356–60.

165 Ibid., pp. 483–7.

166 Ibid., p. 35.

167 Bellaman H (1940) *King's Row*. Dymocks, Sydney, 1945, pp. 445–61.

168 Shreve A (1999) *Fortune's Rocks*. Abacus, London, 2000.

169 Ibid., pp. 15–21.

170 Ibid., pp. 42–56.

171 Bernières L de (1994) *Captain Corelli's Mandolin*. Vintage, London, 1998, pp. 119–22.

172 Ibid., pp. 1–5.

173 Ibid., p. 57.

174 Ibid., pp. 44–5.

175 O'Brian P (1992) *The Truelove*. WW Norton, New York.

176 Ibid., p. 56.

177 Ibid., pp. 14–17.

178 Ibid., p. 200.

179 Ibid., pp. 67–73.

180 Ibid., pp. 146–8.

181 Garcia Marquez G (1985) *Love in the Time of Cholera* (translated by Grossman E). Jonathan Cape, London, 1988.

182 Ibid., pp. 12–14.

183 Ibid., p. 40.

184 Ibid., p. 47.

185 Ibid., p. 196.

186 Ibid., pp. 110–11.

187 Munthe A (1929) *The Story of San Michele*. John Murray, London, 1950.

188 Winick C (1963) The psychiatrist in fiction. *J Nerv Ment Dis*. **136**: 43–57.

189 Lewis S (1920) *Main Street*. Harcourt Brace and Company, New York, 1948, pp. 176–9.

190 Slaughter F (1942) *That None Should Die*. Jarrolds, London, 1958, p. 7.

191 McEwan I (2005) *Saturday*. Jonathan Cape, London.

192 Ibid., pp. 199–200.

193 Williams WC (1932) Mind and Body. In: *The Doctor Stories*. New Directions, New York, 1984, pp. 6–7.

194 Percy W, op. cit., pp. 14–20.

195 Lee H (1960) *To Kill A Mockingbird*. Popular Library, New York, 1962, pp. 108–9.

196 Coombs M (1990) *The Best Man for This Sort of Thing*. Black Swan, Sydney.

197 Ibid., pp. 251–2.

CHAPTER 5

Frustration, boredom, burnout

Our vocations are likely to be badly chosen since few persons are fit to choose them for us and we are at the most unreasonable stage of life when we choose them for ourselves.[1]

There has to be more to life than merely saving lives.[2]

Fictional physicians, like their counterparts in real life, have to endure a variety of annoyances. These include excessive workloads (*see* Volume 1, p. 63–8), bureaucratic constraints,[3-5] inadequate remuneration (*see* Volume 1, p. 35–6), uncooperative colleagues (*see* p. 82), argumentative nurses (*see* Volume 4) and fear of litigation (*see* Volume 1, pp. 240–6). Except under conditions of extreme fatigue, most such frustrations are handled efficiently and with only temporary disturbances to the doctor's outward composure. Episodes involving 'exasperating' patients or the most recent mindlessness of a Health Maintenance Organization's cost-cutting exercise[4,5] may do no more than elicit expressions of mock regret ('Why did I ever become a doctor?'). Such minor irritations may even serve as amusing anecdotes for the entertainment of colleagues and family members.

A chronic inability to cope causes a small number of doctors, mostly general practitioners, to complain of boredom, especially after many years of practice. They express feelings of vague disillusionment and a sense of impotence in the face of death and suffering, hinting that they might have been happier in a branch of medicine other than the one they actually practise. Individuals afflicted by this syndrome tend to remain in medical practice because they have no other training, although some make drastic lifestyle changes in order to provide their colourless existence with some excitement. Total demotivation and a state of burnout may lead, as in real life,[6,7] to irrational behaviour, use of addictive drugs (*see* Chapter 6), early departure from practice, suicide and, in isolated instances, criminal acts.

Doctors who leave for reasons other than lack of job satisfaction

Not all doctors who leave the medical profession (in literature or in real life) have become disenchanted with their work. In countries such as Mexico[8] and Spain,[9] large numbers of medical doctors have been forced by economic circumstances to engage in non-medical activities. In countries where medical unemployment is not a problem, a few 'truants'[10] abandon their medical careers for what they consider to be more challenging activities, especially literary work.[11] During the 1960s the *New*

England Journal of Medicine published a series of biographical sketches about former physicians who deserted medical practice in order to take up posts as diplomats,[12] architects[13] or revolutionaries.[14] Such career changes are relatively rare in the real world, and when they occur in works of fiction they are almost invariably reviled. Medical graduation is regarded as a kind of ordination,[15] with the profession forming a priestly caste.

> Dr Raste would sometimes say with a dry, brief laugh 'we medicos', thereby proclaiming a caste, an order, a clan, separated by awful, invisible, impregnable barriers from the common remainder of mankind.[15]

The ordination is indelible – 'once a doctor always a doctor'[16] – and those physicians who 'step beyond the barriers', abandon the privileges and obligations inherent in their profession and join the laity become the counterparts of unfrocked priests, objects of pity and contempt.

One particular fictional doctor who abandons his career to become a writer is spectacularly unsuccessful in his new endeavours. This misguided character,[17] who should have stayed with his first trade, abandons his calling and impoverishes himself and his family in his futile attempts to become a serious writer. Somerset Maugham treats him with a great deal of disdain:

> Years ago . . . I knew a man who was a doctor, and not a bad one either, but he didn't practise. He spent years burrowing away in the library of the British Museum and, at long intervals, produced a huge pseudo-scientific, pseudo-philosophical book that nobody read and that he had to publish at his own expense. He wrote four or five of them before he died, and they were absolutely worthless.[17]

In the days when the status of doctors was lower than in the early twenty-first century,[18] a departure from the medical profession was almost essential for those wishing to move upwards on the social scale. When *Roderick Random*,[19] a competent ship's surgeon, unexpectedly comes into a sizeable fortune, he is instantly transformed into a Scottish estate owner and there is no further mention of any medical activity. Thackeray's Dr John Pendennis, who has become wealthy through parsimony and share speculations, sells his practice and proceeds to set himself up as a country squire.[20] He wants to forget that 'his hands had ever been dirtied by the compounding of odious pills or the preparation of filthy plasters' and, presumably, by even 'filthier' activities. 'It was now his shame as it formerly was his pride to be called doctor.'[20] Thackeray describes this career change without praise or blame.

Walter Scott, on the other hand, regards the exchange of medicine for careers in commerce or politics as a betrayal. In *The Surgeon's Daughter*,[21] Scott contrasts the decent, unimaginative but competent Adam Hartley, who is proud of his profession, with the scheming, selfish Richard Middlemas, who abandons medicine and instead chooses the career of an entrepreneur. In the process, Middlemas becomes entangled in Indian politics and comes to a very sticky end.[22]

Likewise, Henry James clearly disapproves of Dr Jackson Lemon, who has studied medicine at Harvard, Heidelberg and Vienna.[23] Lemon is about to marry into an English aristocratic family and has managed to convince his future father-in-law, Lord Canterville, that he is 'beastly rich.'[24] Canterville still harbours some old-fashioned prejudices and cannot understand why an independently wealthy individual like Dr Lemon would want to study medicine in the first place.

> 'What the deuce in that case possessed you to turn doctor?' 'Why, my simply having a talent for it.' 'Of course, I don't for a moment doubt your ability. But don't you,' his lordship asked, 'find it rather a bore?' 'I don't practice much. I'm rather ashamed to say that.'[24]

Lemon does not actively dislike medicine, but his aristocratic marital connections make it impracticable for him to work as a doctor. He drifts into a life of idleness and dissipation[25] while his former colleague, the symbolically named Dr Feeder, continues to work in medical research (*see also* pp. 12–13).

Francis Brett Young's Dr Harold Dakers,[26,27] a medical social climber, enters medical school mainly because his older brother (Jonathan) is a doctor. He gains his military rank by virtue of his medical qualification but, as he aspires to a career as an officer and a gentleman, he feels embarrassed by his profession and by his regimental badge, which indicates that he is 'only' an army doctor. Young does not inform his readers of Harold's post-war career, but it seems highly unlikely that this character who aspires to be a 'real' army officer will ever practise 'real' medicine.

Sinclair Lewis's *Arrowsmith*,[28] the story of a dedicated physician hero, also contains accounts of several doctors who are lured away from medicine by the temptations of money and political power. Dr Roscoe Geake, a professor of otolaryngology, comes to the conclusion that there are better ways of getting rich than by removing nasal septa (*see* Volume 1, pp. 164–5). Geake is 'called from his chair to the Vice Presidency of the . . . New Idea Medical Instrument and Furniture Company',[28] and when he delivers his farewell address to the students, his key message concerns the importance of modern office furniture. Dr Almus Pickerbaugh, another renegade, receives due recognition for his undoubted political talents when he is elected to Congress.[29] At least one of these apostates prospers in his new career, but Lewis leaves his readers in no doubt that individuals such as Geake and Pickerbaugh are to be held in profound contempt.

At the other end of the social spectrum we find the unemployable Dr Henry Wilbourne in Faulkner's *The Wild Palms*.[30] Like Jackson Lemon,[23–25] Wilbourne does not express an active dislike of medicine, but his lifestyle makes it almost impossible for him to practise. Wilbourne has completed 20 months of an internship programme in New Orleans when he is seduced by a married woman and elopes with her.[30] The two of them ultimately destroy each other, but for a year they live together in various parts of the USA, mostly in appalling squalor. Henry tries several times to obtain medical appointments, but he interviews badly and he remains unemployed for many months. Faulkner hints that Wilbourne's years of penury in medical school have 'castrated' him[30] so that he is now either unwilling or unable to practise as a 'proper' physician. At one point he even denies holding a medical degree.[30]

Minor irritations and frustrations

Patients who are classified by their physicians as 'uninteresting', 'unpleasant' or even 'repulsive'[31] are well represented in literature. Even the most dedicated doctor looks after occasional patients with whom he is unable to establish rapport, but few of these make him wish that he had entered a different profession, and when such sentiments are expressed, they are generally insincere.

In institutional settings, physicians come into conflict with administrators who see themselves as policy makers rather than facilitators. Such characters may decide to allocate a small room to the nursing staff for storage of Christmas decorations, rather than to a medical research fellow. Other frustrations include a lack of promotional opportunities. These and similar annoyances are likely to lead to a departure for another establishment rather than dissatisfaction with medicine as a career.

The patient with 'a little learning'

Semi-knowledgeable patients have irritated fictional doctors for at least 100 years. At the beginning of the twentieth century, when clinical thermometers became widely available, women who used these instruments to take their children's temperatures on a daily basis became a particular source of annoyance to doctors. 'Since the mamas have begun to keep thermometers, the doctor has no peace',[32] declares Weir Mitchell's Dr Archer in 1901.

Another offending appliance is the sphygmomanometer. As late as 1981 Dr Ethridge in Wharton's *Dad* is unable to suppress his irritation when he discovers that a patient's son (a man with a PhD in psychology) has acquired this apparatus and is using it to monitor his father's blood pressure[33] (*see* Volume 1, p. 197).

Even a self-assured and well-established physician may resent patients who consider themselves familiar with medicine and who imply that they are in possession of 'inside information', especially if that information is incorrect or superficial. Such patients may also attempt to chat about the doctor's colleagues, who are referred to by their first names and in disparaging terms (*see* p. 88). Doctors may feel and display irritation when a patient 'presumes' to use medical terminology in order to converse with them in their own language. An early example of that syndrome is provided by Michael Arlen's *The Green Hat*.[34] Iris Storm, Dr Conrad Masters' patient, has developed 'septic poisoning' in dubious circumstances, and one of her fashionable friends inquires 'I suppose this is the crisis, Masters?' The questioner's refusal to call him 'Doctor' and/or the question itself clearly annoy Dr Masters, who snorts:

> 'Crisis! The way you people talk of crisis this and crisis that! Hear a word once and stick to it through life. . . . There is no crisis in most of these infernal things. . . . The patient just continues ill, two, three, four weeks, might live, might not. . . . Crisis!'[34]

In the twenty-first century, physicians have to cope with 'clued-up' patients and family members who obtain their information from the Internet[35] and from self-help books. Dr Jay Reese[36] spends

> fifteen minutes . . . explaining to two very well-read but misinformed parents that their little girl's herpes simplex – she had a lipful of cold sores – did not necessarily mean she would come down with genital herpes.[36]

Dr Werner Ernst, the medical hero in Dooling's *Critical Care*,[37] has to interview patients' relatives who are filled to capacity with misinformation. While the occupant of Bed Five in the intensive-care unit has been lurching from one disaster to the next, his older daughter has been reading books on 'holistic' medicine.[37]

> Werner knew there was no arguing with family about the validity of the latest medical best-seller. Forget about practicing medicine according to studies published in reputable medical journals; those data had been contaminated by conspiracies of science in the medical establishment. Family wanted its doctor to be enlightened and to practice medicine according to the bibble-babble found in its self-help books.[37]

The poor and the simple

Medical practice among poor, dirty and ignorant patients does not appeal to all doctors (*see also* Volume 1, pp. 223–5). Dr Ezra Wendell in Weir Mitchell's *In War Time*,[38] a deeply flawed homosexual character (*see* pp. 212–13), is too fastidious to see indigent patients.

> The poor whom he had attended he did not like, because their houses were often uncleanly and their ways rough. Indeed he disliked all that belonged to poverty, as he disliked other unpleasant things. He saw this class of person knowing that he must, but made brief visits and found true interest impossible where his senses and taste were constantly in revolt.[38]

Retribution for Wendell's disdain for the poor and his other medical sins comes at the end of the novel when he is himself 'ill and penniless . . . much broken in health and spirit.'[39]

Similarly, Lloyd Douglas's Dr Hudson, who records his thoughts for the guidance of future doctors, has no wish to emulate Dr Albert Schweitzer, and openly expresses his dislike of 'unclean patients' despite his religious background.[40]

> Ailing indigence bathed and fumigated and in bed clad in a sterilized hospital gown was one thing. Sick poverty on its feet – with black fingernails, greasy clothes, a musty smell and a hang-dog air – was offensive to me . . . I made very little effort to disguise my aversion to the dull and dirty patient who grimly applied for . . . [the] benefits of the Free Clinic.[41]

The 'shiftless' poor also annoy Rinehart's Dr Noel Arden ('Chris'), at least early in his career.[42] He detests the indigent patients who attend his office, accompanied by hordes of undisciplined children whom they allow to 'range the place and slide down the banisters.' He resents the spending habits of one particular family who do not own a blanket to wrap up their new baby because they have recently spent all their savings on a new piano. Chris, who is conducting a home delivery, loses his temper.

> 'By God', he shouted at the husband, 'if I did the right thing I'd stick this child in that piano.' 'She wanted it', said the husband sullenly.[42]

Chris, who is adaptable and ultimately becomes a great surgeon, soon realizes the pointlessness of this kind of altercation. He learns to hold his nose and get on with the job: 'He was paid to attend to these people, not to reform them.'[42]

Dr Werner Ernst, whose problems with 'knowledgeable' individuals[37] are discussed on p. 171, also finds it difficult to interview ignorant family members, especially when the patients are not improving and the relatives are unwilling or unable to understand the information that is being conveyed. One of Werner's patients has developed a brainstem infarct after an aortic valve replacement.[43] The family consists of a wife,

> a squat, round, feeble woman with silver hair and a game leg . . . [and a] son, a beef-bellied old farmer in cowboy boots, Osh-Kosh overalls and a NAPA auto parts cap. Werner . . . had told these people a dozen times exactly what they did not want to hear.[44]

Similarly, Ravin's Dr Benjamin Abrams, despite his voluntary work at the Martin Luther King Jr Clinic in the Washington slums, expresses considerable misgivings about medical practice amongst the clientele of that establishment.[45] In medical school he had learned

> that you can be a drunken bum derelict, stinking to high heaven, but once you presented yourself to the door of the clinic, you were a patient and that was the highest status of all.[46]

In practice he finds that 'it's not fun taking care of people who don't know what their liver is, who want prescriptions, not diagnoses.' One clinic patient presents with a chief complaint of

> 'Don't feel good', and all subsequent answers were 'Dunno' or some variation thereof. . . . She was five feet tall, 210 pounds and she sat on the exam table looking sad . . . I examined her as well as 210 pounds will allow itself to be examined, getting no help from her. I told her she could get dressed and she said 'Can you gimme somethin'?' 'Something for what?' 'Well, sometimes I get this feeling', she said, pressing her temples with both hands. 'In your head?' I said eagerly, hoping she had . . . enough . . . neurons to complain of something I could call a headache. 'Well, sort of. What's good fo' that?' I wasted ten more minutes trying to drag a specific symptom out of her, but she didn't have the vocabulary for it.[46]

The demanding patient

Patients from the fancy side of town set off a different kind of exasperation in Dr Abrams.[47]

> Mr Hughes, a seventy-year-old former deputy director of some agency, now a consultant cum lobbyist [suffers from] . . . high blood pressure. . . . Every time I prescribed a new drug, he'd run right home and look it up in his Physicians Desk Reference and promptly be stricken by every adverse effect listed. Usually he'd start with impotence if that was listed. Mr Hughes feared impotence almost but not quite as much as he feared stroke, because he was a very hot item on the Washington over-sixties

scene ever since he'd retired from the government, divorced and become a consultant with an impressive office and a big desk he once described to me in soporific detail.[47]

Cost-conscious patients who have not been seen for years but do not want to pay for office visits leave annoying telephone messages asking for renewal of their anti-hypertensive prescriptions 'without the benefit of blood pressure measurement.'[48]

Mrs Simpson in Ravin's *Seven North*[49,50] is a classic example – a manipulative 'clinger' as seen from the doctor's point of view.

> Mrs Simpson was five feet tall and weighed two hundred pounds and wanted very badly to have a thyroid problem so I could give her pills and make the fat melt painlessly away. But she did not have a thyroid problem and the pounds did not melt, nor did they go painlessly.

Dr Benjamin Abrams takes on the care of Mrs Simpson at a time when he is starting up in practice and things are quiet in the office.

> I've since learned better about taking on patients like Mrs Simpson. . . . [She] was on an 800-calorie diet, hating every minute of it. She got light-headed, had abdominal pains, diarrhea, nausea, bad breath, hyperventi-lation and a hundred other things. . . . As soon as she noticed a new pain fiber firing off she had her husband call. Mrs Simpson never got on the phone [on these occasions]. . . . She was too sick to hold the phone and speak. She put her husband on and I'd have to ask her through him if she had any chest pain or whatever came into my head to ask her about, until I got tired and demanded that he put her on. The she'd come on with a weak little voice to let me know how close to the brink she was.[50]

Abrams, who has been trained to diagnose insulinomas, hyperparathyroidism and Addison's disease, evidently feels inadequate when interacting with the poor and ignorant, with the rich and educated, and particularly with patients who are looking for something other than the relief of symptoms and who would no doubt have angrily refused to see a psychiatrist. He expresses his frustration with the 'Mrs Simpsons' of this world to his secretary and his colleagues, but he has a sufficient number of diagnostically challenging patients for him to retain some of the enthusiasm he acquired during his residency days.[50]

Nourse's *Intern*[51] also has problems with a 'demanding' patient whom he dislikes on sight. He is called urgently to see

> a rich Americano woman who had flown up from Mexico City, sup-posedly in great pain. . . . Her chief complaint was that she hadn't been given a private room. . . . She was about forty and fat, with enough perfume on to fell an ox.

In addition, this patient complains bitterly that she has travelled 2000 miles to see the chief of surgery and does not wish to be examined by a young doctor (*see also* Volume 1, p. 60). This 'hateful' patient – who has kidney stones – 'raises antibodies' not only in the intern, who walks out on her, but also in the chief of surgery, who arrives the next day, spends 20 seconds with her and promptly refers her to a urologist.[51]

Dr Werner Ernst (*see* p. 171 and 172), who has difficulties coping with both 'well-informed'[37] and 'dense'[43] family members, also has to manage an aggressive business-type hot shot who is not only demanding but deliberately rude.[52] Bed Seven in the intensive-care unit is occupied by a desperately ill, elderly man who is almost certainly going to die.

> Bed Seven's son . . . never lost an opportunity to emphasize that his father was staying here only until he could be transferred to the Mayo Clinic. 'I am a businessman, Dr Resident' Bed Seven's son said, . . . 'and being a businessman . . . I am not accustomed to paying this kind of money without seeing some results. My concern is that we try the right approaches.' 'I'm so glad you are here,' Werner thought. 'Until I ran into you, I was all set to try the wrong approaches'. . . . [The businessman son] questioned Werner closely on the vasopressor dosage and the central venous pressure line readings. Werner gauged the fragility of the man's skull and eyed a fire extinguisher hanging on the wall.[52]

The 'uninteresting' patient

Scott Fitzgerald's interns,[53] who become frustrated when dealing with patients who complain of multiple symptoms but fail to display any objective signs ('cases who aren't cases'), are discussed in Volume 1 (p. 108). Dr Peter Harding, the 1910 internist in *The Corner of Harley Street*,[54] is irritated by 'one of those earnest cadaverous persons whose pride it is that they have never taken . . . a holiday in their lives.' The patient, presumably an obsessive-compulsive type, sees Harding at the request of his wife's doctor, although the reader is not told what precipitated such a consultation after 35 years without vacations. Dr Harding, who can think of no better alternative, prescribes a trip to Brighton, even though he is fully aware that this minor functionary who has no hobbies will not benefit from such an expedition and will return to London as soon as he can.[54] The doctor, who is used to dealing with more tangible disorders, finds this patient's vague symptoms annoying. Furthermore, he despises vulgar workaholics, especially as, during his passage into the upper strata of London society, he has 'learned . . . the art of lingering'[55] and now makes a fetish of regular vacations undisturbed by any hint of work.[56] Harding also dislikes chronic invalids whose entire lives rotate around their perceived ailments. 'Mrs Cholmondeley . . . over-fed and under-occupied, [who] cannot make up her mind between the rival hygienic attractions of Cannes and Torquay', wants the doctor to help her decide. He refuses to make a choice, arguing that the act of coming to a decision will be therapeutic for this woman.[57] In Faith Baldwin's *Medical Centre*,[58] wealthy patients suffering from 'imaginary' disorders bore Dr McDonald to such an extent that he changes careers.

Each of the two general practitioners in Pym's *A Few Green Leaves*[59,60] has an aversion to specific types of patient. The older of the two, Dr Luke Gellibrand, now in his late sixties,[59] is nostalgic for the good old days when patients walked rather than drove to his surgery. He likes to deal with births, deaths and 'real' illnesses, and he is intolerant of patients who suffer from what he considers 'trivial' complaints. Gellibrand loves 'the whole idea of life burgeoning', and particularly enjoys caring for pregnant women. He is therefore disappointed when his next patient turns out to be Adam Prince, a former Episcopalian minister with a dubious sexual orientation, who left his congregation to become a Catholic and a food critic.[60] Adam looks the very picture of health, fat and sleek as a well-living neutered cat. What could be his trouble, [Dr Gellibrand] thought irritably, as he greeted him in his usual genial way.

Adam's symptoms consist of insomnia and bouts of unreasonable fury when, on his professional visits to restaurants, he is offered less-than-perfect food. Gellibrand feels little sympathy for this patient, whom he considers a 'pompous bore.' He interrupts Prince's endless litany of complaints, recommends a greater tolerance towards tea bags and processed cheese, and prescribes 'a warm milky drink at bedtime' as a treatment for insomnia. In his 'bluff and hearty' voice he advises Adam not to worry, and dismisses him, hoping that the next patient will be 'more interesting and rewarding.'

In an adjacent office, the younger man, Dr Martin Shrubsole, has his share of frustrations. Shrubsole, whose interests include 'stress' and geriatrics, 'had been obliged to tell an elderly woman patient that her days were numbered, for in his usual frank way he had not shrunk from the truth.' Dr Shrubsole is completely unable to deal with the woman's next question. Does he believe in 'life after death?' He is embarrassed by this interrogation, and refers the patient to the Episcopalian minister.[59,60] Obviously, the interviews would have been less frustrating for all concerned if the two patients had exchanged doctors.

Therapeutic impotence

Physicians who are dedicated to the art of healing may feel frustrated when confronted by an entire series of patients whose problems do not readily lend themselves to treatment. Weir Mitchell's decisive and energetic Dr Sydney Archer, who normally enjoys his work, feels weary after one particularly unsatisfactory session at his 'out-clinic' when he is unable to exercise his therapeutic talents. That afternoon, he complains, he has seen 'just a series of cases of the poor, needing all kinds of things which no man can give, or else hopeless incurables.'[61] The theme of the physician's frustration by his inability to 'heal' social problems or advanced disease recurs many times in literature, particularly in the writings of Chekhov (*see* pp. 185–8), whose doctors use it to explain their discontent.[62] Paradoxically, one of Mitchell's 'bad' doctors, the 'plump and rosy' Dr Thomas Soper with his platitudes and his indecisiveness,[63] would have been better qualified to deal with these 'unsatisfactory' patients than Archer, the energetic interventionist.

Dr Luke Serocold,[64] who has no family and no friends (*see* pp. 8 and 77), feels depressed and frustrated on the morning of his 65th birthday (St Luke's Day, 18 October 1929*). He has been up late the previous night watching his partner die, and he now wonders whether the time has come for him to retire.[64]

'Why am I going on? What am I slaving for? . . . I could retire comfortably on my savings . . . and have a little peace and rest while I can. There's no reason to work myself to death.' Usually he enjoyed his morning's surgery hour, but today he felt depressed and out of humour, and was merely irritated by a violet-faced, dropsical old woman who

---

* The fact that the Great Depression began 10 days later is not mentioned, and seems irrelevant to the story.

wheezed and panted interminably over her tale of bronchitis and cardiac symptoms.[64]

Dr Serocold's self-doubts on this day encompass his shortcomings as well as the practice of medicine in 1929. He continues to ruminate:

> I wonder how much use I've been. . . . Half the time I'm just patching up the troubles [people have] caused by their own stupidity, and the other half of the time I'm groping in the dark . . . sending them to bed, telling them to keep warm, hoping they'll develop something I can diagnose . . . I'm a solitary, bad-tempered old blunderer.[64]

The 'distaste for his life's work'[65] lessens as the day goes on. He feels flattered when Martha Purefoy declares 'None of your old patients can bear to go to anyone but you.'[66] The Town Council supports Serocold's vaccination campaign.[67] His diagnosis of mastoiditis turns out to be correct,[68] and the old-fashioned chiselling operation is not complicated by major disasters. Best of all, 'the day that had begun with an old man's death . . . ended with the birth of a child.'[69] By the time he goes to bed, Dr Serocold is satisfied with his lot in life. He refers to himself as 'an old cart horse in harness'[70] with only a 'few intervals of dissatisfaction or regret.' Life 'hasn't been so dull as all that', muses the old doctor. 'I've had my compensations.'[70]

Dr Frank Gibbs in Wilder's *Our Town*[71] knows all about the unhappy drunken choirmaster who is not 'made for small town life', and who goes on to hang himself, but there is little the doctor can do, so he 'just leaves it alone.'[71] Dr Gibbs does not seem unduly bothered by his inability to heal.

On the other hand, Miksanek's unnamed doctor[72] becomes obsessed with the treatment of 'Mrs Galdinus', a chronic and voluble complainer who suffers from all kinds of ailments but considers herself unable to take any kind of medication. Conscientious but not well trained in the 'art of medicine', the doctor cannot accept that some patients derive a sense of satisfaction from their doctor's apparent helplessness, and he feels impelled to prescribe some drug for Mrs Galdinus' mild hypertension and her sore shoulder, despite her protestations. The inevitable adverse reaction[72] engenders a great deal of frustration in the doctor.

Unforeseen disasters

Unexpected failures, which may engender a sense of frustration in all professions and trades, produce special effects in doctors. An experienced surgeon may declare with mock envy 'I should have been a dermatologist' when one of his patients dies in the immediate post-operative period. Bulgakov's young doctor,[73] an inexperienced operator, becomes terrified during a surgical procedure for which he has not been trained. Fresh out of medical school, and with no resources except misplaced self-confidence, this man attempts to perform procedures which are beyond his expertise and which rapidly land him in deep trouble. He has never even seen a tracheostomy, but he is now trying to perform this operation on a 3-year-old girl, guided only by a textbook.[73] He encounters unexpected bleeding, and when he has finally managed to clamp the offending vein, 'there was no windpipe anywhere. . . . This wound of mine was quite unlike any illustration.' The doctor blames himself for even mentioning a tracheostomy.

> I needn't have offered to do the operation, and Lidka could have died
> quietly in the ward. As it is, she will die with her throat slit open and I
> can never prove she would have died anyway. . . . I bitterly regretted
> having studied medicine.[73]

The young doctor's bouts of self-reproach are of relatively brief duration. He seems
to enjoy the challenge of performing, for the first time in his life and without the
guidance of experienced colleagues, a variety of dangerous procedures such as
tracheotomies,[73] major amputations[74] and complex obstetric procedures.[75] Miraculously, the patients survive and Bulgakov's doctor is able to describe his chosen
career humorously and with some detachment. Unlike Chekhov's doctors (*see*
pp. 185–8), he has not yet become bored and disillusioned by having to practise
medicine among ignorant people, under primitive conditions and in total isolation.

A different kind of unexpected setback occurs when a doctor suddenly has to
inform a patient or a patient's family not only that the news is bad, but also that they
will have to discard an entire range of firmly held assumptions. When there is no
time to let the patient find this out for himself the doctor may fail miserably. In *A
Drink of Water*,[76] Fred MacCann has been involved in an explosion that blew off all
four of his limbs and destroyed both eyes. After some months of convalescence Fred
knows that he will not see again, but no one has told him that he has no arms or legs.

> One day he asked the doctor very carefully 'When are you going to untie
> me – let me get a little exercise?' There was a long silence and then the
> doctor said 'What you need now is rest . . . yes, rest . . .'. And then with a
> sudden and unexpected pathos, 'We are doing everything for you that we
> can.' [Fred wants more details.] 'How much are you going to cut off me?'
> The doctor was still silent. When he spoke it was with difficulty and all he
> said was something about rest and doing all they could for him. Fred
> MacCann heard the doctor's quick steps as he hurried from the room.[76]
> [A few days later Fred realizes that there is nothing left to cut.]

Obstruction by the bureaucracy

The tribulations inflicted on physicians by health maintenance organizations and
government agencies are described in detail in the contemporary medical literature.[2–5] A few particularly irksome restrictions have found their way into fiction. In
Solemn Oath,[77] the bureaucrats insist on a diagnosis *before* a test is ordered,
whereas in many cases the diagnosis can only be established *after* the test results
have been evaluated. 'Unnecessary' tests are denounced, but the Health Plans
provide no protection from litigation if omission of one of these tests results in a
missed diagnosis.

In *Fatal Cure*,[78] Dr Stephen Young, an obstetrician/gynaecologist who has
declined to sign on with 'Comprehensive Medical Vermont' and its aggressive
marketing schemes, now finds himself somewhat vulnerable because this Health
Maintenance Organization has 'snapped up' most of the local patients.

> 'The whole business has got me depressed', Steve said. 'If I could think of
> some way of supporting myself and my family, I'd leave medicine in the
> blink of an eye.'[78]

All doctors working in hospitals have to endure hospital administrators and hospital rules. Non-medical personnel such as nurses (*see* Volume 4) and laboratory technicians tend to enforce such rules more rigidly than physicians, so that tensions and frustrations become almost unavoidable. Francis Roe in *Doctors and Doctors' Wives*[79] tells the story of a typical doctor–nurse dispute over hospital regulations. A young man has been brought into the Emergency Room of a large New York hospital with a bullet wound in his abdomen. There is evidence of intra-abdominal bleeding and Dr Bob Wesley, the resident, decides to send the patient to the operating room immediately.[79] He asks Aster Hicks (the nursing supervisor) to arrange an urgent transfer, but then he hesitates.

> By the time the transportation people got themselves organized, [the patient] could be in deep trouble. 'No, let's take him up ourselves', he said. . . . 'We can't do that', said Aster. . . . 'we're nurses, not aides, and anyway it's against the regulations.' 'Oh for Christ's sake', said Bob, going to the door and opening it wide. 'Call the OR and tell them we're coming . . . and tell the blood bank to send up six units of whole blood directly to the OR. Or is that the secretary's job?'[79]

Bob is reported to the hospital authorities, but the patient, who has a ruptured spleen, survives.[79]

The work practices of the non-medical staff are a constant source of irritation to exhausted hospital doctors, who are incensed when they discover that not everyone shares their sense of urgency or their dedication. When Dr Martin Philips in *Brain*[80] telephones the hospital admissions department to find out whether a particular patient has been discharged or transferred, he has to wait interminably before his call is answered by a temporary receptionist, who then has to transfer him to someone else. After a further wait, that person turns out to handle only admissions, not transfers or discharges, so Philips is transferred again. Only then does he learn that the person he has to speak to is on a coffee break, so he hangs up, frustrated with bureaucracy, and grumbling 'Why didn't I become a plumber?'[80]

An exceptionally annoying episode in *The Intern Blues*[81] involves an infant's blood specimen, which is emptied down the sink by a laboratory technician because a medical student rather than a doctor has signed the request form.[81] The technician evidently lacks the time, the common sense and/or the inclination to telephone the intern and ask him to come to the laboratory and countersign the request. Much time is wasted over a futile altercation, while the baby, who has particularly difficult veins, has to undergo several further attempts at venepuncture before a fresh specimen is obtained.[81]

Sleep deprivation; patients as enemies; temporary loss of control

Hard work and long hours are generally taken for granted as part of a career in medicine. Indeed, among members of the medical community a capacity for endurance is usually perceived as a positive factor, while colleagues lacking that capacity are regarded as inferior (*see* Volume 1, pp. 66–7). Obviously there comes a point, especially in hospital settings, when chronic sleep deprivation becomes so debilitating that it interferes with the doctor's power to make rational decisions. Minor annoyances turn into catastrophes, which the doctor is unable to handle. He may lose his self-control and shout at patients or at patients' relatives. The gravity of this break-down in professional relations varies, but irretrievable damage is usually avoided.

Throughout *The Intern Blues*[80] the young doctors are so tired that they regard the patients as enemies, especially when their complaints are perceived as trivial. Similarly, in the very first paragraph of *Critical Care*[82] we meet a young resident (Dr Werner Ernst) who has just completed a night shift in the intensive-care unit and now has to work another 12-hour day: 'More than anything else, Werner wanted sleep.' Similarly, an exhausted resident in *The Prisoner*[83] becomes angry as a result of an entirely unimportant remark. A convicted murderer and drug addict has been transferred from jail to a public hospital, where he is dying from sepsis, apparently caused by dirty needles. The family, who presumably know something about the patient's criminal history,

> talked reverently of the good life he had led, how he had suffered, how it was time to let him go where he could rest in peace with the Lord. [This harmless lie infuriates the resident.] My anger was disproportionate but I was tired . . . of staying up all night with bleeding alcoholics, overdosing drug addicts, murderers and gang members, and I was tired of families who remade history for the convenience of personal loss. I was tired of giving my sleep and my thoughts to them.[83]

Arnold Bennett's Dr Raste, a general practitioner in a lower-middle-class suburb of London,[84] regards the relationship between himself and his patients as distinctly adversarial, especially at night.

> He regarded sick people and their relations in the mass as persons excessive in their fears, ruthless in their egotism and cruel in their demands upon himself. . . . To him a night-call was primarily a grievance and secondarily an occasion to save life and pacify pain.[84]

As a rule, Dr Raste keeps these 'forbidden' thoughts to himself,[85] and only on one occasion, when a 'recalcitrant' patient refuses to fit in with his special arrangements, does the doctor drop his habitual mask of inscrutability[86] (*see* Volume 1, p. 73 and pp. 153–4).

Eli Silver MD ('practice restricted to the treatment of infants and children'[87]), who has lost a son and whose wife has left him, is unable to deal with the day-to-day frustrations of running a practice.

> Back at his office the afternoon is itchy with bickering voices. Billie, his nurse, complains that the rolls of paper sheets for the examination tables are a week overdue. Maxine gives him a typed list of patients who haven't paid for six months and mutters about welfare clients in Cadillacs. A child's arm swells up immediately after her allergy shot, she begins to wheeze, Silver spikes her with Benadryl* to stop the reaction and her mother complains. . . . Two weeping parents carry in a . . . child with a broken arm and Silver bellows with rage that they should have gone to the hospital. . . . A tired father waiting for his infant to be given a DPT booster argues that the injured child was tended out of

---

* *See* footnote on p. 203.

turn. Silver tells him to find another doctor, and Billie takes the father into Silver's office for coffee and some calming down. 'This isn't practicing medicine', Silver snarls at Maxine. Billie, coming from his office, chants 'Oh yes it is, Doctor', and Maxine nods.[88]

Chronic boredom and disenchantment; geographical relocation

Physicians who have become bored by the apparently repetitive nature of their work complain about the monotony and uselessness of their daily activities, but they remain at their posts, using a variety of coping mechanisms that enable them to continue in practice. Charles Bovary,[89] a particularly limited character (*see* pp. 11 and 141) whose work is compared with that of 'a mill-horse who goes round and round with its eyes bandaged, not knowing what work it is grinding out', provides himself with some variety. At medical school he becomes so obsessed with domino games and other time-wasting pursuits that he fails his examination and has to repeat a year. In practice he diverts himself with an ill-considered excursion into surgery,[90] which turns into a disaster and contributes to his ultimate destruction.

A few bored physicians leave their profession temporarily and go a-roving in search of change or adventure, or both, but such characters tend to continue or resume some form of clinical practice when the opportunity presents itself, especially during crisis situations. Dr Thomas Thurnall in Charles Kingsley's *Two Years Ago*,[91] whose medical qualifications are listed as 'FRCS London, Paris and Glasgow'[92] (*sic*), has no wish to 'settle down in [an English] country practice',[93] and goes off intending to teach anatomy at some South American college.[93] He ends up prospecting for gold in Australia[94] and participating in a variety of adventures, but he never loses contact with medicine and 'doctors gunshot wounds' in various wars and revolutions.[92]

Robert Louis Stevenson's Dr Livesey[95] goes off on a treasure hunt as soon as he has found 'a physician to take charge of his practice.' Despite his itchy feet and itchy palms, Livesey retains his medical skills and, during a mutiny on board, he behaves like a true physician both towards the loyal members of the crew and towards the mutineers.

> He must have known that his life, among these treacherous demons, depended on a hair; and he rattled on to his patients as if he were paying an ordinary professional visit in a quiet English family. His manner, I suppose, reacted on the men; for they behaved to him as if nothing had occurred – as if he were still ship's doctor, and they still faithful hands before the mast.[96]

Another 'medical rolling stone' is described in Henry Handel Richardson's *The Fortunes of Richard Mahony*.[97] Dr Mahony, an Irishman with Scottish degrees (FRCS, MD, Edinburgh), migrates to Australia and keeps a store at Ballarat for a while.[98] At one stage he believes it is 'too late . . . to bemoan the fact that he had broken with his profession',[99] but as soon as the opportunity occurs he sets up as a medical practitioner.[100] Mahony, a restless and impulsive character, moves backwards and forwards between Australia and England, and retires from practice for a time in order to lead the life of a gentleman of leisure and devote himself to various dilettantish activities, including music[101] and spiritualism[102] (*see* p. 127). Towards the end of the story, financial troubles force Mahony to resume practice yet again, but he is no longer able to cope physically or intellectually (*see* pp. 209–10).

The intern in Albee's *The Death of Bessie Smith*[103] considers himself 'stranded' in the emergency ward of a 'second-rate hospital in . . . [a] second-rate state', and fantasizes about involving himself in more romantic activities. The option of remaining in the uncongenial environment of Memphis may not be available to this doctor. The nurse he lusts after detests both him and his liberal ideas, and threatens to denounce him to the hospital and city authorities as a dangerous radical.

Relocations from larger to smaller centres may be used in an attempt to relieve job dissatisfaction. Balzac's Drs Benassis[104] and Martener[105] leave Paris, with its iniquities and temptations, and go off to practise medicine in less polluted environments. Martin Arrowsmith, a researcher, resigns from a large institute in New York City to continue his activities in an isolated area of Vermont.[106] Cronin's Dr Andrew Manson[107] transfers his clinical endeavours from the corrupt atmosphere of London's Harley Street to a small town in the English Midlands.

Robert Herrick devotes two entire novels[108,109] to the peregrinations of medical doctors who find it impossible to practise 'pure' medicine in conventional medical centres where patients pay for their treatment. These dissatisfied idealists become hermits in the desert tradition of John the Baptist, dressing themselves in outlandish clothes and dispensing unorthodox remedies. They turn into fringe doctors, treating society's outcasts[109] as well as psychiatric patients who are not curable by conventional measures.[108] The two hermit doctors have somewhat different backgrounds. The Master of the Inn, whose name is never disclosed, opens his establishment after his fiancée leaves him to marry another doctor, who subsequently makes her unhappy. The recluse never emerges from his hideout, where he 'treats' a variety of patients by making them dig potatoes and swim in the local stream. He even 'cures' his old rival, Dr Norton, who stole his girlfriend, and now, 26 years later, finds that he can no longer operate. In the end, the establishment burns down, with the Master becoming a martyr and perishing in the fire.[108]

In *The Healer*,[110] Dr Frederic Holden has come to recognize the deep flaws inherent in

> the commercial methods of healing, . . . [which contaminate] the hospitals . . . and . . . private practice [with their] pretence and charlatanry . . . [with] the enormous fees charged, [and] the trickery of the trade.

During his 'revolt' against the medical establishment, Holden becomes physically ill and subsequently develops a drug addiction. He 'had gradually sunk into the muck of human degradation [but] . . . he had found the courage to flee back to the wilderness, there to fight his enemies alone, in silence.'[111] He acquires a family and wealthy friends,[112] but he manages to free himself from these entanglements and to return to his wilderness to practise 'true' medicine.[110]

A different desert destination awaits Straub's Dr Michael Poole,[113] who embarks on a medical career after fighting in Vietnam (and participating in a massacre). At the age of 42 he is going through a mid-life crisis. Thoroughly bored by his 'pampered, luxurious' suburban paediatric practice, where he comforts children 'who would never really have anything wrong with them', he leaves the suburbs but continues to practise medicine in a city slum.[114]

Less severely affected doctors express disappointment with their specialty and nostalgia for the career they might have chosen, but they stay on in their practices and continue to grind out what they see as repetitive work. CP Snow's Dr Charles March,[115] who comes from a wealthy family of bankers and stockbrokers, abandons his career as a successful trial lawyer. He studies medicine in his thirties and enters general practice because his ambition to be 'good' and 'useful' is evidently not being satisfied by court work. After some years in his second profession he finds family practice monotonous. However, he continues to work because he believes he is performing a valuable social function.

> Doctoring is tedious for nine hours out of every ten. Anyone who tells you it isn't either doesn't know what excitement is or suffers from an overdose of romantic imagination.[115]

March, who displays a good deal of intellectual arrogance, voices a second complaint about general practice as a career – his talents are underutilized.

> It doesn't give me anything hard to bite on mentally. I've got a taste for thinking, but I shouldn't be any worse a doctor if I were a much more stupid man. [The narrator inquires:] 'Charles, if you had your time again, would you make the same choice?' 'Without a doubt', he said. 'If I had my time again, I might not even take quite so long to make up my mind.'[115]

Another bored general practitioner, Dr Alan Beresford in *Doctor Jo*,[116] had as a young man harboured ambitions to become a neurosurgeon. He fails to obtain the appropriate training and he now resents the fact that he has no admitting rights at the local hospital. Moreover, most of his patients suffer from what he considers trivial complaints. After a brief and disturbing visit by his sister-in-law, a 'successful' tropical diseases doctor whom he has loved since their medical-school days (*see* pp. 15–16), Beresford continues to stagnate in his general practice. He stays married to his dependent wife and he expresses the hope that his 12-year-old son will succeed where he has failed.[116]

Dr Keith's frustrations[117] do not surface until the end of his life. In his final letter (*see also* p. 131), he confesses to his son that he has 'accomplished so little.' Keith, who has spent his working life in general practice on Long Island, ruminates on his deathbed that, in retrospect, he would have preferred a career in cancer research.[117]

Intending to become 'just a good small-town doctor',[118] Dr Bernard Dinteville is side-tracked into medico-historical researches (which are subsequently plagiarized by a senior academic) and devising new cookery recipes.[119] At the time we meet him he 'writes prescriptions with a look of complete indifference', and it is hinted that his patients are inadequately disrobed during physical examinations.[118] 'People don't like him much, thinking he lacks warmth, but they appreciate his efficiency and punctuality and stay with him.'[118] By this stage Dinteville has lost his hair as well as his enthusiasm, and we read with apprehension about his cut-throat razor, which resides on his washbasin next to a bottle of hair restorer.[120]

Dr Joe Derry in *The Healers*[121] is another doctor who remains in general practice even though he is not happy with the work. Unlike his brother Kevin, who has married a rich woman and is now busily climbing the academic and administrative ladders, Joe, whose wife is a policeman's daughter, finds his work tedious and poorly paid. He earns less in a day than his brother earns in an hour,[122] and he feels therapeutically useless.

> Listening to old guys with shortness of breath, neurotic kids, housewives with pains in the womb. All the cases that specialists don't want.[123]

He does not relish the thought of looking after this type of patient until he is ready to retire: 'My practice doesn't just bore me . . . it isn't going anywhere.'[123] However, when his brother Kevin's marriages disintegrate (see p. 35), Joe comes to realize that life in general practice has its rewards.[121]

Yet another disgruntled general practitioner manages to cope with his work through his ability to view the world as a kaleidoscope and through a 'vulgar talent for compassion.'[124] Dr Pincus Silver is acutely conscious of his almost complete impotence when it comes to making his patients 'well.'

> Among these people there were surprisingly few physical diseases. An old Sicilian had a cataract. An adolescent girl . . . who came in clinging to her aunt had a tiny cyst at the margin of the breast tissue. But the most ordinary complaints were headache, backache, sleeplessness, fatigue, obscure travelling pains. It was the old recurrent groan of life. It was the sound of nature turning on its hinge . . . everyone had a story to tell him. What resentments, what hatreds, what bitterness, how little good will! Wives and husbands despised one another, grandchildren were spiteful, the money went on liquor, the children were marrying haughty strangers, the daughter-in-law was a cold-hearted wretch, the fathers left home in the middle of the night. Bedlam, waste, misery – it was humanity seething in its old pot.[124]

Every once in a while Dr Silver speculates that the 'worthlessness of everything' represents a 'divine overwhelming exquisite beautiful irrationality',[124] but most of the time he is 'a GP in the sticks' and very aware of his personal and professional limitations.

Both doctors in Arthur Schnitzler's *Dr Graesler*[125–130] practise on the fringes of real medicine, both are apparently discontented, but both decide in the end to continue in their profession. Old Dr Frank says he intends to sell his sanatorium.

> 'The sooner I can get rid of the place', he said, 'the better pleased I shall be. I haven't many years to look forward to, and I should like to spend them as far away as possible from real or imaginary invalids. I have had to tell a hundred thousand lies during my professional career, and I'm sick of it.'[125]

Dr Frank's plans come to nothing. Instead, he decides to have his sanatorium refurbished and to continue running it.

Dr Emil Graesler, a rootless, indecisive character, has spent many years as a ship's doctor.[126] At the age of 47 he divides his time between two 'ridiculously little' health resorts[127] where he sees 'no cases of exceptional gravity.'[128] He makes half-hearted attempts to keep in contact with 'real' medicine, joining some old colleagues on their ward rounds and displaying an interest that 'was gratifying to himself at least.'[129] Graesler, who is independently wealthy, entertains thoughts of a long holiday. 'He might even give his practice up altogether. The thought alarmed him. He was incapable of living without his profession.'[130]

Kundera's *The Farewell Party*[131] revolves around the activities of Dr Skreta, a cheerful rogue who leads a very enjoyable existence, despite his lack of interest in general practice. Skreta thinks nothing of leaving a group of patients sitting in his waiting room while he takes his friends to a restaurant across the street. He enjoys music, he makes money under the nose of a Communist government and he performs illegal eugenic experiments that include the use of his own semen to impregnate unsuspecting patients. He shows no signs of relinquishing his medical practice, which endows him with a certain status in a small resort town.[132]

Burnout and disillusionment

The most severely affected physicians become totally disenchanted with their profession, and see no purpose in relieving the sufferings of the human race. They say with St Paul 'I do not do what I want but I do the very thing I hate',[133] they imply 'What's the use of it all?' and they either cease practising or perform as little medical work as possible. The reasons for the doctors' rupture with clinical work are not always clear. Some who have managed to soldier on despite chronic boredom, a sense of frustration at medicine's limitations or a loss of faith in their own abilities, are pushed over the brink by a particular event. Others realize, when it is too late, that they have chosen or have been made to choose the wrong career.[134]

Reluctant doctors

Crichton[135] clearly distinguishes between medical malcontents who continue to practise, and would-be drop-outs who detest their entire field of endeavour. He goes on to suggest that at least one member of the second group entered his medical studies unwillingly.

> Doctors are [dissatisfied] for various reasons. . . . Jones because he is hooked on research and can't make as much money as he'd like. Andrews because urology cost him his wife and a happy family life. Telser because he is surrounded in dermatology by patients whom he considers neurotic, not sick. If you talk to any of these men, the resentment shows itself sooner or later. But [Arthur Lee] is resentful against the medical profession itself.[135] . . . I suppose in any profession you meet men who despise themselves and their colleagues. But Art is an extreme example. It is almost as if he went into medicine . . . to make himself unhappy and angry and sad.

Crichton does not explain how Arthur Lee, a Chinese American, had come to be a doctor and then a gynaecologist, but he hints that Arthur had been expected by his family to enter university and to prepare himself for one of the professions. Arthur 'fought his upbringing, which was essentially conservative. He swung the other way, becoming radical and leftist.'[135]

Individuals who embark on a medical career under the duress of family pressures and expectations may develop the burnout syndrome while still in medical school. Vicki Baum's Fritz Rainer,[136] the son of a doctor father and a depressive mother, enters medical school at his father's behest. Dr Rainer, a general practitioner in a small German town, intends Fritz to take over his practice,[137] whereas the young man would much prefer a career in music. Unfortunately, the doctor suffers from stomach cancer so Fritz will have to be the breadwinner before long, and the music option is not open to him. Fritz is 'quiet, shy, [and] somewhat lifeless . . . a child of sorrow with whom things were always going wrong, who failed so often to meet the demands of study and of everyday life.'[138]

In addition, Fritz expresses some distinctly 'anti-medical' sentiments. He detests life, which he describes as a pit, a nightmare and a mistake.[139] Moreover 'he was clumsy . . . and even Horselmann, the attendant in the Anatomy Department, . . . realized that Fritz would never make a doctor.'[140]

Horselmann's predictions come true. Fritz Rainer cannot face life, and he kills himself with an overdose of morphine before he has completed his studies, abandoning his family whom he is supposed to support, and Helene, the girl whom he has made pregnant[141] and who plans to die with him, although at the last minute she changes her mind. If Fritz had survived this particular suicide attempt, he might well have killed himself during his internship. If he had made it as far as his father's practice, he would have joined the ranks of the disgruntled or impaired physicians.

Fifty years later, in a different country and from a completely different cultural background, Bahia Shaheen[142] is also driven into a medical career by her father, a minor public servant in the Egyptian Ministry of Health,[143] whose eyes, like those of other ambitious parents, gleamed 'at the mere mention of the word doctor.'[144] Bahia, an artistic, disturbed teenager who cannot even come to terms with her own sexuality, 'does not want to be a doctor',[143] and engages in activities that guarantee the early termination of her medical studies.[142]

Chekhov's doctors

Several scholarly papers[62,145,146] discuss Chekhov's doctors in detail. For the most part these characters are unmarried (*see* pp. 5–6) and poorly educated (*see* pp. 141–2) general practitioners, who have lost whatever youthful enthusiasm they once possessed,[147–153] and have become convinced that their capacity to benefit the local population is zero. 'What can they do when there isn't any food and when food is needed more than medicine?'[148]

Dr Andrew Yefimovich Ragin,[147] the undistinguished son of a distinguished surgeon, intends to enter the priesthood, but is forced to abandon that idea by his overbearing father (*see* pp. 106–7). As a result, Dr Ragin Junior has spent most of his working life in a filthy, dysfunctional provincial hospital infested by cockroaches, bed bugs and a lazy, corrupt staff: 'The entire hospital boasted only two scalpels and not a single thermometer.'[147] Dr Ragin, like several other physicians in Chekhov's stories and plays,[148,149,151] lacks the political skills to alter his medical environment. At first he

> worked very hard, seeing his patients daily . . . performing operations, attending confinements. . . . But in due course he has . . . become bored with the monotony and palpable futility of his job. He will see thirty patients today, and tomorrow, like as not, thirty-five will roll up, then forty on the next day, and so on. . . . But the town's mortality does not decline, the patients don't stop coming. To give serious help to forty out-patients between breakfast and lunch is a physical impossibility, and the

upshot can only be total fraudulence. . . . The crying need was for hygiene and ventilation instead of dirt, for healthy food instead of stinking sour cabbage stew, and for decent subordinates instead of crooks. . . . And then, why stop people dying if death is every man's normal regular end? Who cares if some huckster or bureaucrat survives an extra five or ten years? And then again, if one sees medicine's function as relieving pain with drugs, the question naturally arises why pain should be relieved. . . . Depressed by such considerations, Dr Ragin let things slide and ceased to attend hospital every day.[147] [When he does attend] he soon wearies of his patients' . . . muddled talk . . . and of his own questions which he has been asking for over twenty years without variations. So he leaves after seeing half a dozen people, and his assistant receives the rest after he has gone.

Ragin's assistant, who professes to be religious, copes much better under these primitive conditions. He contributes to Ragin's ultimate destruction and his admission to *Ward Number Six*.[147]

Unlike Dr Ragin, Dr Sable in Chekhov's *My Wife*[148] is still active in medical and communal affairs. However, his attitude towards his 'vocation' is very similar to that of Ragin. Sable,

a feeble, slovenly, unhappy creature with dreadful table manners, grew tipsy on three glasses . . . and . . . notified me that he had been separated from his wife for some time. 'It's ten years since I read anything. And as for things material, there are times when I can't afford tobacco.' 'But, you do have moral satisfaction' I said. 'Eh?' he asked, screwing up one eye. 'Oh, do let's have another drink.'[148]

Yet another of Chekhov's doctors, Dr Michael Astrov in *Uncle Vanya*[150] (*see* p. 5), exemplifies the transition from boredom to burnout. Astrov has been a general practitioner in a country town for 11 years. He still works hard, but he is beginning to show signs of frustration and disillusionment: 'On my feet from morning to night with never a moment's peace, and then lying under the bed-clothes at night afraid of being dragged out to a patient.' He resents having to deal with argumentative, non-compliant people. 'Please don't ask me to attend your father again', he remarks to Sonya Serebryakov, the daughter of a retired university professor. 'I tell him it's gout, he says it's rheumatism. I ask him to lie down and he sits up.' These are not Astrov's principal complaints. As the play progresses, it becomes clear that he has come to dislike medical practice altogether. He resents having to treat poor peasants who are 'uncivilized and live in filth.' He dislikes seeing educated people who are either too shallow or too intense for him. He has no friends, and towards the end of the play he is well on the way towards chronic alcoholism.[150]

Dr Ivan Chebutykin in *Three Sisters*[151] (*see also* pp. 5 and 142) is almost proud of his ignorance and his indifference. He declares 'I knew a thing or two twenty-five years ago', but he has not opened a medical textbook (or any other book) in years and 'it's all gone.' There are bouts of alcoholic remorse when a patient dies,[151] but in general Chebutykin has ceased to care. 'Nothing matters', he mutters just before the final curtain.

Even Dr Eugene Dorn in *The Seagull*[152] (*see also* pp. 5–6), who at the age of 55 can look back on an enjoyable and satisfying medical career, expresses regret at having chosen an 'earth-bound' profession, and nostalgia for a life as a creative artist: 'If I'd ever experienced the uplift that an artist feels when he's creating, I think I'd have scorned my material environment and all that goes with it and I'd have taken wing and soared away into the sky.'[152]

Chekhov's *The Enemies*[153] contains a unique account of a doctor's outburst of rage, and although we do not hear about his subsequent behaviour, the episode may well have driven him from the ranks of the disgruntled into those of the totally demotivated. The story was written at a time when doctors in provincial Russia were socially inferior to the wealthy landowners of the district and generally resentful of their own status, their powerlessness and their poverty (*see also* p. 141 and Volume 1, p. 42).

The encounter takes place at a particularly distressing moment in Dr Kirilov's life.[153] His only child has died of diphtheria a few minutes earlier, when Aboghin, the local squire, rings the doorbell in a highly agitated state claiming that his wife is dangerously ill and demanding Dr Kirilov's immediate attendance. The doctor demurs. Quite apart from his own and his wife's overwhelming grief, he is physically so exhausted after three sleepless nights that he considers himself incapable of any kind of medical activity. Aboghin pleads with the doctor.

> 'You are bereaved, I understand that, but I'm not asking you to treat a toothache. . . . I'm begging you to save a human life.' Kirilov stood there silent. After Aboghin had said a few more words about the high vocation of a physician, about self-sacrifice . . . the doctor asked morosely 'How far is it?' 'Just about thirteen or fourteen versts. I have excellent horses, Doctor. I give you my word that I'll convey you there and back within an hour. Just one hour.' These last few words produced a greater effect on the doctor than all the references to mankind and the vocation of a physician. He thought for a moment, then said 'All right, let's go.'

As soon as the two arrive at Aboghin's mansion they discover that the wife is not sick at all. Her 'seizure' was a trick intended to send her husband off for medical help, thereby giving her the opportunity to elope with her boyfriend. The doctor is full of hatred, despite Aboghin's genuine distress.

> 'My child's just died, my wife's in agony, quite alone in the house, I myself can hardly keep on my feet . . . and . . . I'm forced to take part in some vulgar comedy, to act as a sort of prop. . . . I don't want to know your vulgar secrets. . . . What have I in common with your romances?'

The doctor considers Aboghin's misery to be trivial, and compares it to the unhappiness of a capon 'burdened with superfluous fat'. And then the real reason for his resentment bursts out.

> 'I'm a physician and you regard physicians and all working people who don't smell of scent and prostitutes as inferior.' [The doctor refuses to accept any payment.] 'You don't pay a man for insulting him.'. . . [He] was . . . gazing at Aboghin with that deep, somewhat cynical and ugly contempt which is shown only by the unsuccessful and bereaved when they see before them elegance and repleteness.[153]

In other circumstances Dr Kirilov might well have behaved more professionally. He would have listened sympathetically to Aboghin 'revealing all his family secrets . . .

apparently even glad that these secrets had at last burst out from his breast.' Instead, the doctor's grief, his physical exhaustion and his perception that Aboghin suspected the real state of affairs all along make him act like a resentful employee confronted by his superior in a commercial establishment.

Céline's doctors

Exceptionally virulent medical self-hatred is expressed by the fictional doctors of Louis Ferdinand Céline,[154,155] who was himself trained as a physician. The medical history, the physical examination and even superficial human contact with patients seem to disgust Céline's doctors. 'Doctor Ferdinand' in *Death on the Installment Plan*[154] gives the impression that he has hated the practice of medicine since he first set foot in a hospital. He declares 'I've not always been a doctor . . . crummy trade.'[154] Almost all the patients, he states,

> ask such tedious questions. It's no use trying to hurry, you've got to explain everything in the prescription twenty times over. They get a kick out of making you talk, wearing you down. . . . They're not going to make any use of the wonderful advice you give them. But they're afraid you won't take trouble enough, and they keep at you to make sure. They want suction cups, X-rays, blood tests . . . they want you to feel them from top to toe . . . to measure everything, to take their blood pressure, the whole damn works.[154]

Ferdinand's activities at the clinic provoke not just boredom but positive disgust with sick people, particularly their secretory and excretory processes, regardless of whether these generate solid, liquid or gaseous material.

> I'm fed up with sick people; I've been patching up those pests all day, thirty of them . . . I was all in. Let them cough. Let them spit. Let their bones fall apart. . . . Let them bugger each other. Let them fly away with forty different gases in their guts! To hell with them.[154]

(Despite these sentiments, Ferdinand lets himself be persuaded to go out of his way to see a sick child.)

Ferdinand's cousin, Dr Gustin Sabayot, is equally cynical and disenchanted.

> Do you think they're sick? . . . They moan . . . they belch . . . they stagger . . . they fester . . . the trouble with those poor bastards isn't their health, what they need is something to do with themselves . . . they want you to entertain them, cheer them up, fascinate them with their belches . . . their farts . . . their aches and pains; they want you to find explanations . . . fevers . . . rumblings . . . new and intriguing ailments . . . they want you to get interested . . . that's what you've got your diplomas for. . . . They cling to their clap, their syphilis, their TB. They need them. And their oozing bladders, the fire in their rectums. . . . But if you knock yourself out, if you know how to keep them interested, they won't die until you get there. That's your reward.[154]

Céline's physicians, like the other characters in his works, divide themselves into two sets. Those who are totally disenchanted, have lost all sense of purpose, and are devoid of any hope for humanity. Members of a second group have retained a clear sense of purpose, but their intentions are evil and their efforts laughable. Both types are completely impotent in terms of making any positive impact on society or even on individual sufferers.

Dr Ferdinand Bardamu, the main character in *Journey to the End of the Night*,[155] initially appears as a cynical medical student who joins the army at the beginning of the First World War, and then drifts around Africa and the USA before resuming his studies. Bardamu graduates and actually sets up in practice,[156] but his disenchantment with medicine ('plenty of jars and very little jam'[156]) is so overwhelming and his contempt for the entire human race so corrosive that he finds it impossible to practise 'normally.' He allows a girl to bleed to death after a bungled abortion because he lacks the energy to stop the girl's mother bleating histrionically about the honour of the family.[157] He becomes a mere spectator after his friend Robinson is shot in the abdomen by a disappointed girlfriend.[158] Bardamu wants to run away from the police inquiry, but turns up in the end. 'Did you get lost, doctor?' a police secretary asks symbolically.[159] To Bardamu, medical practice is no more satisfying than a walk-on part in a musical play.[160] In each case he is a silent bystander and voyeur.

Dr Baryton, also in *Journey to the End of the Night*,[155] starts off purposefully enough. Despite his 'instinctive antipathy' towards mental patients[161] and his dislike of their 'demanding' families, 'always insisting on newer and newer methods of treatment, more electrical, more mysterious, more everything',[162] he runs a financially successful private mental hospital. He is sufficiently interested in the theory of mental illness to fulminate against 'the prurient . . . minions of modern psychiatry.'[163] However, Baryton gradually moves from the ranks of the purposeful to those of the purposeless. He begins to identify with failure, 'no longer knowing what he pretends.'[164] He would be 'glad to go away but no longer knows whither or how to escape.' Baryton leaves his hospital and, like his mentor Bardamu, he becomes a drifter.[164]

Gradual alienation or defining event?

In a few instances a traumatic episode is perceived to put a previously functioning doctor out of action, although more often the burnout process is gradual and no precipitating events can be identified. The majority of disenchanted doctors appear as fully developed cynics, with little or no indication of how they turned out that way.

'Doctor' Sinuhe[165] practises around three millennia earlier than Céline's characters, but his sentiments are very similar to those expressed by Dr Ferdinand Bardamu.[155] Sinuhe, who is diverted from a military into a medical career, enjoys a meteoric rise in the profession[165] and, through his position at court and his readiness to kill a patient, he is able to assist in the suppression of a 'communist' revolution.[166] Sinuhe evidently imbibes some of the new ideas and becomes disenchanted both with the ensuing reactionary governments and with his own activities as a physician.

> I shut myself in my house and received no patients save for a neighbour now and again and the very poor who had no presents to give the regular physicians. I had another pool dug in the courtyard and filled it with

> coloured fish, and I sat all day beside it . . . [gazing] at the fish that swam
> lazily about in the cool water.[167]

In his idleness, Sinuhe even conceives an urge to re-introduce the same revolutionary system that almost caused the total destruction of Egypt. He disguises himself as a member of the 'working classes' and becomes an agitator.

> I dressed myself secretly in the coarse garment of the poor. . . . I went to
> the quays and bore heavy burdens among the porters until my back hurt
> and my shoulders were crooked. I went to the vegetable market and
> gathered its trampled refuse for my food. . . . I did the work of slaves and
> porters; I ate their bread and drank their beer.[167]

Having assumed the garb of poverty, Sinuhe becomes a preacher. His message is obviously seditious: 'There is no difference between one man and another, for all are born naked into the world. A man cannot be measured by the colour of his skin or by his speech or by his clothes and jewels, but only by his heart.' When Sinuhe and his message are received with suspicion and hostility by rich and poor alike, he returns home, 'perceiving that all my labour was in vain', and resumes the practice of medicine. His profession brings him no satisfaction, and he becomes a 'wearisome, bitter man' living 'in continual discontent, [finding] fault with everyone.'[167]

One of the best-known fictional doctors of all time, Lemuel Gulliver,[168] chooses a career in medicine as a means to an end – he wants to travel. After serving a medical apprenticeship and graduating in medicine from the University of Leyden, Gulliver sets up in practice, but 'business' does not prosper and he accepts various posts as a ship's surgeon.[168] By the time he sets out on his fourth major voyage, he has 'grown weary of a surgeon's employment at sea',[169] and on this occasion he starts out as the captain of a 'stout merchant man.' Gulliver's career as a ship's captain is short-lived. He is incapable of selecting or controlling his crew,[169] and after a shipboard mutiny the rebellious sailors put him ashore and leave him marooned in the country of the Yahoos.[169] Gulliver does not resume the practice of medicine after his return to England. On the contrary, he develops a violent dislike of the entire homo sapiens species, particularly those of its members suffering from 'diseases in body and mind'[170] and, like Doctor Dolittle 200 years later,[171] he feels more comfortable in the presence of animals than with humans.

Lofting's Dr John Dolittle,[171] who holds a doctorate in medicine, gives up treating human patients in order to become an animal doctor. All of the Dolittle stories revolve around the notion that animal patients are individuals with their own personalities, and that there are greater rewards in treating these simple folk than in looking after demanding and depraved members of the human race.[171]

Goethe's Faust, a physician and the son of a physician,[172] had been devoted to his patients in his younger days (*see* p. 154).

> And you yourself, a young man then, in every stricken house were found
> and corpse on corpse was carried forth but you came out aye safe and
> sound.[172]

Despite the villagers' adulation, Faust becomes disenchanted with medicine and with his own helplessness. Even though 'conscientiously and in punctilious wise, the art he practice[d] taught him by tradition, . . . the patients still expired.'[172] Although Faust's motives are obviously more complex than a mere lack of satisfaction with his therapeutic efforts, he certainly becomes a medical 'drop-out', and by the time the play opens, he is in the process of selling himself to the devil in the hope of finding the happiness and power that he was unable to achieve as a practising physician.[172]

The reasons for Dr Joseph Womack's gradual disillusionment with his chosen career[173] are not readily apparent. Womack, a junior resident in neurology at a San Francisco city hospital, and hero of Hejinian's *Extreme Remedies*,[173] has decided before his thirtieth birthday that he can no longer handle his work. He talks about quitting and 'applying for a job in a slaughterhouse',[174] though he may not have to bother. By the time he is halfway through his first year of residency, his chief has come to regard him as emotionally unstable,[175] and while Womack is still on the hospital payroll when the book ends, the reader senses that his appointment will not be renewed. What went wrong?

Womack's privileged background is no different from that of thousands of other medical students. His reasons for choosing a medical career are no better and no worse than those expressed by many other medical school applicants:

> A colonial home in the shady suburbs of Connecticut, tennis, sailing, debutante parties, sports cars, the best prep schools, the Ivy League, culture. . . . He believed in goals, in the future. . . . Perhaps he wanted to help people. Perhaps he wanted prestige, respect, money. Perhaps he was only living out his father's wishes. [His father is a successful insurance salesman.] So he worked hard for the future, shunning the delights of the present.

The mechanism of Womack's decline from an optimistic believer in 'the future' to a discontented and finally disgusted resident is not made clear. In college he hates organic chemistry and physics, 'but of course he got his A's and told himself that medical school would be better.' He hates the first two years of medical school – 'so many drab facts' –but he hopes for better things once he starts clinical work. Most doctors learn to cope with the vicissitudes of medical school, internship and residency, but these prove too difficult for Dr Womack. Thirty-six-hour shifts, terminal patients, neurosurgical disasters, poor city hospital facilities and the appalling social situation of the inner-city poor all overwhelm Womack.[174,175] He envies those of his colleagues who have become emotionally detached and/or genuinely interested in research, but he is unable to emulate them.

In Dr Ralph Anderson's case[176] there is a crucial event: an unexpected disaster during the First World War. Anderson, a surgeon, copes with 'ten amputations a day', but suffers a 'nervous breakdown' when he misses a major arterial tear and a patient suddenly bleeds to death ('it pumped out of him') in his presence. He develops nightmares, a morbid fear of blood[177] and a distaste for medical practice, even though he has no other income and may have to settle for an unglamorous desk job in public health.[176]

A sudden, unexpected death also reshapes the career of Dr Hugh Franciscus, Selzer's ferocious chief of plastic surgery.[178] Franciscus regularly travels to one of the banana republics in Central America, where he performs operations on pre-selected patients. On this occasion, he is scheduled to repair the cleft lip of Imelda, a 14-year-old girl, but he has to watch helplessly as the child dies of malignant hyperthermia before he can make his first incision. After this disaster and the subsequent dramatic events in the mortuary, Dr Franciscus becomes an altered man.

> [He] operated a good deal less, then gave it up entirely. It was as though he had grown tired of blood, of always having to be involved with blood, of having to draw it, spill it, wipe it away, stanch it. . . . There were no more expeditions to Honduras or elsewhere.[178]

In the case of Dr Mara Fox, the defining event that precipitates a drastic career change is much more trivial. Mara, the central character in Goldsworthy's *Honk If You Are Jesus*,[179] a brilliant, cynical, ugly and asthmatic virgin of 48, has never been comfortable with clinical work. She has always preferred the 'inhuman' atmosphere of the operating room, with its 'scrubbed floors and walls, its stainless steel trays and trolleys', to the consulting room.[180] As a student she considered careers in anaesthesiology ('asleep they can't answer back'[181]) or pathology ('even better dead than asleep'[181]), and she 'ended up in fertility research for the same reason: I came to prefer the company of human eggs to human beings.'[181]

Despite her aversion to clinical work, Mara holds an academic post in the Department of Obstetrics and Gynaecology, but she is bored by repetitive procedures such as hysterectomies, ovarian wedge resections and especially abortions. She has become weary of 'that race of people who clog waiting rooms with endless shopping lists of complaints', and she has lost whatever sympathy she may have felt in the past for victims of sexual assault.[182] The patient who finally brings Mara's clinical career to a close is a 14-year-old girl who has been gang-raped.

> I had met her many times before in the smallest hours of many other nights – or if not her, her clones. Black jeans bought several sizes ago; a single small tattoo on the cheek or shoulder; crude eyeliner ruined by tears. 'All the other boys in the car seemed so nice', she said, sniffling. Or if not those words, something similar; something I had also heard too many times before. Over the years these stories had ground me down. I sought escape in the paperwork; precise measurement of the bruises, exact descriptions of the torn tissue, the ticking of small neat boxes in neat square case folders. . . . 'Will this hurt?' 'I'll try to be gentle.' 'Bobby – he was driving – he promised to pay for my leg wax.' . . . I had heard more stupid stories on the Assault Roster. I had seen far younger girls in far worse shape. But suddenly it was too much.[182]

Mara decides to accept a Research Chair in Reproductive Biology, but she lasts only a few months in her new environment and ends up, like some other disgruntled female physicians, trying a career in motherhood before it is too late.[183]

Until a few weeks before his sudden and unexpected resignation,[184] the thought that he might have made the wrong career choice never enters Dr Oliver Selfridge's mind. He and his guardian aunt decide independently that he ought to study medicine, and both reach the conclusion, also independently, that he 'might do well to look ahead to specialization in surgery.'[185] Oliver seems to possess all the right virtues – 'self-restraint, kindness, . . . courtesy, privacy.'[185] Above all he is completely in control of his emotions. By the age of 31, Oliver has been appointed to an assistant professorship in clinical surgery at a major university.[186] He puts in unbelievably long hours, but the work seems satisfying and rewarding, with a distinguished surgical academic career as an attainable goal. Then, quite abruptly and without a precipitating event, 'he begins . . . to deplore his work.' He longs for some occupation 'in which control is not a condition of the skill, in which the hands are not concerned with inches and edges.'[187] Within three days of Pearl Harbor he has given up medicine altogether, and he spends the war years in anonymous idleness in New York City.[188] Herbert Wilner implies that Oliver Selfridge is basically an impulsive and violent man, and that no amount of training could have turned him into an efficient and contented surgeon.

Fully developed cynics and failures

Several fictional physicians who have abandoned their profession are presented in their fully developed state and without an explanation for their inability to practise medicine. Some of these characters suffer from latent personality defects which manifest themselves after rather than before graduation, but in several cases no cause is discernible.

Dr Tyko Glas,[189] a medical murderer who abuses a patient's trust and dispenses a lethal poison (*see* pp. 114–15 and 208–9), attributes his amoral behaviour to a badly chosen career. Glas does not see himself as a Good Samaritan or even as one of the bystanders who refuse to become involved. Quite the reverse, he is an adventurer who would have participated in beating up the traveller on the road to Jericho.

> What a profession! How can it have come about that, out of all possible trades, I should have chosen the one which suits me least? A doctor must be one of two things: either a philanthropist, or else avid for honours. True, I once thought I was both. . . . Position, respectability, future. As if I were not ready, any day or moment, to stow these packages aboard the first ship to come sailing by laden with action.[190]

The account of Konner's brief medical career[191] is autobiographical rather than fictional, but it provides a convincing explanation for the disillusionment of this would-be physician. Konner, who studies medicine in his thirties, chooses not to practise because he never acquires the art of partial detachment without which the practice of medicine is impossible (*see* Volume 1, p. 173). *Becoming a Doctor*[191] begins with a description of an emergency room scene. A young blood-soaked woman is screaming 'Oh my God. He knifed me.' There is no wringing of hands and there are no expressions of sympathy for this 'writhing and yelling' person. Instead, an intrathoracic tube is inserted and a major catastrophe is averted.[192] Konner expresses his admiration for doctors, 'their calm in the face of pain and death, their technical facility and power', but he deplores the physicians' collective inability or unwillingness to become involved with 'the fear, the loss, the dependency, the emptiness [and] the pain' of their patients.[193]

> The medical profession has decided tacitly but firmly that universal happiness is unattainable, that some medical and social problems are incurable, and that it is a waste of time to deplore this state of affairs.[193]

Konner and like-minded individuals who cannot accept this decision and who cannot remain benevolently aloof in the face of suffering either leave the profession or, if they remain, become disgruntled and impaired.

Roy Basch, Rhodes scholar and Harvard MD, the anti-hero of *The House of God*,[194] studies medicine in order to accomplish his father's unfulfilled ambition,[195] but dislikes clinical work from the first day of his internship.[196] He detests the smells, sights and sounds that emanate from sick individuals. He complains about having to see well patients, sick patients, dying patients or patients who refuse to die ('gomers'). He ridicules those of his colleagues who are fond of their patients and/or find the practice of medicine challenging, and he almost succeeds in disaffecting an entire cohort of interns.[197]

Basch makes up for his inadequacy in the wards and clinics by displaying tremendous sexual prowess. Indeed, he gives the impression that the hospital is one vast copulatorium, and that most of the nurses are dedicated to the relief of his erections.[194] Basch, despite his alleged academic brilliance, is an immature egotist who is no more fit to practise medicine than would be Alexander Portnoy[198] (whom he resembles in several respects). Whatever it is that goes into the making of a 'good physician', Basch has not got it, and at the end of the book one is left wondering what kind of disruptive influence he will bring to the psychiatry service, which he deigns to join.[197]

Arabella Kenealy describes an innocent female medical student, Phyllis Eve, confronted by a cynical male physician, Dr Paul Liveing, who is or pretends to be disillusioned with medical practice.[199]

> 'Are you a doctor?' she asked. 'I am, worse luck!' he answered. 'Why do you say worse luck? Do you not like your profession?' 'Does anyone like his profession?' . . . 'Why are you a doctor then?' . . . 'For no better reason than that I am not a lawyer or a parson.' [The young lady objects.] 'I think it is a splendid profession. It is magnificent to be able to cure pain and restore people to health' she said with enthusiasm. 'Ah, you will soon get over that' he replied provokingly. 'All that fine fervour soon resolves itself into a question of fees once you get into practice.'[199]

Paul seems to be posing for the benefit of Phyllis. The two subsequently marry and he continues to practise without undue cynicism.

Dr Salter's disparagement of medicine and the medical profession is more deep-rooted and evidently of long standing. Salter, a small town general practitioner in John Mortimer's *Paradise Postponed*,[200] 'avoids ill people as much as possible.' When asked why he chose to become a doctor, he replies – with mock modesty – that he would have been unable to 'hold down a decent job in a biscuit factory',[200] implying that the two careers are of equal value and that a loafer like himself finds it easier to shirk his duty in medical practice than on a production line.

The fat, alcoholic and 'unclean-looking' Dr Parcival in Sherwood Anderson's *Winesburg, Ohio*[201] has 'but few patients and these of the poorer sort who were unable to pay.' Parcival explains: 'There is a reason for that . . . I do not want patients.' Instead of wearing the symbolic garb of medicine – a spotless white coat – he sleeps in his 'unspeakably dirty' office and he dines at the lunchroom owned by Biff Carter, 'whose white apron was more dirty than his floor.'[201] By the time he arrives in Winesburg, Parcival is already impaired (*see* p. 217), although the reason for his decline is not revealed.

Primo Levi's Uncle Barbarico[202] is another medical drop-out, although alcohol is not a problem in his case. Barbarico, like Dr Parcival, avoids regular work and lives in absolute filth. He

> had studied medicine and had become a good doctor, but he did not like the world. That is, he liked men and especially women, the meadows, the

sky, but not hard work, the racket made by wagons, the intrigues for the sake of a career, the hustling for one's daily bread, commitments, schedules and due dates. . . . He regarded both matrimony and an equipped office and the regular exercise of his profession as too much of a commitment.[202] . . . [He lived] in a filthy and chaotic attic room [spending] the entire day stretched out on his cot, reading books and old newspapers. . . . His patients were the poor people on the outskirts of town from whom he would accept as recompense a half dozen eggs or some lettuce from the garden or even a pair of worn-out shoes.[202]

Yet another medical drop-out, Saul Bellow's Dr Elia Gruner,[203] dislikes his work as a gynaecologist (and abortionist) but waits until he has a heart attack before he decides to give up medical practice. He declares himself unfit for work and makes a disability claim on his insurance policy. 'He had been conscientious. He had done his duty but he hadn't liked his trade.'[200] During his final illness (haemorrhage from an arterio-venous malformation of the brain) this physician displays little interest in his former profession, but instead discusses his family tree and the share market.

Although boredom, depression and burnout are common among physicians in real life,[3] these problems affect only a small minority of fictional doctors. The vast majority remain content despite the long hours and repetitive nature of their work. Very few seriously visualize themselves in other occupations. Romanticized nineteenth-century physicians, who are 'devoted to their profession',[204,205] 'cherish . . . their art with fanatical love and [apply] it with enthusiasm and sagacity.'[206] This fervour, which persists well into the twentieth century, is clearly articulated by Martin du Gard's Dr Antoine Thibault.[207] After successfully (and untruthfully) reassuring a guilt-ridden father that a past history of syphilis is unrelated to his little boy's developmental abnormalities, Antoine feels 'a wave of elation. . . . What a fine profession [medicine] is, he murmured to himself. Yes, by God, the finest in the world.'[207]

More recent fictional physicians do not express themselves in such passionate terms. However, whether they are admired or resented, ignorant or knowledgeable, compassionate or detached,[208] their thinking and their behaviour patterns have been permanently affected by their medical training. Even those who cease to practise tend to become nostalgic about their medical career or actually return to it.

Summary

Works of fiction suggest that most of the annoyances experienced by doctors during the exercise of their trade are of a relatively minor nature. Although frustrations associated with rigid HMO policies, exasperating patients or sleep deprivation may cause some physicians to express mock regret of their choice of profession, such doctors do not seriously intend to cease practising. The problem becomes more severe when a doctor finds that he is irritated not by specific patients but by all patients, and adopts a 'What's the use of it all?' attitude. Such doctors practise an inferior kind of medicine, with the most severely demotivated leaving the profession altogether. Serious disenchantment is rare and, when it does occur, it is due to long-held attitudes and beliefs rather than to isolated events.

References

1 Jewett SO (1884) *A Country Doctor*. Houghton Mifflin Company, Boston, MA, p. 105.
2 McEwan I (2005) *Saturday*. Cape, London, p. 28.
3 Kassirer JP (1998) Doctor discontent. *NEJM*. **339**: 1543–5.
4 Simon SR, Pan RJD, Sullivan AM *et al.* (1999) Views of managed care. A survey of students, residents, faculty and deans at medical schools in the United States. *NEJM*. **340**: 928–36.
5 Manian FA (1998) Should we accept mediocrity? *NEJM*. **338**: 1067–9.
6 Bennet G (1998) Coping with loss. The doctor's losses: ideals versus realities. *BMJ*. **316**: 1238–40.
7 Shanafelt TD, Bradley KA, Wipf JE and Back AL (2002) Burnout and self-reported patient care in an internal medicine residency program. *Ann Intern Med*. **136**: 384–93.
8 Frenk J, Alagon J, Nigenda G *et al.* (1991) Patterns of medical employment: a survey of imbalances in urban Mexico. *Am J Pub Health*. **81**: 23–9.
9 Bosch X (1999) Too many physicians in Spain. *JAMA*. **282**: 1025–6.
10 Moynihan BGA (Lord Moynihan) (1936) *Truants: the story of some who deserted medicine yet triumphed*. Cambridge University Press, Cambridge.
11 Smithers DW (1989) *This Idle Trade*. Dragonfly Press, Tunbridge Wells.
12 Curran WS (1961) Arthur Lee and the secret diplomacy of the American Revolution. *NEJM*. **264**: 240–2.
13 Lindgren KM (1966) Doctor Thornton and his Capitol. *NEJM*. **274**: 790–1.
14 Harper GP (1969) Ernesto (Che) Guevara, physician – revolutionary physician – revolutionary. *NEJM*. **281**: 1285–91.
15 Bennett A (1923) *Riceyman Steps*. Cassell, London, 1947, p. 52.
16 James H (1884) Lady Barberina. In: *The New York Edition of Henry James. Volume 14*. Augustus Kelley, Fairfield, NJ, 1976, p. 23.
17 Maugham WS (1944) *The Razor's Edge*. Penguin, Harmondsworth, 1963, p. 94.
18 Maugham WS (1909) Penelope. In: *The Collected Plays. Volume 1*. Heinemann, London, 1960, p. 17.
19 Smollett T (1748) *The Adventures of Roderick Random*. Dent, London, 1964, pp. 424–8.
20 Thackeray WM (1848–1850) *The History of Pendennis: his fortunes and misfortunes, his friends and his greatest enemy. Volume 1*. Smith Elder, London, 1879, p. 11.
21 Scott W (1831) The Surgeon's Daughter. In: *The Waverley Novels. Volume 25*. Adam and Charles Black, London, 1892, p. 102.
22 Ibid., p. 147.
23 James H., op. cit., p. 23.
24 Ibid., pp. 56–7.
25 Ibid., p. 142.
26 Young FB (1928) *My Brother Jonathan*. Heinemann, London, p. 287.
27 Ibid., pp. 431–6.
28 Lewis S (1924) *Arrowsmith*. Signet Books, New York, 1961, pp. 82–5.
29 Ibid., pp. 244–6.
30 Faulkner W (1939) *The Wild Palms*. Random House, New York.
31 Groves JE (1978) Taking care of the hateful patient. *NEJM*. **298**: 883–7.
32 Mitchell SW (1901) *Circumstance*. Century Company, New York, 1902, p. 404.
33 Wharton W (1981) *Dad*. Alfred A Knopf, New York, pp. 159–62.
34 Arlen M (1924) *The Green Hat*. George H Doran, New York, pp. 180–6.
35 Lightman A (2000) *The Diagnosis*. Pantheon Books, New York, pp. 267–8.
36 Busch F (1984) Rise and Fall. In: *Too Late American Boyhood Blues*. David R Godine, Boston, MA, p. 31.

37 Dooling R (1991) *Critical Care*. William Morrow, New York, p. 108.
38 Mitchell SW (1885) *In War Time*. Century Company, New York, 1913, p. 63.
39 Ibid., pp. 422–3.
40 Douglas LC (1939) *Doctor Hudson's Secret Journal*. Grosset and Dunlap, New York, p. 7.
41 Ibid., p. 32.
42 Rinehart MR (1935) *The Doctor*. Farrar and Rinehart, New York, pp. 91–5.
43 Dooling R, op. cit., p. 17.
44 Ibid., p. 31.
45 Ravin N (1985) *Seven North*. EP Dutton/Seymour Lawrence, New York, p. 145.
46 Ibid., pp. 67–9.
47 Ibid., p. 170.
48 Ravin N (1987) *Evidence*. Charles Scribner's Sons, New York, p. 23.
49 Ravin N (1985) *Seven North*. EP Dutton/Seymour Lawrence, New York, p. 23.
50 Ibid., p. 66.
51 Doctor X (Nourse AE) (1965) *Intern*. Harper and Row, New York, p. 208.
52 Dooling R, op. cit., pp. 192–4.
53 Fitzgerald FS (1932) One Interne. In: *Taps at Reveille*. Charles Scribner's Sons, New York, 1935, pp. 349–73.
54 Bashford HH (1911) *The Corner of Harley Street: being some familiar correspondence of Peter Harding MD*. Constable, London, 1913, pp. 15–17.
55 Ibid., p. 9.
56 Ibid., p. 169.
57 Ibid., pp. 22–3.
58 Baldwin F (1939) *Medical Centre*. Horwitz, Sydney, 1962, pp. 11–12.
59 Pym B (1980) *A Few Green Leaves*. EP Dutton, New York, pp. 18–19.
60 Ibid., pp. 206–9.
61 Mitchell SW (1901) *Circumstance*. Century Company, New York, 1902, p. 276.
62 Coulehan J (1998) Chekhov's doctors. 18. The Zemstvo doctor. *JAMA*. **279**: 270.
63 Mitchell SW, op. cit., pp. 232–3.
64 Ashton H (1930) *Doctor Serocold*. Penguin, London, 1936, pp. 29–35.
65 Ibid., p. 66.
66 Ibid., p. 113.
67 Ibid., p. 136.
68 Ibid., pp. 154–5.
69 Ibid., p. 256.
70 Ibid., p. 122.
71 Wilder T (1938) *Our Town*. Longmans, London, 1965.
72 Miksanek T (2004) An adverse reaction. *Healing Muse*. **4**: 65–70.
73 Bulgakov M (1925–1927) The Steel Windpipe. In: *A Country Doctor's Notebook* (translated by Glenny M). Collins and Harvill Press, London, 1975, pp. 29–37.
74 Bulgakov M (1925–1927) The Embroidered Towel. In: *A Country Doctor's Notebook* (translated by Glenny M). Collins and Harvill Press, London, 1975, pp. 13–25.
75 Bulgakov M (1925–1927) Baptism by Rotation. In: *A Country Doctor's Notebook* (translated by Glenny M). Collins and Harvill Press, London, 1975, pp. 53–62.
76 Brown TK (1956) A Drink of Water. In: Engle P and Harnack C (eds) *Prize Stories 1958: the O Henry Awards*. Doubleday, Garden City, NY, 1958, pp. 179–201.
77 Alexander H (2000) *Solemn Oath*. Bethany House Publishers, Minneapolis, MN, pp. 17–18.
78 Cook R (1993) *Fatal Cure*. Pan Books, London, 1995, pp. 112–13.
79 Roe F (1989) *Doctors and Doctors' Wives*. Constable, London, pp. 89–94.
80 Cook R (1981) *Brain*. Pan Books, London, p. 119.
81 Marion R (1989) *The Intern Blues*. William Morrow and Company, New York, pp. 118–19.

82 Dooling R, op. cit., pp. 11–12.
83 Huyler F (1999) The Prisoner. In: *The Blood of Strangers*. University of California Press, Berkeley, CA, pp. 63–88.
84 Bennett A, op. cit., pp. 213–20.
85 Ibid., pp. 245–64.
86 Ibid., pp. 264–71.
87 Busch F (1979) *Rounds*. Farrar Straus and Giroux, New York, p. 3.
88 Ibid., pp. 80–1.
89 Flaubert G (1857) *Madame Bovary* (translated by Steegmuller F). Modern Library, New York, 1982, pp. 7–9.
90 Ibid., pp. 204–5.
91 Kingsley C (1857) Two Years Ago. In: *The Works of Charles Kingsley. Volume 8.* Reprinted by Georg Olms, Hildesheim, Germany, 1969.
92 Ibid., p. 71.
93 Ibid., p. 26.
94 Ibid., p. 33.
95 Stevenson RL (1883) *Treasure Island*. Dent, London, 1925, p. 34.
96 Ibid., p. 149.
97 Richardson HH (1917–1929) *The Fortunes of Richard Mahony*. Penguin, Harmondsworth, 1990.
98 Ibid., pp. 30–1.
99 Ibid., p. 88.
100 Ibid., pp. 164–8.
101 Ibid., p. 453.
102 Ibid., p. 468.
103 Albee E (1959) The Death of Bessie Smith. In: *The Zoo Story*. Coward-McCann, New York, 1960, pp. 67–137.
104 Balzac H de (1833) *The Country Doctor* (translated by Marriage E). Dent, London, 1923.
105 Balzac H de (1840) *Pierrette* (translated by Ives GB). George Barrie and Sons, Philadelphia, PA, 1897.
106 Lewis S, op. cit., pp. 426–7.
107 Cronin AJ (1937) *The Citadel*. Gollancz, London.
108 Herrick R (1908) *The Master of the Inn*. Charles Scribner's Sons, New York, 1913.
109 Herrick R (1911) *The Healer*. Macmillan, New York.
110 Ibid., pp. 426–7.
111 Ibid., pp. 50–1.
112 Ibid., pp. 244–6.
113 Straub P (1988) *Koko*. Penguin, Harmondsworth, 1989.
114 Ibid., p. 299.
115 Snow CP (1958) The Conscience of the Rich. In: *Strangers and Brothers. Volume 1.* Charles Scribner's Sons, New York, 1972, pp. 702–4.
116 Morgan J (1956) *Doctor Jo*. Samuel French, London.
117 Wouk H (1951) *The Caine Mutiny*. Jonathan Cape, London, 1954, p. 61.
118 Perec G (1978) *Life: a user's manual* (translated by Bellos D). Collins Harvill, London, 1987, p. 47.
119 Ibid., p. 209.
120 Ibid., pp. 474–80.
121 Green G (1979) *The Healers*. Melbourne House, London.
122 Ibid., p. 234.
123 Ibid., pp. 221–2.
124 Ozick C (1971) The Doctor's Wife. In: *The Pagan Rabbi and Other Stories*. Penguin, New York, 1983, pp. 181–90.

125 Schnitzler A (1917) *Dr Graesler* (translated by Slade EC). Thomas Seltzer, New York, 1923, p. 53.

126 Ibid., p. 8.

127 Ibid., p. 50.

128 Ibid., p. 11.

129 Ibid., p. 94.

130 Ibid., p. 148.

131 Kundera M (1976) *The Farewell Party* (translated by Kussi P). Knopf, New York.

132 Ibid., p. 36.

133 The Bible, Revised Standard Version. Oxford University Press, New York, 1977, Romans, 7: 15.

134 Hyppola H, Kumpusalo E, Neittaanmaki L *et al.* (1998) Becoming a doctor: was it the wrong career choice? *Soc Sci Med.* **47**: 1383–7.

135 Crichton M (Hudson J, pseudonym) (1968) *A Case of Need*. Signet, New York, 1969, pp. 210–12.

136 Baum V (1928) *Helene* (translated by Bashford F). Penguin, Harmondsworth, 1939.

137 Ibid., p. 107.

138 Ibid., p. 42.

139 Ibid., pp. 61–2.

140 Ibid., pp. 24–6.

141 Ibid., p. 183.

142 El Saadawi N (1975) *Two Women in One* (translated by Nusairi O and Gough J). El Saqi Books, London, 1985.

143 Ibid., pp. 60–4.

144 Ibid., p. 23.

145 Grecco S (1980) A Physician Healing Himself: Chekhov's treatment of doctors in the major plays. In: Peschel ER (ed.) *Medicine and Literature*. Neale Watson Academic Publications, New York, pp. 3–10.

146 Pedrotti L (1981) Chekhov's Major Plays: a doctor in the house. In: Barricelli JP (ed.) *Chekhov's Great Plays*. New York University Press, New York, pp. 233–50.

147 Chekhov AP (1892) Ward Number Six. In: *The Oxford Chekhov* (translated by Hingley R). *Volume 6*. Oxford University Press, London, 1971, pp. 121–67.

148 Chekhov AP (1892) My Wife. In: *The Oxford Chekhov* (translated by Hingley R). *Volume 6*. Oxford University Press, London, 1971, pp. 21–58.

149 Chekhov AP (1888) An Awkward Business. In: *The Oxford Chekhov* (translated by Hingley R). *Volume 4*. Oxford University Press, London, 1980, pp. 99–115.

150 Chekhov AP (1897) Uncle Vanya. In: *The Oxford Chekhov* (translated by Hingley R). *Volume 3*. Oxford University Press, London, 1964, pp. 15–67.

151 Chekhov AP (1900–1901) Three Sisters. In: *The Oxford Chekhov* (translated by Hingley R). *Volume 3*. Oxford University Press, London, 1964, pp. 71–139.

152 Chekhov AP (1896) The Seagull. In: *The Oxford Chekhov* (translated by Hingley R). *Volume 2*. Oxford University Press, London, 1967, p. 246.

153 Chekhov AP (1887) The Enemies (also titled Two Tragedies, or Antagonists). In: *Short Stories* (translated by Fen E). Folio Society, London, 1974, pp. 58–72.

154 Céline LF (1936) *Death on the Installment Plan* (translated by Manheim R). New Directions, New York, pp. 15–25.

155 Céline LF (1932) *Journey to the End of the Night* (translated by Manheim R). New Directions, New York, 1983.

156 Ibid., pp. 204–5.

157 Ibid., pp. 224–7.

158 Ibid., pp. 426–9.

159 Ibid., p. 433.

160 Ibid., pp. 306–7.

161 Ibid., p. 358.
162 Ibid., p. 363.
163 Ibid., p. 365.
164 Ibid., pp. 374–80.
165 Waltari M (1945) *The Egyptian* (translated by Walford N). Panther Books, London, 1960.
166 Ibid., p. 298.
167 Ibid., pp. 340–7.
168 Swift J (1726) *Gulliver's Travels*. Clarkson Potter, New York, 1980, pp. 4–6.
169 Ibid., pp. 210–11.
170 Ibid., p. 285.
171 Lofting H (1923) *The Voyages of Doctor Dolittle*. Jonathan Cape, London.
172 Goethe JW (1808) *Faust. Part 1* (translated by Latham AG). Dent, London, 1948, pp. 30–31.
173 Hejinian J (1974) *Extreme Remedies*. St Martin's Press, New York.
174 Ibid., pp. 221–5.
175 Ibid., pp. 288–93.
176 Barker P (1991) *Regeneration*. Penguin, Harmondsworth, 1992, pp. 28–32.
177 Ibid., pp. 135–7.
178 Selzer R (1982) Imelda. In: *Letters to a Young Doctor*. Harcourt Brace, San Diego, CA, 1996, pp. 21–36.
179 Goldsworthy P (1992) *Honk If You Are Jesus*. Angus and Robertson, Sydney.
180 Ibid., p. 17.
181 Ibid., pp. 45–6.
182 Ibid., pp. 48–9.
183 Ibid., pp. 289–90.
184 Wilner H (1966) *All the Little Heroes*. Bobbs-Merrill, Indianapolis, IN.
185 Ibid., p. 130.
186 Ibid., p. 482.
187 Ibid., p. 258.
188 Ibid., p. 305.
189 Söderberg H (1905) *Doctor Glas* (translated by Austin PB). Chatto and Windus, London, 1963.
190 Ibid., pp. 17–19.
191 Konner M (1987) *Becoming a Doctor*. Viking, New York.
192 Ibid., pp. 2–4.
193 Ibid., p. 376.
194 Shem S (Bergman S) (1978) *The House of God*. Richard Marek, New York.
195 Ibid., pp. 167–83.
196 Ibid., p. 25.
197 Ibid., pp. 354–9.
198 Roth P (1969) *Portnoy's Complaint*. Random House, New York.
199 Kenealy A (1893) *Dr Janet of Harley Street*. Digby Long, London, 1894, pp. 117–18.
200 Mortimer J (1985) *Paradise Postponed*. Penguin, Harmondsworth, 1986, p. 57.
201 Anderson S (1919) *Winesburg Ohio*. Viking Press, New York, 1964, pp. 49–57.
202 Levi P (1975) *The Periodic Table*. Abacus, London, 1990, pp. 13–15.
203 Bellow S (1969) *Mr Sammler's Planet*. Penguin, Harmondsworth, 1977, pp. 66–8.
204 Scott W, op. cit., p. 3.
205 Martineau H (1839) *Deerbrook*. Virago Press, London, 1983, p. 39.
206 Flaubert G, op. cit., p. 363.
207 Martin du Gard R (1922–1929) *The Thibaults* (translated by Gilbert S). John Lane, The Bodley Head, London, 1939, pp. 571–6.
208 Posen S (2005) *The Doctor in Literature. Volume 1. Satisfaction or resentment?* Radcliffe Publishing, Oxford.

CHAPTER 6

The impaired doctor

Ridgeon: 'The most tragic thing in the world is a sick doctor.'
Walpole: 'Yes, by George, it's like a bald-headed man trying to sell a hair-restorer.'[1]

Doctors are just people born to sorrow, fighting the long grim fight like the rest of us.[2]

In the medical literature,[3-6] descriptions of sick doctors focus almost entirely on one specific problem – the identification, notification and rehabilitation of colleagues suffering from drug and alcohol dependency. By contrast, fictional doctors, like their counterparts in real life, become impaired for a multiplicity of reasons. These include, in addition to alcohol and drug abuse, chronic physical and psychiatric disorders and the inability or unwillingness of some physicians to recognize the infirmities of old age in themselves. Authors of fictional works seem fascinated by the paradox of these physically and emotionally impaired doctors, almost all of them male, who cannot 'heal themselves.'

The typical physician, who is in good health and in control of the situation, is able to help and advise less fortunate individuals whereas the inevitable preoccupation of a 'wounded healer' with his own problems is likely to weaken his effectiveness. Admittedly, the sick doctor may be more tolerant and sympathetic towards his patients than are his healthy colleagues. His own suffering may even give him a special flair for dealing with patients, particularly psychiatric patients.[7] In Pat Barker's trilogy, William the Patient (Billy Prior) expresses his conviction that the healing powers of William the Doctor (WHR Rivers) originate 'directly from some sort of wound or deformity in him.'[7] Such sentiments may accurately describe the state of affairs in a few psychiatric cases, but in the vast majority of clinical situations they are clearly inappropriate. Rivers himself, at an earlier stage of his career, suffering from extensive burns to his legs, unable to walk, seeing patients from his sick bed and 'shuffling from the patient to the dispensing cupboard and back again on his bottom',[7a] is obviously less effective as a healer than he would be if he were sitting at his desk and able to walk normally.

This is one of the reasons why physicians (particularly male physicians) in the real world go to extraordinary lengths to hide their physical failings and to assume an air of invulnerability that lasts almost to the end of their lives. They are notorious for their unwillingness to seek or accept medical advice.[8] Writers of fiction tend to perpetuate the myth of the resilient doctor, and applaud his 'heroic' behaviour in the face of sickness and death. Medical hypochondriacs, preoccupied with their real or imagined illnesses, come across as freaks rather than as 'proper' doctors. Heller's Doc Daneeka,[9] who continually broods over his health, instructs the medical orderlies to take his temperature on a daily basis, and feels bitterly disappointed because it is always normal, scarcely merits even his abbreviated title.

Physical illnesses, past and present, acute and chronic

Past illnesses, provided the doctor has fully recovered from them, may indeed give him additional insights into a particular disease, its symptoms and its course. Plato believed that 'the most skilful physicians are those who . . . have had all manner of diseases in their own persons.'[10] Martin du Gard, the 1937 Nobel laureate, makes his hero, Dr Antoine Thibault, express very similar sentiments in his diary two months before his death:

> Health and happiness are blinkers. Illness removes them. I am convinced that the most favourable condition for a sound knowledge of oneself (and of one's fellow-men) is to have been through an illness and recovered one's health. Half-inclined to write [that] the man who 'has never known a day's illness' is bound to be a fool.[11]

An acute illness, like a respiratory infection, is regarded as a minor nuisance, and the consultation with a colleague (if it occurs at all[8,12]) may become a combination between a charade and a social occasion.[8] Advice is sought from colleagues who are selected for their status in the medical hierarchy vis-à-vis the doctor-patient rather than their clinical ability.[8] The two young physicians in Conan Doyle's *Behind the Times*[13] consult old Dr Winter (*see also* p. 227) not because of his skill with the stethoscope (which he does not possess), but on account of his old-fashioned ideas, which will presumably enable them to disregard his advice if it fails to suit them.

Old Dr Gridley in Dreiser's *The Country Doctor*[14] goes in the opposite direction and amuses himself by seeking (and accepting) advice from medical striplings.

> When he felt the least bit ill . . . [Gridley] refused to prescribe for himself, saying that a doctor, if he knew anything at all, was never such a fool as to take any of his own medicine. Instead, and in sequence to this humorous attitude, he would always send for one of the younger men of the vicinity.[14] On this occasion he called in a very sober young doctor . . . who . . . had very little practice as yet, and saying 'Doctor, I'm sick today', lay back on his bed and waited for further developments.[14]

The young man, acutely conscious of the discrepancy between his own experience and that of the old man, is too flustered to perform even a standard physical examination.

> 'Well, Doctor', he finally said, after looking at his tongue, taking his pulse and feeling his forehead, 'you're really a better judge of your own condition than I am. . . . What do you think I ought to give you?' 'Now, Doctor', replied Gridley sweetly, 'I'm your patient . . . and I'm going to take whatever you give me.' . . . The young doctor . . . decided . . . that just for variation's sake he would give the doctor something of which he had only recently heard, a sample of which he had with him.[14]

Dr Gridley, who has never heard of this newly described 'treatment', takes the novel medication, congratulates the young man on keeping up with 'the latest medical developments', and comments good-humouredly that 'medicine was changing and perhaps it was just as well that old doctors died.' The treatment 'works' and Gridley recovers.[14]

Not all physicians are as relaxed with their colleagues as Dr Gridley.[14] When Scott Fitzgerald's Dr Bill Tulliver,[15] a very junior intern, develops acute abdominal pain he irrationally refuses to submit to a laparotomy. He has no faith in his colleague, Dr George Schoatze, who has made a diagnosis of volvulus, but an element of professional jealousy is also intruding. Tulliver is secretly afraid that Schoatze might be right 'and get a lot of credit.'[15] In the end, he is persuaded in the nick of time to have an operation. The person who makes him change his mind is not Schoatze or Dr Norton the 'diagnostician', but Thea Singleton, the nurse whom he is trying to detach from Dr Howard Durfee, the surgeon. The story ends happily. Durfee resects a loop of bowel, Thea gives the anaesthetic and Bill Tulliver makes a full recovery.[15]

Chronic ailments, so long as these are not apparent to colleagues and patients, generally present no problems. The underlying pathology is denied and the symptoms are ignored. Dr Owen Deane in Moore's *The Doctor's Wife*[16] has peptic ulcers. He has had two haemorrhages over the years, and is supposed to be careful. 'Being careful to Dr Deane meant taking two "Gelusil"* tablets after a double Scotch.' He also suffers from intermittent tachycardia, but he reassures himself that 'It's just nerves, my heart's all right.'[16]

Katherine Anne Porter's Dr Schumann,[17] who is atypical in more ways than one (*see* p. 125), also behaves uncharacteristically in the face of a potentially lethal illness. Schumann does not ignore, deny or self-treat his symptoms. He 'had always tried to avoid diagnosing and treating himself. . . . He made a habit of consulting doctors more able than he . . . but he had not needed to be told what his trouble was' (ischaemic heart disease).[18] He accepts with 'fated calm [the]danger of death from one moment to the next',[18] and while he 'longed deeply to live' he is not afraid of death. During angina attacks, he feels his pulse, takes his nitroglycerine, crosses himself and remains quietly reconciled to his fate. He signs on as a ship's doctor, 'hoping for a little repose',[19] but if he entertains subconscious longings to die at sea, his hopes are not fulfilled. Despite a great deal of physical and emotional turmoil during the voyage, he eventually returns to Heidelberg.[17]

When a doctor's affliction becomes common knowledge, or when the signs of his illness are obvious for all to see, his medical work may come to an end. In some instances, he is simply no longer able to cope. Charles Bovary,[20] after his wife's suicide, becomes so depressed that 'he no longer went out, had no visitors, refused even to call on his patients. . . . Now and again someone more curious than the rest would peer over the garden hedge and would be startled at the sight of him, wild-eyed, long bearded, clad in sordid rags . . . and weeping aloud.'[20]

The situation becomes more complex when an overtly sick doctor continues to practise despite his illness. Thomas Mann discusses this paradox in great detail. Dr Behrens, the superintendent of the tuberculosis sanatorium in *The Magic Mountain*,[21] was

---

* See footnote in Volume 1, p. 124 concerning the use of proprietary rather than generic names of drugs.

one of the physicians who are companions in suffering to the patients in their care; who do not stand above disease . . . but who themselves bear her mark – an odd but by no means isolated case and one which has its good as well as its bad side. Sympathy between doctor and patient is surely desirable, and a case might be made out for the view that only he who suffers can be the guide and healer of the suffering. And yet can true spiritual mastery over a power be won by him who is counted among her slaves? Can he free others who himself is not free? . . . May not his scientific knowledge tend to be clouded and confused by his own participation rather than enriched and morally reinforced? . . . Can . . . a man who himself belongs among the ailing . . . give himself to the cure or care of others as can a man who is himself entirely sound?[21]

Thomas Mann provides no answers to these vexed questions, which have obviously troubled many other writers both before and since his time. Most of them say or imply that illnesses and deformities constitute severe handicaps to the practising doctor. Hippocrates[22] is quite firm in his belief that doctors have to be in good health:

The dignity of a physician requires that he should look healthy and as plump as nature intended him to be, for the common crowd consider those who are not of this excellent bodily condition to be unable to take care of others.[22]

John Halle[23] echoes these sentiments during the Elizabethan period: 'All that should be admitted to that art (surgery) should be . . . well formed in person.'

Vincent Van Gogh, a depressive patient, expresses extreme scepticism about his physician, Dr Gachet, when he discovers that the doctor is 'as discouraged about his job as a country doctor as I am about my painting.'[24] He uses the biblical metaphor of 'the blind leading the blind'[24] to describe the doctor's feeble therapeutic efforts. The devastating result of these efforts, whatever their nature, is part of history.

Philip Carey, the principal character in Somerset Maugham's *Of Human Bondage*,[25] a sensitive medical student with a congenital club foot, is persuaded by one of his surgical teachers to have the deformity corrected before he goes into practice: 'The layman is full of fads and he doesn't like his doctor to have anything the matter with him.'[25] AE Ellis's *The Rack*,[26] like Mann's *The Magic Mountain*,[21] is set in an Alpine sanatorium, but, unlike Mann, Ellis is clearly of the opinion that chronic disease does not improve a physician's capacity to care for the sick. Dr Bruneau, a promising young surgeon when he develops tuberculosis, becomes bored and frustrated by his prolonged stay at the sanatorium, and acquires a corroding pessimism which he transmits, consciously or subconsciously, to his patients.[26]

WH Auden[27] expresses the minority view, and regards his doctor's pituitary tumour as a positive factor. To Auden, the diseased doctor is more dependable than his healthy colleague.

For my small ailments
you, who were mortally sick
prescribed with success . . .
Was it your very
predicament that made me
sure I could trust you . . . ?[27]

Crippled and disfigured physicians

Unlike some other disabilities, complete loss of sight is perceived as incompatible with medical practice, in both the nineteenth and twentieth centuries. Kingsley's Dr Edward Thurnall,[28] 'doctor of medicine and consulting physician of all the country round [Whitbury],[29] . . . a gentleman and a scholar and a man of science',[30] totally ceases to function as a physician when he becomes blind.[31] Instead he plays the role of the noble white-haired old father, supported financially by his peripatetic medical son[31] and fussed over by aspiring daughters-in-law.[32]

Saramago's *Blindness*[33] tells an allegorical story of a mysterious epidemic which causes sudden and complete loss of sight and which afflicts an unnamed ophthalmologist as well as several of his patients. Before his illness, the doctor is diligent and conscientious. He takes detailed histories, he performs thorough examinations and he possesses sufficient insight to recognize when 'he is an intruder in a field beyond his comprehension.'[34] At the onset of the unusual epidemic he consults a colleague and peruses the relevant literature.

As soon as he is stricken by the mysterious blindness, the doctor has to join all the other sightless individuals and their contacts, who have been quarantined in a disused asylum. Here the doctor turns into a helpless cripple. Not only is he incapable of functioning as a healer, but whatever moral authority he may have possessed vanishes completely. The hardened criminal who has also become blind, and with whom the doctor has to share a dormitory, snarls at him 'Listen to me, doctor, we're all equal here and you don't give me any orders.'[35] The 'first blind man',* formerly a law-abiding citizen and a patient of the ophthalmologist, does not issue any open challenges, but even he is dubious about the doctor's medical expertise. He reasons that as the doctor has failed to prevent his own blindness, 'he doesn't even know about eyes'[36] he is therefore likely to be even more ignorant about diet and nutrition. Only once during his illness does the doctor recover a vestige of his former stature. He is guided back to his former office[37] where he conducts a mock consultation with an imaginary patient, who is fatuously advised to remain patient.

> He sat down at the desk, placed his hands on the dusty top, then with a sad ironic smile as if he were talking to someone sitting opposite him, he said 'No my dear doctor, I am very sorry but your condition has no known cure.'[37]

Vicky Baum describes several physically and emotionally impaired physicians[38–54] who either do no medical work at all or occupy positions considerably below those commensurate with their training. Dr Otternschlag in *Grand Hotel*[38] has sustained severe injuries during the First World War and has been left with

> half a face. The other half . . . was not there. In place of it was a confused medley of seams and scars, crossing and overlapping and among them was set a glass eye. 'A souvenir from Flanders', Dr Otternschlag was accustomed to call it when talking to himself.[39]

---

* No one in *Blindness* has a name. The symbolic characters are referred to as 'the girl with the dark glasses', 'the boy with the squint', 'the car thief', 'the doctor' and, most importantly, 'the doctor's wife' (*see* p. 44).[33]

Otternschlag's injuries, his subsequent operations and his repulsive appearance have isolated him to such an extent that he not only ceases to practise medicine, but also breaks off all contact with friends and relatives.[40] Otternschlag, who has sufficient means to move from one luxurious hotel to another in various European cities, is a morphine addict,[41] convinced of the futility of life and constantly contemplating suicide: 'One of these days I shall take ten of these ampoules . . . and inject them into my veins.'[42] Despite his multiple flaws, Dr Otternschlag retains some vestiges of medical behaviour. He recognizes that one of the hotel guests (Otto Kringelein) is seriously ill,[40] and he acts with surprising energy when Kringelein's condition suddenly deteriorates.[43] He also has sufficient common sense to identify the thief who stole Kringelein's wallet.[44]

Wilkie Collins in *The Moonstone*[55] describes another disfigured medical man. Dr Ezra Jennings, like Vicky Baum's Dr Otternschlag,[41] has become a morphine addict, although this English doctor of the 1860s does not express his feelings about the futility of life as strongly as the German doctor of the 1920s. Jennings'

> complexion was of a gypsy darkness, his fleshless cheeks had fallen into deep hollows over which the bone projected. . . . His marks and wrinkles were innumerable. . . . [His] eyes . . . [were] deeply sunk in their orbits. . . . Add to this a quantity of thick, closely curling hair which, by some freak of nature, had lost the colour in the most startling and capricious manner. Over the top of his head it was still of the deep black which was its natural colour. Round the sides of his head – without the slightest graduation of grey to break the force of the extraordinary contrast – it had turned completely white. The line between the two colours preserved no sort of regularity. At one place the white hair ran into the black. At another the black hair ran down into the white.[56]

Ezra Jennings' physical appearance 'was calculated to produce an unfavourable impression' and to make him 'unpopular everywhere.' Collins does not explain Jennings' 'female constitution' or 'the cloud of [the] horrible accusation . . . which had rested on [him] for years', but he leaves the reader in no doubt about the contemptuous treatment Jennings receives at the hands of his own servant girl.[57] Despite his vitiligo, his unpopularity and his 'incurable internal complaint'[57] (possibly autoimmune Addisonism), Jennings retains his medical insight, and he is able to throw some light on the disappearance of the moonstone.[55]

Yet another disfigured doctor, Warwick Deeping's Dr Simon Orange,[58] over-comes the handicap of his multiple deformities and his grotesque appearance by sheer ability. Orange, who is known among the student comedians as 'the orang' and 'Septic Simon', is 'swarthy and misshapen.' He has a cleft palate, a squeaky voice, a 'sunken head' and a bulgy forehead. He is prone to severe attacks of 'migraine'. During his student days, when he is desperately poor, some of his loutish classmates attempt to use him as a target for their practical jokes, and are only dissuaded from their intentions 'by the creature's fierceness and its extraordinary simian strength.'[59] Remarkably, this 'misshapen little man' gains the confidence of patients, whom he handles with 'a peculiar abrupt tenderness', and the trust of general practitioners, who admire his reliability and refer patients to him. Above all, his surgical skills impress the power brokers in his class-ridden London hospital to such an extent that despite his 'unsuitable' background and his obvious infirmities, they appoint him to a senior position on the surgical staff.[59]

Bashford's medical amputee is not disfigured, and although his disability obviously prevents him from working, he is nevertheless able to occupy a useful, semi-medical position in the community. Dr Rogers, London's leading neurosurgeon, who 'lost a hand in consequence of a post-mortem infection'*,[60] retires to a small coastal town in northern England where he endows and runs a 'cottage hospital' (*see* p. 112 for Dr Rogers' attitude towards religion[60]).

The unnamed hotel doctor in Baum's *Berlin Hotel*[45] has, like Dr Otternschlag,[38] been injured in the First World War. He has acquired a stiff leg and he feels frustrated because the German army has rejected him for service in the Second World War. He is not as hideously deformed as Otternschlag, and has managed to obtain a position in a hotel, where he spends his time playing solitaire[36] and taking care of drunks, while every now and again 'he had . . . brief lovely vision(s) of abdominal wounds and smashed legs.'[47] Like some other impaired fictional physicians, this hotel doctor has his brief moment of glory during an emergency. During an air raid

> his hands were warm, his mind clear, his fingers sure and nimble and the stiff leg did not seem to hamper him in the least. . . . Merrily he inhaled the stench of disaster in which he felt at home as he had not [felt] since another disaster twenty-five years ago had torn him out and thrown him on to the trash heap.[48]

The exiled physician

Dr Emanuel Hain, another of Vicky Baum's medical characters,[49] is devastated by the murder of his only son during the Berlin 'Night of the Long Knives' (*see also* p. 48). The distinguished surgeon is driven into exile by the Nazis a few days later, and ends up in Shanghai, where he believes he may be able to practise without having to pass an examination.[50]

Once out of Germany, Dr Hain joins the ranks of the medically castrated refugee doctors. His clientele in Shanghai consists of opium-addicted 'coolies'[51] and expatriate alcoholics,[52] and he becomes so isolated and frustrated that he even longs for an outbreak of hostilities: 'If war should start here, I should at least have an aim in life, for they will organize ambulance work and my old war experience will stand me in good stead.'[53] Just before his death, Hain briefly regains some of his medical acumen and integrity. He recognizes that an inebriate British aristocrat has been suffocated by his wife, and refuses this woman's offer of a large sum of money if he will sign an 'appropriate' death certificate.[54] Despite this final flicker of the 'medical candle', Hain, who dies during the bombing of Shanghai, is considered at the end 'a shell without content. . . . The bomb that annihilated him spared him the exercise of courage required to swallow a dose of cyanide.'[54]

'Ravic', the medical hero in Remarque's *Arch of Triumph*, another medical refugee from Nazi Germany,[61] is not quite as marginalized as Hain.[51,52] Ravic has ended up in Paris rather than Shanghai, and although he has no licence to practise medicine in France, he is able, because of his operative skills, to perform 'ghost surgery' for incompetent local colleagues. The arrangement is simple. The

---

* *See* footnote on p. 19.

officially responsible, certified doctor visits the patients before and after the operation, accepts thanks for 'saving their lives' and charges a colossal fee. However, once the patient is anaesthetized, the refugee surgeon takes over and performs the more difficult parts of the procedure, or all of it. He then disappears and receives a fee commensurate with his colleague's generosity.[61] This arrangement, which provides an income for Ravic, is totally unsatisfactory from a medical point of view. The surgeon never examines the patients pre-operatively, he frequently does not know their names, and he has to rely heavily on the diagnostic skills of his licensed colleagues.[62] The nursing staff treat him with contempt, refusing even to call him 'Doctor.' The incompetent members of the 'qualified' fraternity exploit him by using his surgical skills, although they sometimes show signs of pity.[62] Some of the scraps of work that are thrown at this former chief of surgery are thoroughly degrading. He has to perform the weekly vaginal examinations at the local whorehouse, an activity that provides him with some amusement but no intellectual stimulus.[62]

Under these conditions, Ravic rapidly joins the ranks of the impaired doctors. He drinks heavily, he spends his spare time playing chess, and although he uses his previously acquired skills, he makes no attempt to read medical journals or otherwise further his medical knowledge. If, on the last page of the book, instead of being sent off to a concentration camp, Ravic had been given the chance to escape to a free country, he would no longer have been fit to hold down a position of 'chief surgeon in a great hospital'.[62]

Personality dysfunction; organic dementia; irrational and bizarre behaviour; an early case of homophobia?

More sinister than doctors with physical deformities are those with sociopathic behaviour problems, especially if their aberrations are well encapsulated. Bellaman's *King's Row*[63,64] contains descriptions of two such characters. Dr Alexander Tower, a physician without patients, appears merely eccentric to the citizens of King's Row. However, after Tower kills himself and his daughter in a murder suicide, he turns out to have been an incestuous child molester who 'fed on the bitterness of his own solitude and who consoled himself with assurances of his own superiority'.[63]

Unlike Dr Tower, Dr Henry Gordon, also of *King's Row*,[64] is a highly respected surgeon with a large and lucrative practice. After his death, Gordon is unmasked as a sadist and a religious fanatic who regards himself as an avenging angel in the service of the Lord, and who uses his scalpel to punish individuals whom he and his wife consider immoral.

> Sadism was common enough in many forms, but sadism coupled with religious fanaticism was particularly dangerous. Such a person with a surgeon's knife in his hands. . . . Ludie Sims [was] a pretty, flighty quasi-prostitute – a subject of town talk. And then . . . a disfiguring operation. Facial paralysis. What kind of operation had that been . . . and for what?[64]

Söderberg's Dr Tyko Glas,[65] 'a shining light at school' who enters university at the extraordinary age of 15, suddenly loses interest in further studies when he is only 23.

'I was tired. I felt no desire to specialize further. All I wanted was to earn my daily bread.'[66] Dr Glas, who considers himself 'a careful and conscientious doctor',[66] is not simply a case of the early 'burnout' syndrome. Some of his notions are so bizarre that they disqualify him from any form of medicine that requires contact with patients. (*See also* pp. 114–15.)

> A pregnant woman is a frightful object.* A newborn child is loathsome. A deathbed rarely makes so horrible an impression as childbirth, that terrible symphony of screams and filth and blood.[68] [Worst of all is the sexual act.] Why must the life of our species be preserved . . . by means of an organ we use several times a day as a drain for impurities? Why couldn't it be done by means of some act composed of dignity and beauty?[69] [Dr Glas worries that] people would not have so much confidence in me if they knew how badly I sleep at nights.[66]

His patients might have had even less confidence in him if they knew the nature of his nocturnal ruminations. It comes as no surprise that 'life passes by' this perverted voyeur, who can only become aroused by women with lovers. Such women, of course, are not interested in him.[66] Glas' total rejection of the value of human life[68] and his contempt for right and wrong lead him to murder Pastor Gregorius, one of his patients. Gregorius is middle-aged and ugly, and his sexual attentions have become obnoxious to his wife. The pastor is compared to a spider, and the wife, who has acquired a lover, to a 'beautiful little insect with shimmering golden wings.' The doctor poisons Gregorius 'for I do not believe it is forbidden to kill spiders.'[68]

Dr Glas, victim of physical and possibly sexual abuse,[70] a depressive and lonely creature,[68] bored by his work, disgusted by the act of copulation and its results, is obviously unfit for any kind of clinical activity. Yet even this character is portrayed sympathetically, and the reader feels scarcely any revulsion when the doctor deceives, mistreats and finally murders the unsuspecting cleric, 'cut[ting] off the rotten flesh which is spoiling the healthy.'[68]

Taylor Caldwell's Dr Claude Brinkerman,[71] like Bellaman's Dr Henry Gordon,[64] is a surgical psychopath who uses his scalpel to revenge himself on the world. Brinkerman hates 'women and their functions. . . . To him, . . . all pretty young women [are] secret whores',[71] and he takes great pleasure in tormenting them in his examination rooms. He also enjoys performing 'punitive' hysterectomies. When he terminates the pregnancy of the estranged wife of a colleague, the procedure ends in her death, not because of his incompetence but because he behaves like a 'savage madman' in the operating room, deliberately perforating the uterus in several places and lacerating the vagina.[72]

Richardson's *The Fortunes of Richard Mahony*,[73] arguably the best-known Australian novel, describes in harrowing detail the mental and physical decline and finally the death of an expatriate Irish physician. At the beginning of the story Dr Mahony is portrayed as a competent doctor, although always a fussy individual with a 'wayward, vagrant' disposition. Inappropriately idealistic, he displays an exaggerated sense of what constitutes gentlemanly behaviour,[74] he acquires and rapidly discards new gadgets, and he is totally unable to accept criticism. Mahony has an unfortunate inclination to make hasty decisions, many of them clearly

---

* This idea was also expressed by St Jerome, who wrote 'Women big with child are a revolting sight.'[67] It should be said in St Jerome's defense that he was not trying to practise medicine.

disastrous and against the advice of Mary, his loyal and practical wife, whom he blames for 'never . . . understand[ing] things.'[74] He drifts in and out of medicine several times and sets up practice in half a dozen localities in Australia and England.

Unfortunately for Mahony and his family, and fortunately for his patients, his eccentricities make him unpopular long before symptoms of his illness* become apparent. In 'Buddlecombe', England, the locals prefer Dr Robinson drunk to Richard Mahony sober.[74] Robinson has 'the right admixture of joviality and reserve to [hide] his failings', whereas Mahony 'grimly cogitating . . . prepared in advance for further snubs and slights, going about with his chin in the air, looking to the last degree stiff and unapproachable.'[74] In 'Barambogie', Australia, where Mahony is totally alienated from the local community, his practice disintegrates completely.[76] By this time his judgement is so impaired that instead of reprimanding his house-keeper for forgetting to tell him 'the names of those who had called while he was absent' (there had been no callers), he gives her a lecture on the disgraceful state of her teeth. When after three weeks of total inactivity he is summoned to bandage the stationmaster's foot, he 'found himself unable to articulate.'[76] In one of the book's most poignant scenes, little Cuthbert Mahony witnesses his father's slow deterioration, from physician to sick physician, to a sick and querulous patient. 'Papa cried and cried . . . he could hear him through the surgery door.[76] . . . [He] didn't like to be with Papa since he couldn't speak right; when you heard him say a spoon and he meant a chair, it made you feel sick inside.'[77] Mahony becomes a danger to himself and his family, and within a few months of mistreating a fractured femur, he has to be placed in an institution.*[78]

Duhamel's Dr Coupé,[79] chief of surgery at a French military hospital, disintegrates in less than 12 months, under the stresses of old age, a gruelling work schedule and army politics. In his prime, Coupé holds hospital and academic appointments,[80] and although always a little eccentric, he is regarded as a competent, likeable and shrewd surgeon ('vieux chirurgien madré'[79]) – shrewd enough, at any rate, to decline the good offices of his surgical colleagues who want to remove his prostate. 'He liked people and he liked his profession.'[81] During the terrible days of August 1914, Coupé, aged 65 at the time, is brought out of retirement.

His frustrations with the military bureaucracy become focused on the hospital superintendent, an old veteran like himself, whom he comes to regard not as the purveyor of bad tidings from Army Headquarters, but as the enemy. He bombards the superintendent with a stream of dispatches requesting permission in writing to perform even the most minor procedures. He threatens that he will ask for written permission to visit the latrine every time he needs to empty his bladder ('Je jure bien . . . de n'aller même plus pisser sans réclamer une autorisation écrite'[80]). In order to frighten 'a certain person' (the 'evil' superintendent[82]), Coupé applies for a transfer to Gallipoli, and when his request is unexpectedly granted he starts rambling about a new crusade and the need to reconquer Constantinople.[82] Despite his paranoia, Coupé does not achieve martyrdom fighting against the infidels. He becomes ill at Gallipoli and is shipped back to France, but instead of being allowed to die peacefully in his own bed, or at least in the bed of his mistress, he dies in a monastery cell on the way home.

---

* The account of Richard Mahony's decline is based on the life of Dr Walter Richardson, the author's father. Walter Richardson was believed to have suffered from neurosyphilis,[75] a diagnosis which, by modern criteria, must be regarded as highly suspect.

The erratic behaviour of Ravin's Dr Thomas McIlheny, chief of surgery at 'St George University Hospital',[83] leads to the establishment of a committee of inquiry but not to his suspension. McIlheny, 'the best chief resident . . . ever seen at Mass. General',[84] and author of a surgical textbook, has invented 'more procedures than half the guys on the staff [are able to perform]', though his colleagues suspect that he is 'better with the pen than the knife.'[85] Outside the operating room McIlheny seems an intelligent and decent man.[84]

During operations, McIlheny is prone to develop a particularly sinister form of 'OR rage' that turns him into an aggressive and dangerous monster. His behaviour involves more than the usual surge of high-handedness, such as throwing instruments around the operating room,[86] abusing the nursing staff[87] or threatening residents with dismissal.[88] McIlheny commits all of these misdemeanours,[89,90] but in addition he makes abrupt, irrational and life-threatening decisions.[91] Subordinates who advise a more cautious approach are treated as traitors and saboteurs. '"Can't do surgery without someone spying on you", he muttered.' On one particular occasion he has to be treated like a dangerous lunatic who is holding hostages and who can only be induced to release his captives by a mixture of flattery and threats.

McIlheny's surgical career, which begins brilliantly but then deteriorates disastrously, does not come to an abrupt end. When he dismisses an untenured associate professor for 'insubordination',[91] the university sets up a committee of enquiry which fully catalogues McIlheny's surgical misdeeds. The committee recommends the associate professor's reinstatement, but

> McIlheny stayed on as chief of surgery for another year. He still operated most days, but then they made him a provost of the university and gave him some post in the medical school [so that] he had less and less time for surgery and more and more committee meetings to attend.[92]

Compared with Tyco Glas[65,66,68-70] and Thomas McIlheny,[83-85,89-92] Graham Greene's Dr Crombie[93] seems a harmless eccentric with curious views about the association between sexual activities and cancer. He writes long articles for the *Lancet* and the *British Medical Journal*, which are never published. Unfortunately, Crombie's knowledge of medicine is so inadequate, even when it concerns his chosen subject of sexual purity, that when one of the senior-school students develops painful testicles after a sexual encounter with a street prostitute, Dr Crombie diagnoses 'acidity' and advises avoidance of tomatoes. After Dr Crombie resigns from his school position (at the request of the governors), 'his practice was reduced to a few old people almost as eccentric as himself.'[93] (*See also* Volume 1, p. 161.)

A brilliant account of medical impairment is provided by Andrew Miller in *Ingenious Pain*.[94] The miraculous transformation that turns the uncaring but highly competent Dr James Dyer into a compassionate individual who is now capable of comforting sufferers, also brings about the loss of his sanity and his surgical skills (*see* p. 23). In the memorable venesection scene,[95] Dyer not only mismanages the procedure, but also violates some elementary rules of medical behaviour.

The Reverend Julius Lestrade, who has himself 'bled' on a regular basis (the year is 1771),[96] asks Dyer to use a temporal rather than an antecubital vein. Initially the doctor objects but, unlike his former self, he is no longer firm with his advice, and when Lestrade insists, he tries to comply. He accidentally opens an artery rather than a vein, and a torrential haemorrhage results. At this point Dyer behaves like a schoolboy who has injured a friend – he runs away. When he finally returns, he manages to stop the bleeding, but he then sits down next to the clergyman 'sobbing like a child.'[95] The Reverend is in no doubt about the meaning of Dyer's behaviour: 'Finished as a doctor, of course.'[97]

Weir Mitchell's Dr Ezra Wendell[98–111] constitutes a special case. Wendell does not suffer from any overt physical or psychiatric handicap. He is intelligent,[95] extremely good-looking[100] and fond of poetry.[101] However, his 'defects of character'[101] are so severe that his rapid decline is almost predictable: 'He was designed by nature to illustrate . . . the certainty of failure.'[102]

His 'first failure was as a teacher',[101] presumably because of his inability to maintain discipline in the classroom, although there are other possibilities. He then studies medicine and sets up as a 'practicing physician' in his home town, but 'the experiment failed.' The reasons for Wendell's failure are not stated but, judging from subsequent events, his inability to inspire confidence among his patients[102] is due to lack of forcefulness rather than lack of skill. A brief army career during the American Civil War ends abruptly and ignominiously when he leaves a group of wounded soldiers to their fate in the face of 'heavy fire.'[103] Subsequently Wendell seems to flourish for a brief period in Philadelphia, but then once again his practice falls apart.[104] At the end of the story, this medical loser leaves hurriedly for 'the West',[105] barely escaping criminal charges for manslaughter[106] and financial peculation.[102,107] Just before his departure he takes 'a good deal of opium.'[105]

The modern reader who scrutinizes *In War Time* finds it difficult to understand what exactly is lacking in Wendell and what it is that makes Weir Mitchell declare 'he should never have been a doctor.'[100] Wendell may lack the courage to attend to the wounded under enemy fire,[103] but he is sufficiently brave to visit a farmhouse where four members of a family are suffering from smallpox.[104]

What we hear from one of his disgruntled patients hardly reflects adversely on Dr Wendell. He has been summoned to examine young Sarah Grace, who is suffering from the after-effects of 'much furtive ingestion of bon-bons.'[100] Sarah's mother, who holds strong views on many subjects, considers it is 'all liver and malaria.'[104] Wendell does not openly disagree with Mrs Grace's 'diagnosis.' Instead, 'he . . . advised her impassive and sallow daughter to eat less and walk more and he prescribed some of the mild remedies which neither help nor hurt.'[102]

A few weeks later he is told that his services are no longer required. 'He never was of much account about liver', remarks Mrs Grace, a malicious busybody,[108] to her friends on the Orphans' Aid Committee. Mitchell does not explain why Mrs Grace finds Wendell inadequate as a doctor, although it is likely that his friendship with Alice Westerley, a wealthy widow, is resented.[102]

Another manifestation of Wendell's 'mental unstableness' consists of 'too frequent changes of opinion.'[102] As every medical student is aware, diagnoses are not fixed and immutable, even with all the technical aids available in the twenty-first century. 'Firm' opinions would have been almost impossible to justify in 1865. So what is wrong with Dr Wendell?

One is forced to conclude that Mitchell is describing a homosexual who is held in contempt not because of his activities in the bedroom (there may not be any such activities), but because he displays the stereotyped characteristics commonly attributed to this group. Wendell looks effeminate. His mouth is 'too regular for manly beauty.'[109] He carries a 'sun-umbrella' to protect his skin, much to the amusement of two sunburnt soldiers.[109] He is also moody and 'sensitive to all reproof.'[109]

> He was always planning some valuable research but was never energetic enough to overcome the incessant obstacles which make research so difficult.[109] . . . He was naturally a refined and . . . sensitive man, . . . he liked sympathy and as is common with such natures, women pleased him more than men; nor indeed was he well fitted on account of his self-regard and his girl-like tenderness to contract strong and virile attachments to men.[100]

Wendell performs particularly badly when young Edward Morton, who suffers from progressive weakness of his legs, questions him about the prognosis (*see* Volume 1, pp. 126–7).

> Had he been a true woman he would have been touched by the manliness and moral courage of the young fellow's questions. Had he been a more masculine man he would have met them with sympathetic appreciation.[110]

The word 'homosexuality' does not occur in *In War Time*, and the term 'homophobia' did not exist in 1885. However, Mitchell clearly describes (with considerable distaste) a doctor whom he considers to be impaired on account of his lack of manliness. Far from recognizing that such a 'refined and sensitive man' may be particularly suited to looking after certain types of patients, Mitchell becomes moralistic and blames the doctor's 'weakness' for his financial irregularities,[102] his attempts to cover up his fatal mistakes[111] and his drug addiction.[105]

Drug abuse

Unlike medical sadists[64,71,72] and physicians with organic dementia,[73] who are rare both in real life and in literature, doctors suffering from drug or alcohol abuse are common. In general, writers treat addicted doctors with a great deal of sympathy.

Arthur Hailey's Dr Noah Townsend,[112] chief of medicine at St Bede's Hospital, a 'seasoned, experienced' and conscientious internist with a 'courtly and dignified' manner, has become addicted to a cocktail of stimulant and sedative drugs.[113] An attempt to notify the relevant authorities fails (*see* 'Whistle-blowing', pp. 223–5), and Townsend is left to his own devices.[114] Almost five years later, under the influence of sedative drugs, Townsend inappropriately orders penicillin for a patient with a known penicillin allergy, and then tries to cover up his mistake by attributing the patient's death to 'heart failure.'[115] When Townsend's hospital privileges are withdrawn he becomes violent and incoherent and has to be admitted to a psychiatric institution forthwith.[116] The incident is hushed up and there are no manslaughter charges or claims for damages.[117]

Despite Townsend's direct responsibility for a patient's death, Hailey portrays him as a victim rather than a culprit. The patient who dies as a result of Townsend's negligence is categorized as an 'insignificant loser.'[115] The doctor's colleagues, who have done nothing to help, dump him unceremoniously despite the fact that he has given decades of loyal service to the hospital. The drug detailers, representatives of the 'evil' pharmaceutical companies, keep supplying him with pills even though they are aware of his addiction.[118] Instead of anger and frustration, the reader feels pity for the flawed doctor.

By contrast, Raymond Chandler, who regards the entire medical profession with amused contempt,[119] treats medical drug addicts as pests. Several of them are portrayed as drug pushers as well as drug takers.[120–124]

> In our town quacks breed like guinea pigs. . . . Some are prosperous and some poor, some ethical, others not sure they can afford it. A well-heeled patient with incipient DT's could be money from home to plenty of old geezers who have fallen behind in the vitamin and antibiotic trade.[120]

One of Chandler's drug addicts, Dr Lester Vukanich, ostensibly an Ear, Nose and Throat man, practises on the outer fringes of the medical profession.

> Not too skilful, not too clean, not too much on the ball, three dollars and please pay the nurse[121] . . . [Vukanich] specialize[s] in chronic sinus infections. Rather a neat routine. You go in and complain of a sinus headache and he washes out your antrums for you. First, of course, he has to anesthetize you with Novocain. But if he likes your looks, it don't have to be Novocain. Catch?[122]

Dr Vukanich gives himself intravenous morphine injections between patients,[123] but his clinical judgement is still sufficiently intact for him to recognize that Philip Marlowe's headaches are not due to sinus troubles.[123] Dr Albert Almore in Chandler's *The Lady in the Lake*,[124] another drug pedlar with a medical degree, also elicits disgust rather than sympathy in the reader.

Bulgakov's Dr Sergei Polyakov,[125] a recent medical graduate, receives his first morphine injection (to help him over a bout of biliary colic) on 15 February 1917. Within days he is addicted, and within a year he kills himself. He leaves a diary describing his initial euphoria, his withdrawal symptoms and his lack of sterile techniques (which causes the formation of multiple abscesses). Polyakov claims that his addiction does not interfere with his work as a physician in a remote Russian town, but he is wrong. Despite his assertion that 'I am incapable of inflicting harm . . . on a single one of my patients', Polyakov would cheerfully steal their belongings or their drugs in order to obtain 'those life-giving crystals.'[125] A Moscow psychiatrist who regards him with a mixture of pity and contempt feels tempted to report him to the medical licensing authorities, but desists because of a sense of collegiality.

The hero of Palmer's *Miracle Cure*,[126] Dr Brian Holbrook, is something of an exception. Despite his long-term addiction to opiates, he has managed not only to rehabilitate himself but also to retain his diagnostic[127] and procedural[128] skills. However, Holbrook's impressive talents fail to transform his behaviour from the enthusiastic involvement of a young resident to the compassionate detachment of a mature physician. Instead of evaluating a new drug dispassionately, he becomes so excited that he steals some of the material to inject into his father.[129] When it turns out that the 'miracle cure' is not only worthless[130] but also dangerous,[131] he embarks on a one-man crusade to expose the conspirators who allowed the drug to go to clinical trials. Holbrook, a reformed drug addict, gifted footballer,[132] devoted son and brilliant but unconventional cardiologist, is able to solve the conspiracy that his more mature colleagues either ignore or condone.

The alcoholic doctor: his background, his activities and his ability to cope

The catalogue of alcoholic doctors in fictional literature seems never-ending,[133–193] although the effects of alcohol addiction vary widely from case to case. Some medical drunkards (all of them male) have given up practice altogether, and spend their time quenching their thirst and engaging in non-medical pursuits. Others, although unkempt, still have a few supporters, especially in areas where there are no competitors.[133] Members of a third group retain considerable clinical skills, and function effectively and even skilfully between drinking bouts.

Nineteenth-century fictional doctors with drinking problems include Kingsley's Dr Heale,[133] with his 'shaky hand' and his filthy 'surgery' or in plain English, 'shop', who is held in contempt by the inhabitants of the small English coastal town where he works. In emergencies he has to be 'stirred out of his boozy slumbers and thrust into his clothes.' Fortunately for Heale, the absence of a 'rival in the field' has so far prevented the total disintegration of his practice.[133]

Chellis's *The Old Doctor's Son*[134] is a simplistic temperance tale which, like other stories of this genre, blames moral turpitude and 'the demon rum' for most of the ills of mankind. Howard Foster, who smokes and drinks at 18, is well on his way to perdition at the age of 25 when, under the beneficent influence of his future wife, he concludes that he has already 'wasted too much time.'[135] He decides to follow the family tradition, he studies medicine, he actually graduates and he practises for a while. Regrettably, his clinical activities do not protect him from resuming his sinful habits.[136] One particular afternoon, when Dr Foster has retired to his office after dinner with 'a bottle of wine and a stand of cigars', Skye James comes in with a broken finger. Dr Foster's 'first impulse had been to send this boy to another surgeon', but he is evidently still sufficiently sober to deal with the situation: 'The bruised hand with its broken finger was properly dressed and directions given for its further treatment.' James is the antithesis of the alcoholic doctor. Sober and hard working, he moves up the social scale while Dr Foster, together with his family, move down. The doctor 'beggared himself to gratify a drunkard's insatiable thirst', his habits 'drove away his remaining few patients' and his son declares at the end 'Papa ain't a doctor now.'[137]

As a rule, alcoholic doctors are portrayed as flawed heroes rather than as repulsive town drunks, medical incompetents or moralistic object lessons. One of the medical characters in Havard's *Coming of Age*[138] actually expresses the view that alcohol poses particular dangers to kind-hearted physicians.

> It's the passionate ones who become the drinkers. . . . They say it can happen to anyone, but you don't see it in cold-hearted skinflints, do you? It's as if alcoholism only thrives in the warmth. The pity is that by the time they have become recognized drinkers they have made such an awful nuisance of themselves that people forget what they used to be like.[138]

Francis Brett Young uses the same theme in *My Brother Jonathan*.[139] Dr John Hammond, an untidy, disorganized alcoholic with a chaotic lifestyle, a dysfunctional family (*see* p. 20) and an inability to understand accounts, is portrayed, despite his multiple blemishes, as a kind and honest man who becomes a victim of the machinations of his competent and precise former partner, Dr Charles Craig. Craig, 'energetic, sober, good looking'[140] and no doubt Hammond's professional superior, is revealed as a 'cold, systematic devil'[155] with a 'commanding if sinister personality . . . [and a] capacity for intrigue.'[140] Hammond, like 'Doc Rivers' of New Jersey[142] (*see* p. 218), is trusted by the poor people of Wednesford whether 'drunk or sober', while the more discerning inhabitants of the 'high-class residential neighbourhoods', who are impressed by Craig's 'studied reticence', would not allow Dr Hammond to come anywhere near them.[140]

Reed,[143] like Havard,[138] portrays a doctor whose kind-heartedness is held responsible for his alcoholism and, like Havard,[138] suggests that excessive compassion drives a doctor 'to drink', whereas his hard-hearted colleagues are able to 'detach'[144] and to witness suffering without damage to their own personalities. Reed's Dr Jack Galvin[143] practises

> during the great depression. Not like the country club doctors nowadays. . . . A family doctor. A humble man who made house calls and had no head for business. . . . Somewhere along the way [Galvin's] stamina broke . . . Jack Galvin was too sensitive or too weak. [His son] Frank could never decide which. . . . [He] worried excessively about his patients, particularly those who failed to improve.[143] . . . They came to him, the new patients with their pleading eyes and it became exhausting to lie. A young child would die for no apparent reason and all the medicine . . . seemed a waste. At night he lay in bed, terrified of sleep. Each time he closed his eyes the dead patients would come to visit him. . . . Nothing grotesque. Not accusingly. Just persistently. . . . He started drinking gin to get to sleep. . . . He forgot about office hours. He would start out on a house call and never get there. Colleagues began whispering about his 'problem.' He went from gin to cheap wine and finally straight medicinal alcohol. In the end he was shooting up with Demerol and morphine. They found Dr Galvin one dreary morning in a mud-splattered hallway. . . . [He] was thirty-six years old when he died.[143]

In one of the greatest novels of the twentieth century,[145] Scott Fitzgerald tells the story of the decline of a talented, generous and lovable doctor. Dr Richard Diver, a brilliant young psychiatrist, succumbs to the emotional, physical and financial attractions of a schizophrenic patient (Nicole Warren) and, despite dire warnings from colleagues,[146] goes on to marry her and devote his life to keeping her out of institutions (*see* pp. 21–2). Surprisingly, for the best part of six years he succeeds by leading a life of 'rigid domesticity',[147] but in the meantime the manuscript of his major work gathers dust.[147] As time passes, he becomes physically and emotionally less competent to deal with the periodic exacerbations of Nicole's illness when she develops murderous tendencies.[148] The intolerable domestic tensions dissipate Richard's strength. Formerly possessed of 'inexhaustible energy' and 'incapable of fatigue',[149] this potentially great psychiatrist is transformed into a heavy drinker who loses his ability to remain in control and whose professional career vanishes as a result. In the end he tries to work as a general practitioner in a small town in upstate New York, but 'he became entangled with a girl who worked in a grocery store and he was also involved in a lawsuit about some medical question.'[150] Nicole's family blames Richard for the marital breakdown and spreads the rumour that she 'had thrown herself away on a dissipated doctor'[151] who married her for her money. This malicious slander only reinforces the reader's perception of Richard Diver as a tragic hero.

Most writers present medical alcoholics in their fully developed state rather than during their period of deterioration. Remarkably, even severely impaired characters retain traces of medical behaviour patterns. For instance, Sherwood Anderson's 'unclean' Dr Parcival,[152] whose arrival in a bar is likely to disperse the other patrons, still dabbles in medicine (*see* p. 194).

> Doctor Parcival . . . came from Chicago and when he arrived he was drunk and got into a fight [which] ended by the doctor being escorted to the village lockup. When he was released he rented a room above a shoe-repairing shop at the lower end of Main Street and put out a sign that announced himself as a doctor. . . . He had but few patients.[152]

Parcival, who considers himself a philosopher, is preparing a book 'that may never get written.' It contains the central message (which is also enunciated to any drinking companion willing to listen) that 'everyone in the world is Christ and they are all crucified.'[152]

Other deteriorated alcoholic doctors with vestigial medical employment include several of Chekhov's characters[153–155] (*see* p. 185) and Simenon's Dr Vallabron,[156] who 'spent a good deal of time playing cards in cafés and . . . was slovenly in his appearance.'

Dr Relling in Ibsen's *The Wild Duck*,[157] although not exactly a hero, is the least repulsive male character in the play. Relling formerly practised medicine in a small country town, but now leads a life of idleness and drunkenness in company with his room-mate, a seminary drop-out.[158] Despite his alcoholism, Relling retains some medical traits and he stands out for his common sense among the inhabitants of the Ekdal household, who seem determined to destroy each other. He tries to stop Gregers Werle, a compulsive and thoughtless 'do-gooder', from enlightening Hedvig Ekdal (a 15-year-old girl) about her true ancestry.[159] He encourages Hedvig's non-biological father to invent a new photographic technique even though he is fully aware of Ekdal's limitations.[160] Relling, who has no time for 'purifying' truths ('one can get through life in a wig'[161]), recognizes that Ekdal, with his limited intellect and his ridiculous posturing, will never have an original thought in his head. However, the 'idea of an invention' provides a little happiness both for this weak and selfish man and for his innocent child.[160] When the tragedy occurs, Relling's medical training enables him to recognize that Hedvig has killed herself,[162] and he predicts that her self-centred fool of a father will continue to behave like a pretentious buffoon. He hisses at his sentimental ecclesiastical drinking companion 'Shut up, you fool; you're drunk.'[162]

Ellen Glasgow's Dr Jason Greylock,[163] medical drunkard and son of a medical drunkard,[164] epitome of the ineffectual, whining male[165] in an early feminist novel is a considerably less attractive character than Dr Relling.[157] Naturally, his patients soon abandon him in favour of the town's other doctor, a physically repulsive but hard-working and dependable individual.[166] Dr Greylock spends his life complaining and drinking, although we see him practising medicine reasonably competently at various stages of his career.

Young Dr Greylock's clinical experience enables him to predict the fatal outcome of Rose Emily Pedlar's pulmonary tuberculosis[167] and to treat her 'correctly' (with fresh air) according to the medical notions of the time. When the patient protests that old Dr Greylock had advised her to stay in her room, Greylock Junior has sufficient common sense to account for the conflicting advice: 'My father was good in his generation, but he belongs to the old school.'[167] Rose Emily is told, untruthfully, that she will be 'up and out before summer', and she allows herself to be deluded (*see also* p. 119). The Pedlars' confidence in Dr Greylock's ability is not unbounded. When he proposes to operate on their baby's club foot (? echoes of Charles Bovary), they decline, fearing that an operation 'may make it worse.'[168] In his later years, 'people said he was still a good doctor when he has his senses about him. The pity was that he was often too drunk to know what he was doing.'[169] Greylock redeems himself to some extent on his deathbed (*see* pp. 232–3).

Some alcoholic doctors, such as 'Ravic' in Remarque's *Arch of Triumph*[61] (*see* pp. 207–8) and Philip Denny in Cronin's *The Citadel*,[170] not only retain their professional skills[171] but are also more competent than their abstemious colleagues. Denny, one of the few likeable medical characters in *The Citadel*,[170] is completely free from hypocrisy. He is not particularly interested in money and he remains a superb surgeon (when sober). Indeed, it is a reformed Denny who assists Dr Andrew Manson in his rehabilitation from a miserable 'Harley Street' charlatan to an honest physician[172] (*see also* p. 181).

Dr Hugh McGuire, the surgeon in Thomas Wolfe's *Look Homeward Angel*,[173] is well on the way to becoming an alcoholic derelict.[174] Unshaven and unwashed, he is treated with contempt by the young men of 'Altamont.' 'By God, if you ever cut me open, McGuire', said Ben [Gant, aged 20], 'I'm going to be damned sure you can walk straight before you do.'[174] Despite his alcoholism, McGuire is still consulted by the other doctors in the town when difficult operations have to be performed (*see* p. 150), and he still has some loyal admirers among the townsfolk. Joe, who works behind the counter of the 'Uneeda Lunch' establishment, regards McGuire as a magician who performs better drunk than sober: 'He ain't worth a damn until he's got a quart of corn liquor under his belt. Give him a few drinks and he'll cut off your damn head and put it on again without your knowing it.'[174]

A relatively recent addition to the series of alcoholic doctors is Dr Thomas More, the psychiatrist and principal character in Percy's *The Thanatos Syndrome*.[175] More has just been released from jail, where he spent two years for writing illegal prescriptions (*see* pp. 127–8). He describes himself as an 'addled' old drunk,[176] barely fit to practise orthodox psychiatry, but events prove otherwise. He is a shrewd observer of society in general, the local Louisiana community in particular and psychiatric patients most of all. When a provisional licence to practise is issued to him, More teams up with an alcoholic priest, and the two of them 'look after' terminal AIDS patients.[176] They try to relieve the anguish of the 'haggard young men' in the hospice for the dying by simply chatting to them as equals, and in this setting Dr More, the impaired psychiatrist, is perceived as more useful than unimpaired interventionists.

Some fictional medical inebriates appear to regard their chronic alcohol intake as one of their hobbies. They continue to practise, but somehow avoid doing harm to patients. William Carlos Williams' *Old Doc Rivers*,[142] despite his addiction to a variety of substances including alcohol, is regarded as a genius by his patients, who consider him superior to other medical practitioners regardless of his blood alcohol levels. This category also includes Chevallier's Dr Mouraille,[177] who has been a heavy drinker since his university days. The citizens of *Clochemerle* do not idolize

Dr Mouraille, who cannot even diagnose the cause of an old woman's constipation, but despite the doctor's obvious failings, no serious debacles occur on his watch.

Sinclair Lewis's Doc Vickerson[178] (Martin Arrowsmith's negative role model) and Robertson Davies's Dr Ogg[179,180] of 'Sioux Lookout', Northern Ontario* (Jonathan Hullah's early mentor), both of whom are habitual drunkards, also seem to avoid major catastrophes. Dr Ogg's medical bootlegging activities during the Prohibition period are described in a spirit of tolerant disapproval rather than fierce condemnation.

> Dr Ogg was not an ornament of the medical profession and he was rarely called to our house except in extreme emergencies. Dr Ogg was a drunk and a failure. His wife had run away long ago to pursue a life of shame in Winnipeg, which must certainly have been more lively than life with Dr Ogg. Since her departure the doctor had declined into dirt and moral squalor. His livelihood was earned chiefly by writing prescriptions for bottles of gin, whisky and brandy required regularly by the few hundred citizens of the village for ailments that Dr Ogg identified. This was an era when the sale of intoxicating liquor was forbidden by law in Canada but a qualified physician could prescribe them when they were imperatively needed, and qualified physicians regularly did so, though rarely on the scale of Dr Ogg. As there was no pharmacy in the village, he kept the stocks in his own professional premises and thus had the advantage of being able to sell them at his own prices. He was in fact a bootlegger raggedly cloaked in a physician's gown, but when there was an emergency it was remembered that he was also a doctor.[179]

After recovering from scarlet fever Jonathan Hullah develops an interest in medical matters (*see* Volume 3) and attaches himself to Dr Ogg.

> It did not take me long to discover that the Doc did not really know very much and had not added anything to his knowledge since he received his degree. That degree from the University of Toronto was attested to by a framed certificate which hung, always crooked, on his office wall.[180]

Subsequently, when Hullah himself attends medical school at the University of Toronto, he discovers that Dr Ogg, even in his student days, had not been an academic achiever. But, despite his drunkenness and his ignorance, Dr Ogg teaches the future Dr Hullah the most important principles of medical practice:

> I must not be ungrateful to the Doc. I cannot say that he taught me pharmacy because he was himself too shaky-handed and slovenly to mix anything with real accuracy, but he showed me how to teach myself a few of the elements of it. He made it possible for me to look at sick people professionally and without either pity or contempt.[180]

Scott Fitzgerald's Dr Forrest Janney[181] of 'Bending', Alabama, is also treated convincingly but sympathetically. Janney, aged 45, was formerly a source of pride to his poor relatives. 'One of the bess [*sic*] surgeons up in Montgomery, yes, suh.' Unfortunately, the doctor 'had committed professional suicide by taking to cynicism

---

* In the study by Talbott *et al.*,[4] family physicians practising in professional and geographical isolation were over-represented among substance abusers.

and drink.' He retains enough insight to evaluate his proficiency and his emotional state, and he admits 'I am thoroughly anesthetized the greater part of the day [but] I only undertake work that I know I can do when I'm in that condition.' He also acknowledges that as his compassion for his fellow-drunks and for mankind in general has intensified, his professional competence has declined.

> My pity no longer has direction, but fixes itself on whatever is at hand . . .
> I have become an exceptionally good fellow – much more so than when I
> was a good doctor.

The objects of the lonely doctor's affections are eight-year-old Helen Kilrain, an orphan whom he thinks he might adopt, and 17-year-old Mary Decker, whom he 'loves' in an asexual way until she runs away with one of his nephews.[181] This worthless character is subsequently brought into the local hospital after being shot in the head, but Dr Janney refuses to treat him: 'My decisions are not reliable, and if anything went wrong it would seem to be my fault.' However, when a disastrous hurricane makes communications with larger centres impossible, he changes his mind and, fortified by corn whisky, decides to remove a bullet from his nephew's brain under local anaesthesia. The patient dies.[181]

Full rehabilitation of impaired physicians, once they have been identified as such, is rare. Arthur Miller's Dr Walter Franz returns to practice as an 'important scientist' despite his mental breakdown, which is recognized during a murderous attack on his wife (*see* p. 34).[182] Cronin's Philip Denny[171,172] manages to stop drinking and join a group practice in a small English town (*see* p. 218). By contrast, Dr Paddy Rice's spectacular attempt to restore his reputation fails completely, and he continues his life as a drunken drifter.[183]

Dr Rice, the eye surgeon in Brian Friel's *Molly Sweeney*,[183] constitutes an exceptional case of impairment because he starts off at the pinnacle of the profession. At the age of 31, a meteor on the ophthalmological horizon, Rice has already worked in some of the best eye hospitals in the world and leads the frenzied lifestyle of an internationally acclaimed medical academic: 'Work. Airports. Dinners. Laughter. Operating theatres. Conferences. Gossip. Publications. The professional jealousies and the necessary vigilance. The relentless devouring excitement.'[183] Rice not only jets around the conference circuit ('Oslo last month, Helsinki next week, Paris the week after'), but is also summoned to various parts of the globe to operate on the rich and powerful. His Icarus-like ascent comes to an abrupt end when his beautiful and glamorous wife leaves him for one of his colleagues, after which his life 'no longer cohered.' He abandons medicine altogether for some years, working as a labourer in Bolivia, then running a pub in Glasgow, and finally returning to work at a fourth-rate provincial hospital in County Donegal. By this time he is an established drunkard.

Despite considerable misgivings, Dr Rice performs a lens extraction on Molly Sweeney, who has been blind for 40 years. His motives are complex. Naturally he hopes to restore her sight but, in addition, he sees a successful operation as a means of rescuing his own career. Surprisingly, there is no surgical catastrophe, even though Rice sits up the night before the operation imbibing considerable quantities of whisky. However, his attempt to imitate Christ in restoring sight to the blind (he actually quotes the relevant biblical passage) ends in disaster. Molly, who had been blind but independent before the operation, now not only cannot see, but also becomes withdrawn and confused and has to be placed in a psychiatric institution.

Rice, conscious of his failure and his shortcomings, packs his bags and departs for an unknown destination.[183]

Some alcoholic physicians who continue working or return to work after an enforced vacation end up in 'sheltered workshops' such as sanatoria, hospices for the dying and government agencies where their opportunities for doing harm are relatively limited. In the days when abortions were illegal, many abortionists were drunkards.[184,185] Dr Gustin Sabayot in Céline's *Death on the Installment Plan*,[184] who is 'building up to . . . cirrhosis', is appointed to a municipal job soon after graduation, as a reward for performing 'a little abortion [on] a girlfriend of a city councilor. . . . It had come off smoothly, his hand hadn't begun to shake'.[184]

Dr Matthew O'Connor, the central figure among the freaks of Djuna Barnes' *Nightwood*,[186] has had to relocate from San Francisco to Paris because of his 'interest in gynecology.'[187] O'Connor, a highly talented but unstable, immature individual, a 'middle-aged medical student',[187] harangues his audiences at parties or in bars[188] on such diverse topics as the difference between legend and history, the Jews' sense of humour or the tattoos on a bear-fighter's genitalia. O'Connor has enough insight to realize that his alcoholism[188] and his secret transvestism[189] consign him to the category of the 'scorned and the ridiculous',[188] and he describes himself as 'an instrument that has lost its G-string.'[188] Naturally, O'Connor no longer has a licence to practise,[190] and although rumour has it that he still performs abortions,[189] it is doubtful whether he is mentally or physically fit even for this degraded form of medicine (*see also* p. 152).

A few medical alcoholics tend to become professional witnesses, presumably because the required bouts of sobriety are relatively brief.[191] These 'experts', who will testify to anything in court, are a constant source of worry to their employers in case their capacity for temporary abstinence has been overestimated. When Grisham's attorney Jake Brigance[192] is introduced to a key medical witness,

> the doctor was lying on his back with his shirt unbuttoned and his mouth wide open. He snored heavily with an unusual guttural gurgling sound. . . . A rancid vapor emanated with the snoring and hung like an invisible fog over the end of the porch. 'He's a doctor?' Jake asked, as he sat next to Lucien. 'Psychiatry', Lucien said proudly.[192]

Government departments (federal, state and local) are perceived to provide suitable employment for medical inebriates. Hailey's Dr Gideon Mace, who works for the Food and Drug Administration, is described as 'a failed doctor.' He did not like other doctors and 'he . . . didn't like his patients.'[193] Mace, an alcoholic in constant financial trouble because of his alimony commitments, supplements his meagre salary by moonlighting evenings and weekends in a private practice. He also engages in 'insider' share transactions, using confidential information acquired at the FDA, where he is hired because 'they have trouble getting anybody.'

> The agency contained many highly qualified dedicated professionals. But inevitably there were others. The unsuccessful, the soured and alienated, who preferred comparative solitude to meeting many people. The dedicated self-protectors, avoiding difficult decisions. Alcoholics. The unbalanced. Clearly . . . Dr Gideon Mace was one of these.[193]

Another alcoholic physician who finds refuge in a government job is described in Freedman's *Key Witness*.[194]

> The jailhouse doctor, a genial hack, made his rounds in the morning. He was a private physician who couldn't sustain a normal practice if it was handed to him on a silver platter, so he worked on contract to the city and various insurance companies, drank his lunch and was useless for the rest of the day.[194]

Kornbluth's Dr Bayard Kendrick Full[195] is essentially noble and redeemable even after he has reached the 'skid-row' stage. At the start of *The Little Black Bag*,[195] Dr Full sits 'in the filth of the alley' drinking cheap wine out of a broken bottle. He ignores a little girl who has cut herself on a piece of glass, because all he can think about is his next drink. Miraculously, Full, who had been expelled from the County Medical Association, finds a futuristic doctor's bag, which helps him to treat the little girl as well as numerous other patients. He gives up drinking, establishes a successful practice and retains or regains a sufficient degree of altruism to propose handing over the magic bag to the College of Surgeons.[195] Doctor Full's associate, 'Angie', who started life as a 'gaunt-faced, dirty blonde sloven' of the slums, has no such ideals. Her 'infancy had been spent on a sour and filthy mattress, [her] childhood had been play in the littered alley and [her] adolescence had been the sweatshops and the aimless gatherings at night under the glaring street lamps.' Doctor Full's 'love for humanity' has not been transmitted to Angie, who only wants to be rich and who ends up murdering the doctor.

Kornbluth does not hold the intelligence of doctors in very high esteem. They function well because a moron with a computer and other modern equipment is more efficient than an intelligent medieval physician who had 'to count on his fingers.' However, even moronic and drunken doctors retain some vestige of 'noblesse oblige', a sentiment which remains alien to Angie the 'guttersnipe'.[195]

Dooling's Dr Randolph Hiram Butz, like Friel's Dr Paddy Rice (*see* pp. 220–1), has an unusual background for a medical alcoholic.[196] Butz graduated from the Yale Medical School *magna cum laude*, and he is a co-author of a standard medical textbook which is still being updated every five years. Butz' alcoholism is severe. His short-term memory is non-existent, he confabulates incessantly, and he is totally and aggressively incoherent after lunch. The state medical licensing board has received numerous complaints against Butz, who is evidently facing deregistration although, amazingly, he still has admitting privileges at the University Medical Center where his problems and his patients are managed by the resident staff.

Despite his multiple failings, Butz is a more pleasant character than the cold chief of medicine who knows more clinical facts than anyone 'within five hundred miles',[197] but is totally devoid of sympathy towards his patients or his staff. One cannot help being amused by Butz attributing his lecherous behaviour (which results in a complaint of sexual harassment) to 'atypical priapism'[196] and by his thinly disguised racist remarks about an imaginary 'Leroy Washington' (who wants free medical care but refuses to mow Butz' lawn unless he gets paid). Most importantly, despite his addled brain and his simplistic approach, Butz retains the true physician's attitude towards any form of euthanasia, and warns young Dr Ernst against withholding treatment from dying patients.

> Butz appeared on the verge of apoplexy. 'You want to starve a man to death just because he might die soon? . . . Why should any of us eat? We're all gonna die!'[197]

Whistle-blowing:* the reaction of the relevant authorities

Attempts to notify the appropriate authorities that a particular doctor is no longer fit to practise usually result in a reprimand for the person lodging the complaint. The alleged offender immediately attains a degree of collegiate sympathy while the exposure of an incompetent or an alcoholic doctor is perceived as detrimental to the entire profession. When Dr Lucas Marsh, the idealistic young medical hero in *Not as a Stranger*,[198] reports Dr Alpheus Snider for gross incompetence, his suggestion that Dr Snider be deprived of his licence to practise is not well received. The Chairman of the County Medical Society, who knows all about Dr Snider's misdeeds, adopts a 'There but for the Grace of God' attitude and refuses to recommend the old man's suspension. Instead, he warns Luke against casting the first stone.

> Dr Snider is old. . . . (He) is not the doctor he once may have been . . . no man is perfect. . . . You have a long life ahead, Dr Marsh. Perhaps you have not yet made an honest mistake. Perhaps you have not yet in a moment of fatigue or tension or human weakness been careless. . . . The public has . . . faith in us and it is our duty to keep that faith whole.[198]

In *Nothing Lasts Forever*,[199] Sheldon describes a very similar scene.[200] Dr Arthur Kane, a particularly obnoxious and incompetent surgeon, has removed a patient's only normal kidney. Dr Paige Taylor, an enthusiastic surgical resident (and target of Kane's clumsy attempts at sexual harassment), rushes into the office of Dr Wallace, the hospital administrator, to report the disaster. Wallace adopts a 'take it easy' attitude – Kane's mistake is regrettable but not intentional: 'If he were removed there would be bad publicity and the reputation of the hospital would be hurt.' He advises Paige to act like a 'team player' and not like a 'maverick . . . blowing the whistle on her fellow doctors.'[200] A peer review evaluation is set up, but it takes several more years (and presumably further surgical catastrophes) before Kane finally loses his licence to practise.[201] Paige is less keen to report Dr Campbell, 'a likeable grey-haired man in his fifties' who has developed Parkinsonism and frequently asks her to take over during operations.[202] She confronts him and tries to persuade him to give up surgery.

> He smiled wanly. 'I guess I'll have to quit now, won't I? You're going to tell Dr Wallace.' 'No', Paige said gently. 'You're going to tell Dr Wallace.'[202]

When Dr Noah Townsend's partner in Hailey's *Strong Medicine*[109] tries to acquaint the hospital authorities with Townsend's problems of addiction (*see* pp. 213–14), he also comes up against an administrator who has no time for whistle-blowers, particularly whistle-blowers against Dr Townsend, who 'knows everybody and is a genius at fundraising.'[109]

By contrast, Dr Edward McIntosh, the Chairman of the Committee that is hearing the 'Impairment Case' in Frank Slaughter's *Doctors at Risk*,[203] is less considerate towards a young colleague. Dr Mark Harrison, a promising surgeon, has became

---

* The terms 'whistle-blower' and 'team-player' suggest a game between opposing sides (doctors and patients).

addicted to alcohol, amphetamines and finally increasing quantities of 'Demerol.' No convincing explanation is provided for Harrison's drug abuse. He decides at the end of his Baltimore residency to join a private surgical clinic in Southern Alabama rather than stay on as an Assistant Professor, but such decisions are not unusual. Although the transition is somewhat traumatic, the tensions are no worse than those experienced by other doctors entering a group practice. A jealous colleague reports Harrison to the State Licensing Board and to the 'Medical Society Disabled Doctors Committee.'

Slaughter obviously sympathizes with the drug-addicted surgeon[203] rather than with Dr McIntosh, who is suspected of harbouring political ambitions and of using the committee

> as a stepping stone towards the presidency of the State Medical Association. . . . With all the furore nowadays over doctor impairment I suppose that's one of the best ways for a politically minded doctor to get ahead.[203]

In addition, McIntosh holds a personal grudge against Harrison, so the hearing is conducted with considerable acrimony. Instead of 'helping' a fellow physician, McIntosh contacts Harrison's employer, who promptly terminates Harrison's contract.

Slaughter's 'Impaired Doctors' Committee' goes on to debate the balance between the doctor's right to practise and the right of the community to be protected against dangerous individuals. One of the fair-minded members deplores the adversarial attitude of some of his colleagues: 'We're here to help another doctor, not sitting in judgment on him.' However, the committee has the power (and uses it) to destroy this doctor who, in retrospect, should have availed himself of the right to 'bring counsel.'[203] Slaughter resolves the situation by having his committee make the 'right' decision for the wrong reason. Harrison, whose addictive habits have indeed impaired his ability to function as a doctor, does not protest against the lack of due process, but instead tries to kill himself. When his suicide attempt fails, he submits to the recommendation that he should enter a designated rehabilitation facility for a minimum period of four months.

Dr George Bull in *The Last Adam*[204] comes to the attention of the 'New Winton, Connecticut' authorities not on account of substance abuse but because of his laziness and incompetence, which have been a byword in the town for 40 years.[205–208] The doctor's misdeeds are numerous. His indiscriminate use of castor oil is responsible for a number of deaths,[205,206] his neglect of a young woman who dies of eclampsia is scandalous even in the early 1930s,[207] and the final straw is a typhoid epidemic directly attributable to the doctor's indolence. Bull, who is also the town's Health Officer, has failed to inspect the water reservoir, which is being contaminated by camp latrines.[207]

Several leading citizens of New Winton decide that Dr Bull has done too much harm to be tolerated any longer, and they discuss the options of having him removed from office, indicted before a grand jury, or both. Matthew Herring, one of the doctor's detractors, believes that it would be a mistake to leave Dr Bull in peace

> under the guise of mercy and not casting the first stone. . . . That's doing to others what you hope they will do to you if at any time you decide to

take advantage of the situation. That can go on until there are no duties, no standards, no responsibilities left.

A town meeting is called, but Dr Bull's supporters win and he is allowed to continue his medical practice or malpractice.[208]

The hero of Havard's *Coming of Age*,[209] the virtuous and virginal Dr Jonathan Brookes, encounters two impaired colleagues, but for different reasons he reports neither of them. The first of the pair, Dr Robert Bannerman, is the standard male, middle-aged, medical inebriate. Fat, dishevelled and disillusioned, Bannerman is a surgeon who at one stage is on the way to a senior orthopaedic position in a major British hospital.[209] The appointment does not materialize, although it is not apparent whether Bannerman's alcoholism is the cause or the effect of his blocked career. He ends up in charge of the emergency department of the district hospital in a coal-mining town,[210] and by the time he appears in the novel, he has become a dangerous drunkard.[211,212] Brookes, a surgical resident temporarily attached to Dr Bannerman's emergency department, discusses the problem of whistle-blowing with his medical father. What is the correct course of action for a junior resident when the potential 'blowee' is an experienced medical specialist?[209] Brookes' father offers to whisper a few words in someone's ear, but in the end the Drs Brookes (senior and junior) decide to remain silent: 'It's up to the other consultants there to do something about it if it gets too bad. They're bound to know about his drinking.'[209] When Bannerman's futile surgical efforts during a bout of inebriation lead to the death of a patient,[212] he is at last persuaded to get himself 'dried out.'[138]

Jonathan, who blames himself for not reporting Dr Bannerman to the appropriate authorities, has no such guilt feelings about Dr Susannah Ridgeway, a 28-year-old resident in anaesthesiology, a reformed cocaine addict[138,213] and the spoilt daughter of 'one of the richest men in Lancashire.' During her last year at medical school, Susannah has spent 'fifteen thousand pounds' on cocaine alone, 'and that was without the trimmings. God knows how much . . . [she] spent on pot and vodka. And, of course, the odd amphetamine.'[213] Remarkably, she not only survives but she also graduates with high marks. Physically and emotionally scarred by her experiences, Susannah, with the help of Daddy Ridgeway's money, spends several months in an expensive detoxification facility,[213] and emerges capable of holding down a demanding job with only temporary lapses into alcoholism.[138] Jonathan decides that this beautiful, rich, somewhat tarnished princess, has 'things under control' and looks forward to becoming the Prince Consort.[138]

Old age

> The village is proud of him in his decline.[242]

The correlation between physicians' ages and the quality of their medical care was recently reviewed by Choudhry *et al.*,[214] who concluded that when assessed by a variety of objective criteria, the young perform better than the old. This finding is not reflected in works of fiction, where elderly doctors fit the Platonic notion of serenity[215] rather than the Shakespearean stereotype of decrepitude.[216] In general, even when clearly in his decline, the old doctor is not represented as a toothless, demanding, irascible pest whose only interest to the reader is the money he may leave to a young heroine. On the contrary, unless obviously in his dotage, he is portrayed as an experienced and tolerant man whose accumulated wisdom and compassion compensate for his lack of higher qualifications and enthusiasm for innovations. He is no longer capable of participating in the smart cocktail-party repartee of the younger members of the profession (*see* p. 94), but that does not make him hanker after his lost youth. 'I am in no hurry to grow young again', Hawthorne's Dr Heidegger,[217] with his 'venerable dignity', informs his four geriatric friends who cannot wait to be turned into teenagers by his magic potion.[217]

Obviously there are exceptions. Old age constitutes a handicap even for a healthy doctor when it comes to dealing with adolescent patients. Hennie Berger in Clifford Odets' *Awake and Sing*,[218] who suffers from morning sickness, is not at all impressed by her mother's suggestion that Dr Cantor should be called. 'Don't call that old Ignatz', says Hennie, 'I won't see him.'[218] Hennie, who has been impregnated by a virtual stranger, evidently feels that Dr Cantor, the family physician who treated her as a child, is not the appropriate person to deal with her current problems.

Lilly Berry in *Hotel New Hampshire*[219] is only ten years old and does not actually refuse to see the old family doctor. However, Lily and her siblings imply that Dr Blaze is too far removed from adolescence to deal with her problem (suspected growth hormone deficiency).

> We had our annual physicals just before Thanksgiving and our family doctor – an old geezer named Dr Blaze, whose fire, Franny remarked, was almost out – discovered during a routine check that Lilly hadn't grown in a year. . . . There were tests that could be run on Lilly, and old Dr Blaze was apparently trying to figure out what the tests were.[219]

In general, age-related illnesses, which constitute an important cause of impairment in fictional (and real) physicians, are tolerated to a remarkable extent by patients and readers. Sick old doctors, whose infirmities may be obvious to their colleagues, continue 'fighting the long grim fight'[2] to the detriment of their patients, who are not troubled by the doctors' ailments until the day of his ultimate degradation. To the people in his village, Elizabeth Gaskell's old Dr Hall[220] is a perfect healer, despite his disabilities.

> Blind and deaf and rheumatic as he might be, he was still Mr Hall, the doctor who could heal all their ailments – unless they died meanwhile – and he had no right to speak of growing old. . . . The good citizens of Hollingford were [therefore] shocked to hear that their 'skilful doctor' . . . could no longer cope with his work and was going to take a partner.[220]

In *The Fortunes of Richard Mahony*,[221] Dr Brocklebank, a family physician whose frailties are described in very similar terms, has in addition developed a degree of senile belligerency and is treated less kindly. Brocklebank

> had all but reached the eighties; and despite one of those marvellous country-bred English constitutions . . . the infirmities of age began to vex him. For some time past his patients had hesitated to call him out by night or in bad weather or for what he might consider too trifling a cause; though they remained his faithful adherents, preferring any day a bottle of Mr B's good physic to treatment by a more modish doctor. Recently,

however, he had let two comparatively simple cases slip through his fingers; while the habit was growing on him of suddenly nodding off at a bedside; what time the patient had to lie still until the old gentleman came to himself again. A blend, too, of increasing deafness and obstinacy led him to shout people down. So that altogether something like a relief went up when one fine day . . . the rumour ran that Mr B was retiring; was being carried off . . . to be wheeled to the grave-brink in the humiliating bath chair to which he had condemned many a sufferer.[221]

The citizens of 'Buddlecombe'[221] are evidently relieved to see the back of this aggressive old man, but until his actual retirement there are no mass desertions.

In *Behind the Times*,[13] Conan Doyle's Dr James Winter is stone-deaf. The younger doctors in the town declare themselves outraged by his total ignorance of bacteriology and pharmacology, and they joke about his inability to hear cardiac murmurs[13] (*see* p. 202). Dr Winter's lack of modern skills is not perceived as a major disadvantage by the townspeople, who continue to seek his advice. Indeed, the two younger doctors who had previously hinted that the old man ought to be compulsorily retired end up consulting him rather than each other when they become ill.[13]

The old and old-fashioned Sir Patrick Cullen in Shaw's *The Doctor's Dilemma*,[2] who expresses himself in a series of grunts, comes across as a considerably more sensible individual than his younger colleagues who practise 'modern' medicine. Cutler Walpole, the fashionable surgeon, performs useless and meddlesome operations for laughable indications. Bloomfield Bonnington, the internist who attends the British royal family, misuses the 'latest' drugs with disastrous results. Sir Patrick, who has seen medical fads come and go, is obviously ignorant of the most recent 'breakthroughs', but nevertheless commands a great deal of respect from the younger men. '"A little chilly? A little stiff? But hale and still the cleverest of us all" . . . [Sir Patrick grunts].'[1]

Seventy-five-year-old Dr John Bradley[222–224] is in the final stages of selling his practice to Dr Harwood, a younger and better-qualified man. Harwood, who uses 'modern' techniques which the old man has barely heard of, is having electricity installed as soon as he takes over, so that he can give his patients 'ionization' treatment.[223] Harwood is also a shrewd businessman, and offers to buy Dr Bradley's 'bad debts' which have accumulated over the years and now total many 'thousands of pounds.'[223] Bradley makes up for his lack of business acumen and his ignorance of modern treatment methods with old-fashioned kindness. While out on his last house call, the old doctor decides to forego a large sum of money rather than allow his former patients to be badgered by debt collectors. He is physically frail and his memory is beginning to slip, but unlike the smart young entrepreneur he remains the 'beloved physician.'[224]

Helen Ashton's Dr Richard Gaunt,[225] whose expired 'use-by' date is revealed by his name, the cracked leather couch in his consulting room and the rack of broken test tubes on the shelf above the stained sink, is yet another doctor who is treated as a loyal old warhorse. Gaunt, in his late seventies, has become 'a frail, indomitable gnome . . . untidy in his habits and impatient of interference.' However,

the old doctor was still trotting round, paying visits to some of his old cronies. Of course he knew quite well that he was past anything serious.

> He'd let all his operating go and we'd managed to stop the night work. . . .
> But he was uncommonly jealous about his old patients. . . . They all
> backed him up, too, wouldn't call in [other doctors] . . . until they were
> absolutely obliged.[225]

The perception of the decayed doctor as a hero rather than a nuisance continues
almost to the present day. At the age of 81, Garcia Marquez' Dr Juvenal Urbino[226]
is still practising and teaching medicine, despite his deafness, his weak legs, his
urinary problems[227] and his impaired memory. The doctor profoundly mistrusts all
forms of treatment, but prescribes a large variety of useless medications for
himself. Urbino's former students, his wealthy patients and Garcia Marquez
himself see nothing abnormal in a state of affairs that allows this relic from an
earlier age to intervene in dangerous situations. On the contrary, Dr Urbino's
distinguished appearance and his aristocratic bearing make him a living national
treasure and perpetuate the myth that 'he could tell what was wrong with a patient
just by looking at him.'[226]

The 'idlers around the court house' in *Parris Mitchell of King's Row*,[228] who form
a kind of Greek chorus, commenting in the local vernacular on the plot as well as on
general topics (*see* p. 158), are divided in their opinion about the correlation
between age and medical skills. One of these amateur philosophers would rather
'have one of these young doctors than the old ones. There's a lot of new medicine an'
cures that the old fellers haven't learned about yet.' Another purveyor of homespun
wisdom argues very convincingly that the latest is not necessarily the best: 'I'll git me
an old-fashioned country doctor ever' time. Did you hear what happened to old Bill
McChesney last fall? One of these new fellers took him to the hospital . . . an' he
died right there on the operatin' table. Like as not there wasn't nothin' more wrong
with him than a stomach ache.'[228]

Doctors who possess sufficient insight and adequate financial resources to retire at
the first warning signal are admired, but those who stay on are treated with pity and
apprehension rather than disapproval. Dr Charles Dornberger, an elderly obstetrician in Hailey's *The Final Diagnosis*,[229] gives up work abruptly and dramatically.
Dornberger is about to perform an exchange transfusion on a neonate when he
experiences

> a feeling of dizziness; his head was throbbing, the room swirling.
> Momentarily he closed his eyes, then opened them. It was all right.
> Things were back in focus, the dizziness almost gone. But when he
> looked down at his hands he saw they were trembling. He tried to control
> the movement and failed. . . . The incubator containing the Alexander
> baby was being wheeled in. At the same moment he heard the intern ask
> 'Dr Dornberger, are you all right?' It was on the edge of his tongue to
> answer 'yes.' He knew that if he did, he could carry on concealing what
> had happened with no one but himself aware of it. In the same moment
> he remembered all that he had said . . . over the years – about old men
> clinging to power too long; the boast that when his own time came he
> would know it and make way. . . . He thought of these things, then
> looked down at his shaking hands. 'No', he said, 'I don't think I'm all
> right.' He paused and, aware for the first time of a deep emotion which
> made it hard to control his voice, he asked 'Will someone please call Dr
> O'Donnell? Tell him I'm unable to go on. I'd like him to take over.' At

that moment . . . Dr Charles Dornberger retired from the practice of medicine.[230]

Soubiran's Professor Louis Hauberger,[231] chief of surgery at the Charité Hospital, is more reluctant to recognize the signs of old age in himself, but ultimately he steps down gracefully. Towards the end of his illustrious career Hauberger has

> become an almost legendary figure. . . . [He] was always in the papers, signing bulletins on the health of distinguished invalids, addressing international congresses on behalf of French surgery, receiving honorary degrees from numerous foreign universities. . . . [He was the] holder of the Grand Cross of the Légion d'Honneur, [a] Member of the Institute and [the] President of the Academy of Medicine.[232]

Professor Hauberger is now approaching the age of mandatory retirement, but the public regard him as 'one of the greatest surgeons of his age',[232] and there is much speculation as to whether his term of office might be or should be extended.[232]

Within his own hospital, the professor's close associates recognize that he has turned into a hindrance to progress. A pioneer in his younger days, he now feels threatened by new procedures, mainly because the old techniques constitute his life's work. He insists on a gastrectomy when a vagotomy would have been more appropriate,[233] and he continues to use the 'Hauberger' technique for the relief of trigeminal neuralgia, even though more effective operations have been developed.[234] 'Hauberger refused to have these [newer] operations mentioned in his block.'[233] One day when Hauberger is believed to be out of town, his first assistant re-operates on one of the old man's patients and performs a 'forbidden' procedure. The professor returns unexpectedly, but fortunately has sufficient insight to recognize the *coup de grâce* for what it is. Instead of making a scene and ruining the assistant's career, he concedes that 'even in the eyes of his pupils he was out of date as a surgeon.' He takes early retirement, declaring 'I want to step down from my Chair, not fall from it.'[233]

Mauriac's Dr Paul Courrèges[235] does not retire, despite his Parkinsonism. He still attends medical congresses, although he lacks the endurance to stay to the end, and he still sees patients who tolerate or ignore his poor health. His advice to Victor Larousselle, a drunken business and horse-racing type who has cut his hand on a broken bottle, sounds strangely old-fashioned even for the 1920s: 'Poultry at lunch and no butcher's meat at night. Do as I say and you'll live to be a hundred.'[235] Larousselle, when he has sobered up a little, sneers:

> 'He's just ripe for the cold stone.' He added that the poor fellow had obviously had a slight stroke. Many of his old patients, who didn't like to abandon him, secretly consulted other doctors.[235]

Mauriac (himself a doctor's son) clearly sympathizes with the old doctor rather than with his cynical detractor.

Even those fictional doctors whose deferred retirement leads to loss of life in the operating room are treated with compassion rather than disgust. Van der Meersch's Professor Géraudin,[236] who was a great surgeon in his younger days, is aware that for some years he has been suffering from transient cerebral ischaemic attacks. Like Mauriac's Doctor Courrèges,[235] Géraudin lacks sufficient insight to give up his university position, but unlike Courrèges, who offers harmless and useless advice to his patients, Géraudin has a further attack of giddiness during a Caesarean section and slices through a major blood vessel.[236] There is torrential bleeding and the patient (a colleague's daughter) dies on the operating table[236] (*see also* p. 71). Even after this disaster Géraudin does not give up surgery, although he is aware that he is 'ageing and losing his talent. . . . More and more often . . . in the midst of an operation, he would be seized with vertigo and hardly able to see clearly.'[237] After several further incidents, including the accidental transsection of a ureter,[237] he at last has the sense to avoid difficult procedures. He no longer attempts to resect rectal carcinomas, but merely provides the patients with a colostomy.[238] Instead of removing gastric ulcers he performs simple gastroenterostomies. Géraudin's reputation declines rapidly, patients are no longer referred to him and he finally kills himself with an overdose of barbiturates.[238]

Dr Joseph Pearson, an ageing pathologist in *The Final Diagnosis*,[229] has received no abrupt warnings about his health, but after 32 years as head of department in the same hospital, he is clearly 'burnt out'. Unable to delegate, he orders all laboratory supplies himself,[239] he cannot bring himself to fire his lazy and slovenly senior technician, and he has become unenthusiastic about 'new ways of doing things.'[239] He has never heard of the Coombs test, and becomes resentful when a junior technician suggests that this test might be required in the investigation of an infant with rhesus incompatibility.

> As Pearson spoke his bitterness came through – the bitterness against all who were younger, who were interfering, trying to deprive him of authority – absolute and unquestioned – which until now had been his. . . . He . . . decided once and for all to put this upstart lab assistant in his place. . . . 'I'm the one in charge of this department . . . I happen to be a pathologist and I know what I'm talking about.'[240]

Pearson's obstinacy cost the infant its life and cost him his job.[241] However, instead of having to endure a humiliating dismissal, he is allowed to resign, and after his departure a hospital endowment fund is named in his honour to commemorate his years of faithful service, which come to an end a little too late.[241]

Obviously, old age does not improve pre-existing ignorance and slovenliness. Dr Alpheus Snider in *Not as a Stranger*[198] is a marginalized character of a type more likely to be found practising as a mid-twentieth-century abortionist than working in a community hospital. He is untidy in his appearance, disorganized in his thinking and totally ignorant of medical principles. This 'bumbling old man' and 'long-ago graduate of a defunct fourth-rate school' orders a purgative for a woman suffering from typhoid fever. The patient's bowel perforates and she dies within a few hours. Remarkably, Snider is allowed to continue to practise, but in his case there are no hints that 'the village is proud of him in his decline'[242] (*see also* p. 223).

There comes a time when even the most devoted followers of an ancient doctor either die or seek medical advice from a physician who will at least stay awake during the consultation. James Hadley Chase's Dr Mallard,[243] who has been practising medicine at Glyn Camp for the best part of 50 years, is a little closer to the grave than Dr Snider,[198] and although Mallard

> still had a handful of faithful patients . . . they were dying off fast and he now spent most of his time playing checkers with Sheriff Jefferson or

sitting on the verandah of his shabby little cabin, staring emptily at the view.[243]

Richard Stern's Dr Rudolph* Cahn[244] is still further away from practice, but his deeply ingrained medical behaviour pattern has not been completely erased. Dr Cahn, aged 91 and thoroughly demented, ceased seeing patients many years ago. He cannot remember that his wife is ill and that she has spent the last two weeks in the Mount Sinai Hospital. He confuses his son Will with his brother George, who died 'the day after Franklin Roosevelt', and he cannot recall the name of the hospital or the fact that he had been on the staff there for 50 years. 'Is it a good hospital?', he asks.

The family members, afraid that the confused old man might create a disturbance in the hospital, are unsure whether to take him to see his wife for the last time. They need not have worried. At his dying wife's bedside, Dr Cahn's medical training briefly reasserts itself so that for a few seconds he behaves and talks like a doctor.

> Dr Cahn . . . came in, looked at the bed, realized where he was and who was there. 'Dolph, dear. How are you, my darling? I'm so happy you came to see me.' The old man stooped over and took her face in his hand. For seconds there was silence. 'My dearest', he said, then, 'I didn't know. I had no idea. I've been so worried about you. But don't worry now. You look wonderful. A little thin, perhaps. We'll fix that. We'll have you out in no time.'[244]

The dying physician

The idealized priestly physician who is portrayed as a romantic hero, having spent his working life 'fighting disease', dies from overwork,[245] preferably during[246,247] or just after[248] a house call. Alternatively, he acquires a lethal infection during an autopsy[249] or while performing a life-saving procedure.[250–252] The patient survives but the doctor dies as a result of sepsis. Delirious and almost moribund, the dedicated physician tries to haul himself off his deathbed in order to attend to imaginary patients.[249] Not quite so romantic but still commendable is the doctor who neglects his health and departs quietly, save for a professional interest in his own pathology and some insight into his impending demise. Suicide is quite acceptable.[238,253,254] The dying doctor who keeps complaining about his symptoms, asks for more treatment, expresses anger at the impotence of the medical profession or deplores the lack of compassion among his colleagues is reduced to the rank of patient and treated as a nuisance who should know better.

Balzac's doctors, of course, are well trained and know how to die. At the age of 88, Dr Denis Minoret[255] has reached the stage where 'his appearance made it obvious to his friends and to his expectant heirs that the end was approaching.' The doctor himself, whose 'intellect remained clear, strong and exact' . . . harbours no illusions about his life expectancy and declares 'I feel that I have not long to stay.'[255] When, a few days later, the old man is mortally ill and a young medical colleague orders mustard plasters to be applied to his feet, the dying man summons Ursule, his 'ward', who is to inherit some of his money. He says 'My darling child . . . my hours,

---

* Dr Cahn's full name is not provided. His wife calls him 'Dolph' which could equally well be an abbreviation for Randolph or Adolph.

my minutes are numbered. I have not been a doctor for nothing; the mustard plasters . . . will not carry me through till tonight.' The doctor asks Ursule to fetch a copy of his will which he has hidden, but he dies before she can retrieve the document.[255]

Similarly, Braddon's Dr George Gilbert,[256] a dull provincial doctor of very limited intellect, displays considerable dignity when he develops fatal typhoid fever. At the onset of the disease, Gilbert, who has 'never before . . . known what it was to have a day's illness', ignores the warning signals and the advice of his colleague and rival to stay in bed. When he begins to deteriorate and his wife asks whether she ought to recall his colleague, who has become exasperated by Gilbert's unwillingness to comply with his instructions, Gilbert replies 'If I should happen to get delirious . . . you can send for him because I daresay you'd be frightened, poor girl, and would feel more comfortable with a doctor pottering about me.' He also instructs his wife that 'she was to fumigate the room in which he was to lie.'[256] Mary Elizabeth Braddon declares herself surprised that Dr Gilbert

> so clever while other people were concerned, was not the best judge of his own case. . . . [He] set . . . at naught those very first principles of health wherein it was his duty to instruct other people.[256]

In fact, Gilbert behaves exactly as one would expect a sick doctor to behave. The initial symptoms are denied, work continues as usual from a sense of duty or, as in this case, a sense of competition, and therapeutic measures of doubtful validity are declined.

Dr Austin Sloper in Henry James' *Washington Square*[257] is a much more intelligent and successful man than George Gilbert, although his family life, like that of Gilbert, is a total disaster (*see* p. 45). Sloper adopts a somewhat different approach to his impending demise. While remaining consistently rational when making medical decisions about his final illness (pneumonia), he evidently believes that it would be unseemly for a medical man not to go through the motions of 'appropriate' treatment. He gives his daughter detailed instructions on how he is to be nursed, although he knows that he will not recover.

> 'I hate an ill-conducted sick room, and you will be so good as to nurse me on the hypothesis that I shall get well.' He told her which of his fellow physicians to send for, and he gave her a multitude of directions.[257]

Francis Brett Young's Dr Marshall,[245] who is also dying of pneumococcal pneumonia, asks for brandy and blankets, and instructs John Ingleby, his young assistant, to take his temperature. Like Dr Sloper, he is sufficiently familiar with the fatal disease to realize that treatment will make little difference. Throughout his five-day illness, Dr Marshall simply gasps for breath, saying very little. On the last day of his life, the solitary old doctor, barely able to speak but still lucid, asks Ingleby to burn his account books and bills. 'I shan't want any more money', he said.[245]

Dr Jason Greylock, Ellen Glasgow's disreputable drunkard in *Barren Ground*,[258] who has not practised for many years (*see* pp. 119 and 217–18), and John O'Hara's Dr George Reed, a distinguished surgeon,[259] represent opposite ends of the spectrum of medical achievement. Both recognize their hopeless prognoses and accept the inevitable, although the settings are different. Greylock, on his deathbed, redeems himself to some extent by retaining sufficient insight to realize that he is beyond medical help. When his carer (a former lover whom he abandoned many years earlier) expresses concern about the non-arrival of his medical colleague, Greylock remarks 'It makes no difference. I am a doctor.'[258]

Dr Reed[259] is still in his office eating sandwiches and drinking coffee when he discusses his impending death with a former sweetheart. He has been too busy to seek the advice of colleagues, but he is now due to have a laparotomy. 'I'm fairly sure I know what they'll find' he declares. The doomed doctor has evidently decided to continue working for as long as he can. Only one thing has changed as a result of his illness: he has begun to read poetry.[259]

Richard Gordon's Sir Lancelot Spratt, the aggressive and totally self-centred surgeon in *Doctor in the House*,[260] handles his own final illness with a minimum of fuss.

> One day . . . he disappeared. He said goodbye to no one. He . . . wrote a letter to the Chairman of the Governors simply stating he would not be back again. The hospital radiologist explained it later with an X-ray film. Sir Lancelot had a cancer in his stomach and had gone off to his cottage in Sussex to die. He refused to have an operation.[260]

The 'heroic' death of a romanticized medical hero may be presented in quite unrealistic terms even in the hands of great authors like Garcia Marquez. Dr Marco Aurelio Urbino,[261] who has contracted cholera as a result of his dedication to his patients, refuses treatment and, alive or dead, avoids contact with his family so as not to infect them. His deathbed letter is so finely timed that he just manages to sign it before his demise. The sordid aspects of the disease, such as the constant diarrhoea, are simply ignored. Urbino

> was a civic hero during [the cholera epidemic] as well as its most distinguished victim. . . . When he recognized in himself the irreversible symptoms that he had seen and pitied in others, he did not even attempt a useless struggle, but withdrew from the world so as not to infect anyone else. Locked in a utility room at the Misericordia Hospital, deaf to the calls of his colleagues and the pleas of his family, he wrote a letter of feverish love to his wife and children, a letter of gratitude for his existence. . . . It was a farewell of twenty heartrending pages on which the progress of the disease could be observed in the deteriorating script and it was not necessary to know the writer to realize that he had signed his name with his last breath. In accordance with his instructions, his ashen body was mingled with others in the communal cemetery and was not seen by anyone who loved him.[261]

Urbino's son, Dr Juvenal Urbino, the principal character in *Love in the Time of Cholera*,[262] is favoured with a sudden and more bizarre death. He breaks his neck when he falls off a ladder while trying to catch his pet parrot.

Guterson's *East of the Mountains*[263] is the story of Dr Ben Givens, a retired cardiothoracic surgeon who suffers from inoperable carcinoma of the colon. Givens, a widower, has so far managed to conceal his illness from the remaining members of his family and to prevent it from becoming 'a pestilent force in their lives.'[263] However, he is aware that over the next few months his condition will become obvious and that the inevitable pain and degradation will only end when he dies. He therefore decides to end his life now 'swiftly, cleanly', rather than to submit to the inexorable ravages of the cancer, which are already beginning to manifest themselves. As the plot evolves, it becomes clear that Dr Givens does not really want to kill himself. Instead of ending his life with an overdose or a gun placed in the conventional position, Givens plans a complex hunting expedition during which he will shoot himself in the neck so that his suicide will look like accidental death.[263] The plan fails in its original design, but other means of dying present themselves. Givens avoids all of them. Instead, he helps a tuberculous illegal immigrant past the inevitable administrative red tape and has him taken off to hospital in an ambulance.[264] His final moment of medical glory arrives when he saves the life of a baby who would have died at birth from a shoulder presentation.[265] There is no further talk of suicide, and Dr Givens allows himself to be driven home, where he will explain the position to his family. Guterson does not describe the demise of his medical hero, but the reader is left with the strong impression that Dr Givens, who is closer to death than he realizes, will bear his final illness with dignity and fortitude[266] until his friend, Dr Ward, gives him a gentle shove into the next world with an overdose of morphine.[254]

Nourse's Dr Paul Merritt,[267] who is bleeding to death from oesophageal varices, needs to be intubated with a gastro-oesophageal pressure bag. The poor man has suffered five previous major haemorrhages and is considerably more conversant with the intricacies of the apparatus than the intern who is telling the story:

> He lay there and patiently told me step by step how to work the thing, which lubricant to use, how to pass the tube so that it was less irritating . . . [and] how much water to let him swallow. Once we got the uninflated bag down, he told me how much air to pump into it to inflate it properly.

Dr Merritt is then subjected to an eight-hour surgical procedure, and dies two days later.[267]

Léon Daudet in *Les Morticoles** contrasts the courageous death of young Dr Misnard, an intern,[251] with the unseemly and messy departure of Professor Wabanheim.[269] Misnard, like Chekhov's Dr Osip Dymov[250] has saved the life of a patient with acute tracheobronchitis by sucking out a blocked tracheostomy. When, a few days later, Misnard dies from the same disorder, he knows exactly how a doctor should behave on his deathbed, and goes 'gentle into that good night.' Wabanheim, a politically powerful academic who 'rages against the dying of the light', becomes a contemptible buffoon and dies a miserable death.[268,269]

Two concerned senior physicians are visiting Misnard, who begins by asking about one of his own patients.

> 'How is the man in bed thirty-four, chief, you know, the one with the fractured skull?' 'He's all right . . . but let's not worry about the others, it's you we're concerned about, my dear fellow.' . . . [One of the consultants] examined Misnard's throat, listened to his chest, felt his pulse and whispered a few words [to the other attending physician. He then declares, aloud] 'You're going to recover – the worst is over.' [Misnard is not taken in quite so easily.] 'But doctor' [he insists] 'do you think the bronchi are affected? I seem to be having breathing problems.

---

* *Les Morticoles* ('The Deadly Charlatans')[268] is a satire on medical practice but contains many realistic scenarios. The book is not available in English, and the translations are mine.

And I've got the irregular pulse you've described.' [The medical patient and his two physicians then proceed to use] technical terms . . . and for several minutes the three of them talked as if they were discussing some [abstract] scientific problem with no particular patient in mind.[251]

The attempt to interest the dying doctor in religion produces only a slight shake of the head, although it is unclear whether this conveys disbelief or astonishment (*see* Chapter 3). Dr Misnard's last words are 'I'm choking. This is the end. You won't be able to feel my pulse. Goodbye and thanks.'[251]

Professor Wabanheim, on the other hand, who has probably sustained a massive myocardial infarction, is treated with profound contempt.[269] Prior to the arrival of his colleagues he is alternately whining about his fears of death and raging against his political enemies, 'his voice changing from moment to moment like a comedian's.' When the physicians arrive he begs them 'Don't tell me if it's something serious – that would kill me.' One of the consultants remarks rather nonchalantly that there might be signs of pulmonary oedema. The old doctor calls out 'I'm going to die! Save me!', and then asks for obsolete treatments such as leeches and cupping glasses. One of his former students tries to be gentle:

'My dear professor, it would be childish to hide things from you. You are seriously ill and possibly in immediate danger. You might recover, but I'm afraid. . . . You can have leeches and cupping glasses but . . . between ourselves these things are completely useless.' He had hardly finished when Wabanheim jumped out of bed with a heroic effort and, swaying on his hairy legs, bellowed . . . 'Get out, you scoundrels, you miserable ungrateful wretches . . . I gave you everything – patients, titles, decorations and . . . you come here announcing . . . [I'm] going to die. What do you know? You know nothing, you idiots. I'm not going to die, do you hear? I don't want to. You'll see.' [One of Wabanheim's colleagues remarks icily:] 'His brain's gone. He'll die sooner than I expected.'[269]

Wabanheim goes on fulminating against his enemies and, at the same time, begging for help for several hours before he finally succumbs. Right up to the end he seems incapable, despite his medical experience, of appreciating that there comes a point when treatment is no longer indicated or possible.

Almost 100 years after the publication of *Les Morticoles*, Susan Cheever describes another senior doctor whose terminal behaviour is perceived as not befitting a physician. In *Doctors and Women*,[270] Cheever traces the transformation of 'Dr Lessons' from a respected doctor to a sick doctor to a dying and querulous patient.

When doctors on the staff of the 'Parkinson Cancer Center' developed cancer, their colleagues treated them with surgery and radiation and chemotherapy. Their colleagues also treated them like freaks. . . . They were solicitous but distant. The doctor who had cancer became an outcast . . . isolated by his colleagues; he knew too well what his chances were. . . . Suddenly he was thrown through the scrim of language, knowledge and power which protects doctors from their patients – he had become a patient. . . . Dr Edward Lessons . . . had been the head of a department, a great teacher, a beloved fellow. A year ago [Drs] Riley and Lessons would stride down the hall together discussing patients and

> treatments. Now, Lessons had lung cancer. He had been relieved of his duties at the hospital but he kept his office. . . . He was being treated in Riley's department with chemotherapy. . . . Everyone wished Ed Lessons would stay home, but he came every day . . . [shuffling] slowly and painfully down the hall that had once been his kingdom. 'Edward, how are you feeling?' Riley said with pretended heartiness – how he was feeling was all too obvious. Riley was afraid that Lessons would come into his office and collapse on the couch. There was a time when Riley was pleased to have Ed Lessons drop by his office. . . . 'These treatments', Lessons croaked, 'these treatments are terrible. I think we underestimate our patients, we don't know what we are doing to them.'[270]

If one of Riley's clinic patients had wandered uninvited into his office, the doctor would have asked his secretary or a member of the security department to escort this person back to where he belonged. Things are more complicated when the patient is a former colleague. 'Riley felt impatient. Most of the doctors wouldn't even stop to talk with Ed Lessons. What on earth was the use of arguing with this sick old man?'[270]

Rosenbaum's autobiographical account describes a physician who suffers from cancer of the larynx[271] and who commits every error that sick doctors have been warned against.[8] After neglecting his symptoms for six months[272] he finally seeks medical advice, but instead of consulting a competent specialist he opts for an old-fashioned doctor friend who comes up with an incorrect diagnosis and whose orders are ignored.[272] The sick physician then obtains a second opinion, also erroneous, during a kerbside consultation[8] (a chance encounter with another colleague). He fails to improve, and returns to his old doctor friend for an exchange of gossip and anecdotes. During the farcical interview he pleads with his 'medical attendant': 'Don't treat me like a patient. Treat me like a doctor.'[272] When a competent doctor with the right equipment finally makes the correct diagnosis and organizes appropriate treatment at the university hospital, the sick doctor finds the role reversal particularly difficult.[8] Like Ed Lessons,[270] he seems unable to make up his mind as to which side of the table he belongs. He ruminates about whether or not he ought to mention his nausea. Silence may lead to yet another missed diagnosis, while complaints may result in unpleasant and potentially hazardous investigations.[273] He recollects his own clinical mistakes and proceeds to worry about the radiotherapy students' ability to position the linear accelerator. Might they have more up-to-date machines at 'Mayo or Stanford or Sloan Kettering'?[274] Rosenbaum's sick doctor complains repeatedly that his treating doctors spend hardly any time with him. One of them actually walks out when the doctor-patient asks 'What caused this [cancer]?'[271] We are not given an explanation for the behaviour of the ENT and radiotherapy specialists, who may have been naturally laconic and uncommunicative types. However, one cannot help speculating that this sick medical man with his stale anecdotes, his ancient reminiscences, his boasts about his children's achievements and his semi-educated medical questions might have sorely tried the patience of his healthy colleagues.

Martin du Gard's description[275] of Dr Antoine Thibault's final illness (exposure to mustard gas followed by progressive pulmonary fibrosis and lung abscess formation) provides what is arguably the best account to date of the transition from physician to mortally ill physician. Thibault retains his medical status to the end, and never becomes a 'simple' patient. During his first few months in the 'Gas Casualty Hospital', Dr Thibault has a somewhat ambiguous role. He is treated as a patient but he also helps as a physician. As long as he believes that he will ultimately recover, Dr Thibault periodically puts on a white coat[275] and

> displayed a keen interest in the case histories of the other patients . . . sometimes even joining in the nightly conferences which took place in Professor Sègre's study.[275] [Antoine] had several times listened to . . . [the] chest [of his fellow patient, Colonel Chapuis] and had formed the opinion that the Colonel before being gassed had suffered from mitral incompetence. He was on the point of mentioning his discovery [to the hospital physicians]. Even more than in the past, his pride was apt to be agreeably titillated by 'catching out' a colleague . . . and pointing out his blunders. It was a mild if slightly malicious compensation for the feeling of inferiority that illness had imposed on him. But talking was an effort and he refrained.[275]

When Antoine's anticipated improvement does not occur, he consults Dr Philip, a senior colleague and one of his medical father-figures.[276] Philip takes infinite pains with his former student and tries desperately to remain optimistic throughout the interview. However, Antoine knows his old teacher too well to be deceived. He recognizes the pulse-taking ritual for what it is – a ruse to allow his senior colleague to think quietly for a minute. The two doctors discuss the climate of various health resorts where Antoine might spend the coming summer.

> Suddenly (Antoine) . . . had a glimpse in the small grey eyes . . . of . . . a vast compassion. Philip's look, his whole expression seemed to be saying: 'What's the good? What difference can it make where you spend the summer? Your case is hopeless.' . . . Antoine all but cried out aloud, so brutal was the shock. But then he told himself: 'In my heart of hearts I too knew it: I knew there was no hope.'[276]

After his return to the hospital, Antoine ceases 'playing doctors' with his fellow patients, and instead concentrates on his own case, discussing it in detail with the physicians in charge.

> Not, as formerly, from the standpoint of a patient who thinks himself on the way to recovery and snatches at every favourable symptom, but as a competent, well-informed colleague who is no longer to be fobbed off with kindly lies. It did not take me long to corner them; I very soon had them shirking direct answers, making partial admissions or relapsing into a silence which told me more than words.[277]

Antoine's diary covers the last five months of his life. The first entry is dated 2 July 1918, a few days after he realizes that his prognosis is hopeless; the last appears on 18 November 1918, the day he kills himself with an overdose of morphine. In between, entries denoting physical suffering, boredom, disappointment and despair provide glimpses of pride in his profession.[278] Despite Antoine's certainty about his imminent demise he submits to all sorts of treatments, including the drainage of a lung abscess six weeks before his death.[278] Remarkably, when the abscess is diagnosed, he says that 'I only had one idea – that the operation should take place at the earliest moment . . . and succeed.' In his last 'medical' entry Antoine writes:

> No, I don't envy the ordinary patient his ignorance, his wishful illusions. Much nonsense has been talked about the 'cruel lucidity' of the doctor watching himself die. On the contrary, I believe this lucidity has stood me in good stead so far. And will, perhaps, help me through the last phase. . . . I know what's going on inside me. I can see my lesions. They interest me. I watch Bardot trying out his treatments. And up to a point this interest . . . is a great stand-by.[279]

Summary

Writers of medical fiction are both fascinated and puzzled by the paradox of sick doctors, almost all of them male, whose illnesses (whatever their nature) are not necessarily perceived as impediments to the practice of good medicine. The doctor's drunkenness, his infirmities and his eccentricities may set him apart from his medical brethren, but he is still in possession of magic that may succeed at the decisive moment. Like Graham Greene's 'whisky priest',[280] whose indelible ordination enables him to work 'miracles' in his impaired state, the 'ordained'[281] physician, even as a cripple, a drunkard or a drug addict, remains a healer.

For the same reason, authors treat out-of-date and severely hypo-competent physicians, who let 'simple cases slip through their fingers'[221] (in other words, 'cause unnecessary deaths'), as tragic King Lear-like figures who retain traces of wisdom and dignity to the end. Unless the doctor has become totally incapacitated, he continues to display, to a greater or lesser extent, the attitudes and behaviour patterns appropriate to his former calling. His medical training remains with him until he dies. 'Once a doctor, always a doctor.'[282]

References

1 Shaw GB (1906) The Doctor's Dilemma. In: *The Bodley Head Bernard Shaw: collected plays with their prefaces. Volume 3*. The Bodley Head, London, 1971, pp. 339–45.
2 Chandler R (1943) *The Lady in the Lake*. Vintage Books, New York, 1976, p. 22.
3 American Medical Association Council on Mental Health (1973) The sick physician: impairment by psychiatric disorders including alcoholism and drug dependency. *JAMA.* **223**: 684–7.
4 Talbott GD, Gallegos KV, Wilson PO and Porter TL (1987) The Medical Association of Georgia's Impaired Physicians Program. Review of the first 1000 physicians: analysis of specialty. *JAMA.* **257**: 2927–30.
5 Hughes PH, Brandenburg N, Baldwin DC *et al.* (1992) Prevalence of substance use among US physicians. *JAMA.* **267**: 2333–9.
6 Aach RD, Girard DE, Humphrey H *et al.* (1992) Alcohol and other substance abuse and impairment among physicians in residency training. *Ann Intern Med.* **116**: 245–54.
7 Barker P (1995) *The Ghost Road*. Viking, London, p. 110.
7a Barker P (1993) *The Eye in the Door*. Penguin, Harmondsworth, 1994, p. 245.
8 Schneck SA (1998) 'Doctoring' doctors and their families. *JAMA.* **280**: 2039–42.
9 Heller J (1955) *Catch 22*. Dell, New York, 1974, pp. 32–3.
10 Plato (4th century BC) *The Republic* (translated by Jowett B). In: Buchanan S (ed.) *The Portable Plato*. Penguin, Harmondsworth, 1979, p. 400.

11 Martin du Gard R (1936–1940) *Summer 1914* (translated by Gilbert S). The Bodley Head, London, 1940, p. 1059.

12 Toyry S, Rasanen K, Kujala S *et al.* (2000) Self-reported health, illness and self-care among Finnish physicians. *Arch Fam Med.* **9**: 1079–85.

13 Doyle AC (1894) Behind the Times. In: *Round the Red Lamp*. John Murray, London, 1934, pp. 1–8.

14 Dreiser T (1919) The Country Doctor. In: *Twelve Men*. Constable, London, 1930, pp. 102–22.

15 Fitzgerald FS (1932) One Interne. In: *Taps at Reveille*. Charles Scribner's Sons, New York, 1935, pp. 349–73.

16 Moore B (1976) *The Doctor's Wife*. Jonathan Cape, London, pp. 4–5.

17 Porter KA (1945–1962) *Ship of Fools*. Little Brown, Boston, MA, 1962.

18 Ibid., pp. 111–13.

19 Ibid., p. 196.

20 Flaubert G (1857) *Madame Bovary* (translated by Steegmuller F). Modern Library, New York, 1982, p. 394.

21 Mann T (1924) *The Magic Mountain* (translated by Lowe-Porter H). Penguin, Harmondsworth, 1960, pp. 132–3.

22 Hippocrates (attrib.) (*c.* 400 BC) The Physician. In: *The Works of Hippocrates* (translated by Jones WHS). *Volume 2*. Loeb's Classical Library, Heinemann, London, 1923, p. 311.

23 Halle J (1565) Preface to the reader. In: *Lanfranc of Milan, the Herball*. John Daye, London, p. 5.

24 Van Gogh V (1873–1890) *Complete Letters* (translated by Van Gogh-Bonger J and de Dood C). *Volume 3*. Thames and Hudson, London, 1958, p. 271 and p. 294.

25 Maugham WS (1915) *Of Human Bondage*. Signet Classics, New York, 1991, p. 512.

26 Ellis AE (1958) *The Rack*. Penguin, Harmondsworth, 1988, pp. 97–8.

27 Auden WH (1972) The Art of Healing. In memoriam David Protetch MD. In: *Epistle to a Godson and Other Poems*. Faber and Faber, London, pp. 13–15.

28 Kingsley C (1857) Two Years Ago. In: *The Works of Charles Kingsley. Volume 8*. Reprinted by Georg Olms, Hildesheim, Germany, 1969.

29 Ibid., p. 18.

30 Ibid., p. 72.

31 Ibid., pp. 34–8.

32 Ibid., p. 492.

33 Saramago J (1995) *Blindness* (translated by Pontiero G). Harvill Press, London, 1997.

34 Ibid., pp. 15–21.

35 Ibid., p. 46.

36 Ibid., p. 224.

37 Ibid., p. 281.

38 Baum V (1929) *Grand Hotel* (translated by Creighton B). Geoffrey Bles, London, 1930.

39 Ibid., p. 3.

40 Ibid., pp. 43–4.

41 Ibid., p. 84.

42 Ibid., p. 249.

43 Ibid., pp. 244–6.

44 Ibid., p. 253.

45 Baum V (1944) *Berlin Hotel*. Angus and Robertson, Sydney, 1945.

46 Ibid., pp. 6–8.

47 Ibid., p. 79.

48 Ibid., p. 240.

49 Baum V (1939) *Nanking Road* (translated by Creighton B). Geoffrey Bles, London.

50 Ibid., pp. 74–85.

51 Ibid., p. 496.
52 Ibid., p. 433.
53 Ibid., pp. 296–359.
54 Ibid., p. 806.
55 Collins W (1868) *The Moonstone*. Perennial Classics, Harper and Row, New York, 1965.
56 Ibid., pp. 317–18.
57 Ibid., pp. 361–71.
58 Deeping W (1925) *Sorrell and Son*. Cassell, London, 1927, pp. 288–9.
59 Ibid., p. 297.
60 Bashford HH (1911) *The Corner of Harley Street: being some familiar correspondence of Peter Harding MD*. Constable, London, 1913, pp. 204–10.
61 Remarque EM (1945) *Arch of Triumph* (translated by Sorell W and Lindley D). Appleton Century, New York, 1945, pp. 178–84.
62 Ibid., pp. 38–48.
63 Bellaman H (1940) *King's Row*. Dymocks, Sydney, 1945, pp. 253–6.
64 Ibid., pp. 393–415.
65 Söderberg H (1905) *Doctor Glas* (translated by Austin PB). Chatto and Windus, London, 1963.
66 Ibid., pp. 29–34.
67 Jerome Saint (Eusebius Sophronius Hieronymus) (403 AD) Letter 107. In: *St Jerome: select letters* (translated by Wright FA). Loeb's Classical Library, Harvard University Press, Cambridge, MA, 1980, p. 363.
68 Söderberg H, op. cit., pp. 93–108.
69 Ibid., p. 21.
70 Ibid., pp. 65–6.
71 Caldwell T (1968) *Testimony of Two Men*. Collins, London, 1990, pp. 345–51.
72 Ibid., p. 385.
73 Richardson HH (1917–1929) *The Fortunes of Richard Mahony*. Penguin, Harmondsworth, 1990.
74 Ibid., pp. 406–9.
75 Ibid., p. 838 (Afterword by Green D).
76 Ibid., pp. 676–703.
77 Ibid., pp. 788–92.
78 Ibid., pp. 819–31.
79 Duhamel G (1928) *Les Sept Dernières Plaies*. Mercure de France, Paris, pp. 16–17.
80 Ibid., p. 92.
81 Ibid., p. 52.
82 Ibid., pp. 105–17.
83 Ravin N (1987) *Evidence*. Charles Scribner's Sons, New York.
84 Ibid., pp. 132–51.
85 Ibid., p. 229.
86 Gordon R (Ostlere GS) (1952) *Doctor in the House*. Michael Joseph, London, 1967, pp. 69–71.
87 Nourse AE (1978) *The Practice*. Futura Publications, London, 1979, p. 36.
88 Cook R (1981) *Brain*. Pan Books, London, p. 42.
89 Ravin N, op. cit., p. 80.
90 Ibid., pp. 241–8.
91 Ibid., pp. 181–7.
92 Ibid., p. 291.
93 Greene G (1965) Doctor Crombie. In: *Collected Stories*. The Bodley Head and William Heinemann, London, 1972, pp. 129–35.
94 Miller A (1997) *Ingenious Pain*. Harcourt Brace, New York.

95 Ibid., pp. 31–3.
96 Ibid., p. 19.
97 Ibid., p. 41.
98 Mitchell SW (1885) *In War Time*. Century Company, New York, 1913.
99 Ibid., p. 45.
100 Ibid., pp. 60–8.
101 Ibid., pp. 19–26.
102 Ibid., pp. 232–44.
103 Ibid., p. 303.
104 Ibid., pp. 323–7.
105 Ibid., pp. 415–19.
106 Ibid., pp. 375–90.
107 Ibid., p. 293.
108 Ibid., pp. 208–15.
109 Ibid., pp. 3–7.
110 Ibid., p. 103.
111 Ibid., p. 363.
112 Hailey A (1984) *Strong Medicine*. Dell, New York, 1986.
113 Ibid., pp. 77–80.
114 Ibid., pp. 82–3.
115 Ibid., pp. 128–30.
116 Ibid., pp. 137–8.
117 Ibid., pp. 139–41.
118 Ibid., p. 143.
119 Posen S (2005) *The Doctor in Literature. Volume 1. Satisfaction or resentment?* Radcliffe Publishing, Oxford, pp. 195–6.
120 Chandler R (1953) *The Long Good-Bye*. Pan Books, London, 1979, p. 85.
121 Ibid., p. 98.
122 Ibid., p. 89.
123 Ibid., pp. 99–101.
124 Chandler R (1943) *The Lady in the Lake*. Vintage Books, New York, 1976, p. 129.
125 Bulgakov M (1925–1927) Morphine. In: *A Country Doctor's Notebook* (translated by Glenny M). Collins and Harvill Press, London, 1975, pp. 113–44.
126 Palmer M (1998) *Miracle Cure*. Arrow Books, London.
127 Ibid., pp. 28–31.
128 Ibid., pp. 122–3.
129 Ibid., pp. 144–5.
130 Ibid., pp. 220–2.
131 Ibid., pp. 262–3.
132 Ibid., pp. 202–3.
133 Kingsley C, op. cit., p. 65.
134 Chellis MD (1870) *The Old Doctor's Son*. Henry A Young, Boston, MA.
135 Ibid., p. 129.
136 Ibid., p. 175.
137 Ibid., pp. 348–52.
138 Havard J (1988) *Coming of Age*. Heinemann, London, pp. 251–6.
139 Young FB (1928) *My Brother Jonathan*. Heinemann, London.
140 Ibid., pp. 228–9.
141 Ibid., pp. 202–9.
142 Williams WC (1932) Old Doc Rivers. In: *The Doctor Stories*. New Directions, New York, 1984, pp. 13–41.
143 Reed B (1980) *The Verdict*. Simon and Schuster, New York, pp. 31–3.
144 Posen S, op. cit., p. 173.

145 Fitzgerald FS (1934) *Tender is the Night*. Penguin, Harmondsworth, 1998.

146 Ibid., p. 156.

147 Ibid., pp. 182–8.

148 Ibid., pp. 210–11.

149 Ibid., p. 323.

150 Ibid., p. 338.

151 Ibid., p. 308.

152 Anderson S (1919) *Winesburg Ohio*. Viking Press, New York, 1964, pp. 49–57.

153 Chekhov AP (1892) My Wife. In: *The Oxford Chekhov* (translated by Hingley R). *Volume 6*. Oxford University Press, London, 1971, pp. 21–58.

154 Chekhov AP (1897) Uncle Vanya. In: *The Oxford Chekhov* (translated by Hingley R). *Volume 3*. Oxford University Press, London, 1964, pp. 15–67.

155 Chekhov AP (1900–1901) Three Sisters. In: *The Oxford Chekhov* (translated by Hingley R). *Volume 3*. Oxford University Press, London, 1964, pp. 71–139.

156 Simenon G (1963) *The Patient* (translated by Stewart J). Hamish Hamilton, London, 1963, p. 78.

157 Ibsen H (1884) The Wild Duck. In: *Three Plays* (translated by Ellis-Fermor U). Penguin, Harmondsworth, 1957, pp. 139–260.

158 Ibid., p. 189.

159 Ibid., pp. 223–4.

160 Ibid., pp. 243–4.

161 Ibid., p. 207.

162 Ibid., pp. 253–60.

163 Glasgow E (1925) *Barren Ground*. Virago, London, 1986.

164 Ibid., p. 6.

165 Ibid., pp. 128–31.

166 Ibid., p. 262.

167 Ibid., pp. 64–71.

168 Ibid., p. 92.

169 Ibid., p. 360.

170 Cronin AJ (1937) *The Citadel*. Gollancz, London.

171 Ibid., p. 93.

172 Ibid., pp. 426–46.

173 Wolfe T (1929) *Look Homeward Angel*. Charles Scribner's Sons, New York, 1936.

174 Ibid., pp. 170–80.

175 Percy W (1987) *The Thanatos Syndrome*. Ivy Books, New York, 1988.

176 Ibid., p. 395.

177 Chevallier G (1936) *Clochemerle* (translated by Godefroi J). Secker and Warburg, London, 1952, pp. 60–1.

178 Lewis S (1924–1925) *Arrowsmith*. Signet Books, New York, 1961, pp. 6–9.

179 Davies R (1994) *The Cunning Man*. Viking, New York, 1995, pp. 26–7.

180 Ibid., pp. 48–9.

181 Fitzgerald FS (1932) Family in the Wind. In: *Taps at Reveille*. Charles Scribner's Sons, New York, 1935, pp. 303–20.

182 Miller A (1968) *The Price*. Secker and Warburg, London.

183 Friel B (1994) Molly Sweeney. In: *Plays*. *Volume 2*. Faber and Faber, London, 1999, pp. 455–509.

184 Céline LF (1936) *Death on the Installment Plan* (translated by Manheim R). New Directions, New York, p. 32.

185 Theroux P (1989) *My Secret History*. Penguin, Harmondsworth, 1990, pp. 164–86.

186 Barnes D (1936) *Nightwood*. Faber and Faber, London, 1985.

187 Ibid., pp. 29–31.

188 Ibid., pp. 223–32.

189 Ibid., pp. 116–64.

190 Ibid., p. 56.

191 Posen S, op. cit., p. 239.

192 Grisham J (1989) *A Time to Kill*. Island Books (Dell Publishing), New York, 1992, p. 228.

193 Hailey A, op. cit., pp. 210–17.

194 Freedman JF (1997) *Key Witness*. Signet, New York, 1998, p. 106.

195 Kornbluth CM (1950) The Little Black Bag. In: Conklin G and Fabricant ND (eds) *Great Science Fiction About Doctors*. Collier Books, New York, 1963, pp. 165–95.

196 Dooling R (1991) *Critical Care*. William Morrow, New York, pp. 110–21.

197 Ibid., p. 93.

198 Thompson M (1955) *Not as a Stranger*. Michael Joseph, London, pp. 648–57.

199 Sheldon S (1994) *Nothing Lasts Forever*. Harper Collins, London.

200 Ibid., pp. 102–5.

201 Ibid., p. 293.

202 Ibid., pp. 120–7.

203 Slaughter FG (1983) *Doctors at Risk*. Hutchinson, London, pp. 196–211.

204 Cozzens JG (1933) *The Last Adam*. Harcourt Brace & Company, New York.

205 Ibid., p. 23.

206 Ibid., p. 166.

207 Ibid., pp. 221–35.

208 Ibid., p. 301.

209 Havard J, op. cit., pp. 183–6.

210 Ibid., p. 21.

211 Ibid., p. 154.

212 Ibid., pp. 220–4.

213 Ibid., pp. 7–8.

214 Choudhry NK, Fletcher RH and Soumerai SB (2005) Systematic review: the relationship between clinical experience and quality of health care. *Ann Intern Med.* **142:** 260–73.

215 Plato, op. cit., pp. 283–5.

216 Shakespeare W (1599–1600) *As You Like It*. Act 2, Scene 7. Signet Classics, New York, 1963, p. 78.

217 Hawthorne N (1837) Dr Heidegger's Experiment. In: Pearson NH (ed.) *The Complete Novels and Selected Tales of Nathaniel Hawthorne*. Modern Library, New York, 1937, pp. 945–52.

218 Odets C (1935) Awake and Sing. In: *Famous Plays of 1935–6*. Gollancz, London, 1936, p. 545.

219 Irving J (1981) *Hotel New Hampshire*. Corgi Books, London, 1984, pp. 135–7.

220 Gaskell E (1864–1866) *Wives and Daughters*. Oxford University Press, Oxford, 1987, p. 27.

221 Richardson HH, op. cit., pp. 369–70.

222 Young FB (1938) *Doctor Bradley Remembers*. Heinemann, London.

223 Ibid., pp. 32–5.

224 Ibid., p. 744.

225 Ashton H (1930) *Doctor Serocold*. Penguin, London, 1936, pp. 10–17.

226 Garcia Marquez G (1985) *Love in the Time of Cholera* (translated by Grossman E). Jonathan Cape, London, 1988, pp. 8–14.

227 Jones AH (1997) Literature and medicine: Garcia Marquez' *Love in the Time of Cholera*. *Lancet.* **350:** 1169–72.

228 Bellaman H and Bellaman K (1948) *Parris Mitchell of King's Row*. Simon and Schuster, New York, p. 96.

229 Hailey A (1959) *The Final Diagnosis*. Bantam Books, New York, 1967.

230 Ibid., pp. 250–51.

231 Soubiran A (1947) *The Doctors* (translated by Coburn O). WH Allen, London, 1954.
232 Ibid., pp. 133–41.
233 Ibid., pp. 235–42.
234 Posen S, op. cit., p. 160.
235 Mauriac F (1925) *The Desert of Love* (translated by Hopkins G). Eyre and Spotti-swoode, London, 1949, pp. 151–7.
236 Van der Meersch M (1943) *Bodies and Souls* (translated by Wilkins E). William Kimber, London, 1953, pp. 232–5.
237 Ibid., p. 309.
238 Ibid., pp. 396–401.
239 Hailey A (1959) *The Final Diagnosis*. Bantam Books, New York, 1967, pp. 141–7.
240 Ibid., p. 175.
241 Ibid., pp. 302–5.
242 Eliot TS (1939) Old Deuteronomy. In: *The Complete Poems and Plays of TS Eliot*. Faber and Faber, London, 1978, p. 220.
243 Chase JH (1959) Shock Treatment. In: *Three of Spades*. Robert Hale, London, 1974, p. 2.
244 Stern R (1980) Dr Cahn's Visit. In: *Noble Rot: stories 1949–1988*. Grove Press, New York, 1989, pp. 134–8.
245 Young FB (1919) *The Young Physician*. Heinemann, London, 1935, pp. 185–6.
246 Marquis DRP (1939) Country Doctor. In: *The Best of Don Marquis*. Garden City Books, Garden City, NY, pp. 444–63.
247 Green G (1956) *The Last Angry Man*. Charles Scribner's Sons, New York.
248 Balzac H de (1833) *The Country Doctor* (translated by Marriage E). Dent, London, 1923, pp. 270–80.
249 Thompson M (1951) *The Cry and the Covenant*. Pan Books, London, 1969, pp. 462–9.
250 Chekhov AP (1892) The Butterfly. In: *The Oxford Chekhov* (translated by Hingley R). *Volume 6*. Oxford University Press, London, 1971, pp. 61–82.
251 Daudet LA (1894) *Les Morticoles*. Fasquelle, Paris, 1956, pp. 142–6.
252 Young FB (1928) *My Brother Jonathan*. Heinemann, London, pp. 575–95.
253 James PD (1971) *Shroud for a Nightingale*. Sphere Books, London, 1988, p. 275.
254 Guterson D (1999) *East of the Mountains*. Bloomsbury, London, pp. 15–16.
255 Balzac H de (1841) *Ursule Mirouët* (translated by Bell C). Dent, London, 1925, pp. 166–73.
256 Braddon ME (1864) *The Doctor's Wife*. Oxford University Press, Oxford, 1998, pp. 309–15.
257 James H (1881) *Washington Square*. Bantam Books, New York, 1959, pp. 150–2.
258 Glasgow E, op. cit., p. 399.
259 O'Hara J (1962) The Properties of Love. In: *Forty-Nine Stories*. Modern Library, New York, pp. 286–96.
260 Gordon R, op. cit., p. 82.
261 Garcia Marquez G, op. cit., pp. 116–17.
262 Ibid., p. 30.
263 Guterson D, op. cit., pp. 4–10.
264 Ibid., pp. 235–8.
265 Ibid., pp. 258–64.
266 Ibid., pp. 276–7.
267 Doctor X (Nourse AE) (1965) *Intern*. Harper and Row, New York, pp. 253–9.
268 Daudet LA (1894) *Les Morticoles*. Fasquelle, Paris, 1956.
269 Ibid., pp. 267–74.
270 Cheever S (1987) *Doctors and Women*. Methuen, London, 1988, pp. 168–72.
271 Rosenbaum EE (1988) *The Doctor* (also titled *A Taste Of My Own Medicine*). Ivy Books, New York, 1991, pp. 40–2.

272 Ibid., pp. 9–12.
273 Ibid., pp. 83–4.
274 Ibid., pp. 130–43.
275 Martin du Gard R, op. cit., pp. 814–24.
276 Ibid., pp. 943–46.
277 Ibid., p. 976.
278 Ibid., pp. 1021–6.
279 Ibid., p. 1071.
280 Greene G (1940) *The Power and the Glory*. Heinemann, London, 1959, pp. 233–83.
281 Bennett A (1923) *Riceyman Steps*. Cassell, London, 1947, p. 52.
282 James H (1884) Lady Barberina. In: *The New York Edition of Henry James. Volume 14.* Augustus Kelley, Fairfield, NJ, 1976, p. 23.

Conclusions

Fictional doctors are essentially solitary figures, and relatively few of them enjoy a normal family life. Like traditional celibate priests, many practitioners of medicine (mostly men) are portrayed as unencumbered by families. Those who have wives and partners chose them badly and treat them badly. A medical degree is a hindrance rather than a help when it comes to communicating with teenage children. Even happy families have to remain out of sight while the doctor 'serves at the altar of Asclepios'.

Doctors are not good team players and compromisers. Quite the reverse, they deal with life and death problems, and have little time for political activities. They are particularly resentful of bureaucrats whose agenda differs from their own. For the same reason, doctors do not fit readily into religious or quasi-religious movements. They have their own ethics, which are based on the relief of suffering rather than obedience to a supernatural being or integration into a particular ideology.

The cultural accomplishments of twentieth-century doctors are narrower than those of their nineteenth-century predecessors. With notable exceptions, the scholarly nineteenth-century physicians are familiar with a variety of subjects, whereas their twentieth-century counterparts are highly skilled 'cavemen' who never read a book.

Most of the frustrations that beset doctors in their professional work are perceived as minor irritations. Doctors complain with mock regret that they wished they had trained for a different trade, but they continue to practise and to believe in their own usefulness. The truly disillusioned doctor is an object of pity because, with his training and his attitudes, he is useless for most other occupations. Likewise, the sick doctor is almost expected to neglect his own illness and to die without fuss. For a doctor to be demoted to the rank of a patient constitutes the ultimate degradation.

Bibliography

Primary sources

The dates in parentheses refer to the original publication of the work being quoted. An additional unbracketed date refers to the date of publication of the edition being used. The volume and page numbers refer to the publication being cited. The numbers in square brackets refer to the pages where the relevant work is cited in this book. For instance, Sherwood Anderson's *Winesburg, Ohio* was first published in 1919. The edition being used for citation appeared in 1964, where the relevant extracts are found on pages 49–57. *Winesburg, Ohio* is cited on pages 194 and 217 in this book.

Adams, Alice (1991) The Last Lovely City. In: Stone, Robert and Kenison, Katrina (eds) *The Best American Short Stories 1992*. Houghton Mifflin, Boston, MA, 1992, 316 pp.; pp. 1–14 [p. 43].

Albee, Edward (1959) The Death of Bessie Smith. In: *The Zoo Story*. Coward-McCann, New York, 1960, 158 pp.; pp. 67–137 [p. 181].

Alexander, Hannah (2000) *Solemn Oath*. Bethany House Publishers, Minneapolis, MN, 351 pp.; pp. 17–18, 26–35, 63, 161, 169, 178, 217, 224–6, 235–7, 244, 262, 283–9, 334–5, 351 [pp. 130–1, 177].

Ambler, Eric (1974) *Doctor Frigo*. Fontana/Collins, Glasgow, 1976, 245 pp.; pp. 130–1 [p. 90].

Anderson, Sherwood (1919) *Winesburg, Ohio*. Viking Press, New York, 1964, 247 pp.; pp. 49–57 [pp. 194, 217].

Ariyoshi, Sawako (1967) *The Doctor's Wife* (translated by Hironaka, Wakako and Kostant, Ann Siller). Kodansha, Tokyo, 1989, 174 pp.; p. 68 [p. 28].

Arlen, Michael (Kouyoumdjian, Dikran) (1924) *The Green Hat*. George H Doran, New York, 350 pp.; pp. 180–6 [p. 170].

Ashton, Helen (1930) *Doctor Serocold*. Penguin, London, 1936, 256 pp.; pp. 10–17, 29, 30–1, 35, 66, 72, 76–80, 113, 122, 136, 154–5, 256 [pp. 8, 77, 112–13, 175–6, 227–8].

Auden, Wystan Hugh (1936) Miss Gee. In: *Selections by the Author*. Penguin, Harmondsworth, 1970, 70 pp.; pp. 43–5 [p. 41].

Auden, Wystan Hugh (1972) The Art of Healing: In Memoriam David Protetch, MD. In: *Epistle to a Godson and Other Poems*. Faber and Faber, London, 72 pp.; pp. 13–15 [pp. 38, 204].

Auden, Wystan Hugh (1972) Lines to Dr Walter Birk on his Retiring from General Practice. In: *Epistle to a Godson and Other Poems*. Faber and Faber, London, 72 pp.; p. 16 [p. 62].

Baldwin, Faith (1939) *Medical Centre*. Horwitz, Sydney, 1962, 226 pp.; pp. 11–12, 24, 41–7, 61 [pp. 16, 174].

Balzac, Honoré de (1833) *The Country Doctor* (translated by Marriage, Ellen). Dent, London, 1923, 287 pp.; pp. 36–7, 270–80 [pp. 5, 156, 181].

Balzac, Honoré de (1836) *The Atheist's Mass* (translated by Bell, Clara). Dent, London, 1929, 291 pp.; pp. 1–20 [pp. 72, 131, 143].

Balzac, Honoré de (1840) *Pierrette* (translated by Ives, George B). George Barrie and Sons, Philadelphia, PA, 1897, 338 pp. [p. 181].

Balzac, Honoré de (1841) *Ursule Mirouët* (translated by Bell, Clara). Dent, London, 1925, 259 pp.; pp. 9, 13–19, 26–9, 39, 53, 166–73 [pp. 104–5, 110, 231–2].

Barker, Pat (Patricia Margaret) (1991) *Regeneration*. Penguin, Harmondsworth, 1992, 252 pp.; pp. 28–32, 135–7 [p. 191].

Barker, Pat (Patricia Margaret) (1993) *The Eye in the Door*. Penguin, Harmondsworth, 1994, 280 pp.; p. 245 [p. 201].

Barker, Pat (Patricia Margaret) (1995) *The Ghost Road*. Viking, London, 278 pp.; pp. 50–1, 110 [pp. 1, 201].

Barnes, Djuna (1921) The Doctors (also titled Katrina Silverstaff). In: Herring, Phillip (ed.) *Djuna Barnes: collected stories*. Sun and Moon Press, Los Angeles, CA, 1996, 477 pp.; pp. 319–26 [p. 22].

Barnes, Djuna (1936) *Nightwood*. Faber and Faber, London, 1985, 239 pp.; pp. 29–31, 56, 115–55, 156–64, 223–32 [pp. 152, 221].

Bashford, Henry Howarth (1911) *The Corner of Harley Street: being some familiar correspondence of Peter Harding MD*. Constable, London, 1913, 271 pp.; pp. 9, 13, 14, 15–17, 18, 21–3, 32–3, 38, 39–41, 41, 49–51, 57, 63, 84, 93–4, 102, 130–9, 147, 168–9, 174–5, 204–10, 212–16, 217, 219–23, 237, 242–5, 246, 253, 254, 265, 268, 270 [pp. 40, 82, 116, 157–8, 174, 207].

Baum, Vicki (Baum, Hedwig) (1928) *Helene* (translated by Bashford, Félice). Penguin, Harmondsworth, 1939, 279 pp.; pp. 24–6, 42, 61–2, 107, 183 [pp. 184–5].

Baum, Vicki (Baum, Hedwig) (1929) *Grand Hotel* (translated by Creighton, Basil). Geoffrey Bles, London, 1930, 315 pp.; pp. 3, 43–4, 84, 244–6, 249, 253 [pp. 205–6].

Baum, Vicki (Baum, Hedwig) (1939) *Nanking Road* (also titled *Shanghai '37*) (translated by Creighton, Basil). Geoffrey Bles, London, 807 pp.; pp. 73–6, 77–85, 296, 359, 433, 496, 806 [pp. 46, 207].

Baum, Vicki (Baum, Hedwig) (1944) *Berlin Hotel*. Angus and Robertson, Sydney, 1945, 249 pp.; pp. 6–8, 79, 240 [p. 207].

Beauvoir, Simone de (1964) *A Very Easy Death* (translated by O'Brian, Patrick). Andre Deutsch and Weidenfeld and Nicholson, London, 1966, 106 pp.; pp. 10–12 [p. 74].

Bellaman, Henry (1940) *King's Row*. Dymocks, Sydney, 1945, 504 pp.; pp. 253–6, 376–80, 393–415, 430–40, 445–61 [pp. 88, 114, 158, 208].

Bellaman, Henry and Bellaman, Katherine (1948) *Parris Mitchell of King's Row*. Simon and Schuster, New York, 333 pp.; pp. 96, 110, 187–8, 292 [pp. 15, 91, 228].

Bellamy, Edward (1880) *Dr Heidenhoff's Process*. AMS Press, New York, 1969, 139 pp.; p. 105 [p. 105].

Bellow, Saul (1956) *Seize The Day*. Penguin, New York, 1996, 118 pp.; pp. 11, 12, 14, 27, 34, 36, 42–4, 45–6, 51, 61–9, 104, 108–10 [pp. 48, 150–1].

Bellow, Saul (1969) *Mr Sammler's Planet*. Penguin, Harmondsworth, 1977, 286 pp.; pp. 66–8 [p. 195].

Benét, Stephen Vincent (1938) Doc Mellhorn and the Pearly Gates. In: *Tales Before Midnight*. Heinemann, London, 1940, 232 pp.; pp. 102–24 [p. 131].

Bennett, Arnold (1908) *The Old Wives' Tale*. Hodder and Stoughton, London, 1964, 544 pp.; pp. 461–3 [pp. 158, 160–1].

Bennett, Arnold (1923) *Riceyman Steps*. Cassell, London, 1947, 319 pp.; pp. 12–15, 51–2, 178–80, 185, 213–20, 245–64, 264–71, 314 [pp. 38, 40–1, 66, 103, 145, 168, 179].

Bernhard, Thomas (1967) *Gargoyles* (translated by Winston, Richard and Winston, Clara). Alfred A Knopf, New York, 1970, 208 pp.; pp. 21–2, p. 24 [pp. 75, 154].

Bernières, Louis de (1994) *Captain Corelli's Mandolin*. Vintage, London, 1998, 434 pp.; pp. 1–5, 44–5, 53, 57, 119–22 [pp. 63, 107, 159].

The Bible, Revised Standard Version. Oxford University Press, New York, 1977, II Chronicles, 16: 12–13 [p. 103].

Ecclesiasticus, 38: 13–15 [p. 103].

Genesis, 30: 16–18 [p. 15].

Hosea, 1: 2 [p. 17].

I Kings, 15: 14 [p. 103].

Luke, 10: 38–40 [p. 15].

Matthew, 13: 44 [p. 128].

Romans, 7: 15 [p. 184].

Blodgett, Ruth (1932) *Home is the Sailor*. Harcourt Brace, New York, 349 pp.; pp. 84–92, 258–66, 239, 287, 325, 337–48 [p. 14].

Boccaccio, Giovanni (1348–1353) *The Decameron (IV, X)* (translated by McWilliam, GH). Penguin, Harmondsworth, 1980, 833 pp.; pp. 392–401 [p. 17].

Braddon, Mary Elizabeth (1864) *The Doctor's Wife*. Oxford University Press, Oxford, 1998, 431 pp.; pp. 6, 108, 114, 183, 199, 221, 224, 308–15, 368 [pp. 32, 74, 232].

Brontë, Charlotte (1853) *Villette*. Penguin, Harmondsworth, 1983, 622 pp.; pp. 82, 148–52, 167–9, 296–302, 463, 532–3 [pp. 39–40].

Brown, Thomas K (1956) A Drink of Water. In: Engle, Paul and Harnack, Curt (eds) *Prize Stories of 1958: the O Henry Awards*. Doubleday, Garden City, NY, 1958, pp. 179–201 [p. 177].

Browne, Thomas (1642) Religio Medici. In: Keynes, Geoffrey (ed.) *The Works of Sir Thomas Browne. Volume 1*. Faber and Faber, London, 1964, 295 pp.; p. 11 [p. 104].

Bulgakov, Mikhail Afanasevich (1925–1927) Baptism by Rotation. In: *A Country Doctor's Notebook* (translated by Glenny, Michael). Collins and Harvill Press, London, 1975, 158 pp.; pp. 53–62 [pp. 176–7].

Bulgakov, Mikhail Afanasevich (1925–1927) The Embroidered Towel. In: *A Country Doctor's Notebook* (translated by Glenny, Michael). Collins and Harvill Press, London, 1975, 158 pp.; pp. 13–25 [pp. 176–7].

Bulgakov, Mikhail Afanasevich (1925–1927) Morphine. In: *A Country Doctor's Notebook* (translated by Glenny, Michael). Collins and Harvill Press, London, 1975, 158 pp.; pp. 113–44 [p. 214].

Bulgakov, Mikhail Afanasevich (1925–1927) The Steel Windpipe. In: *A Country Doctor's Notebook* (translated by Glenny, Michael). Collins and Harvill Press, London, 1975, 158 pp.; pp. 29–37 [pp. 176–7].

Busch, Frederick (1979) *Rounds*. Farrar Straus and Giroux, New York, 243 pp.; pp. 3, 80–1, 90 [pp. 179–80].

Busch, Frederick (1984) A History of Small Ideas. In: *Too Late American Boyhood Blues*. David R Godine, Boston, MA, 275 pp.; pp. 150–70 [pp. 37, 143].

Busch, Frederick (1984) Rise and Fall. In: *Too Late American Boyhood Blues*. David R Godine, Boston, MA, 275 pp.; pp. 17–51, 31 [pp. 34–5, 170].

Cable, George Washington (1885) *Dr Sevier*. James R Osgood and Company, Boston, MA, 473 pp.; p. 62 [p. 118].

Caldwell, Taylor (1968) *Testimony of Two Men*. Collins, London, 1990, 476 pp.; pp. 13–15, 16, 17, 51–7, 61–3, 73, 75–8, 87–8, 107, 129, 132–8, 141–4, 157–67, 216–20, 225, 278, 330, 345, 347, 351, 385, 447–8, 468, 472 [pp. 21, 80–1, 127, 209].

Camus, Albert (1947) *The Plague* (translated by Gilbert, Stuart). Penguin, Harmondsworth, 1960, 252 pp.; pp. 11, 20, 173–9, 237–8 [pp. 29–30, 92, 117].

Cao Xue Qin (also spelt Tsao Hsueh Chin) (1792) *The Story of The Stone* (also titled *The Dream of The Red Chamber*) (translated by Hawkes, David). Penguin, Harmondsworth, 1973, 540 pp.; p. 226 [p. 65].

Čapek, Karel (1929) Giddiness (translated by Selver, Paul). In: *Tales From Two Pockets*. Allen and Unwin, London, 1967, 215 pp.; pp. 177–83 [p. 103].

Cather, Willa (1931) *Shadows on the Rock*. Virago, London, 1984, 275 pp.; pp. 124, 253 [p. 106].

Cather, Willa (1932) Neighbor Rosicky. In: *Five Stories*. Vintage Books, New York, 1956, 214 pp.; pp. 72–111 [p. 63].

Cave, Hugh Barnett (1951) The Doctor's Wife. In: *The Witching Lands*. Alvin Redman, London, 1962, 260 pp.; pp. 62–80 [p. 21].

Céline, Louis Ferdinand (Destouches, Louis Ferdinand) (1932) *Journey to the End of the Night* (translated by Manheim, Ralph). New Directions, New York, 1983, 446 pp.; pp. 204–5, 224–7, 259, 306–7, 358, 363, 365, 374–80, 426–9, 433 [pp. 2, 73, 188–9].

Céline, Louis Ferdinand (Destouches, Louis Ferdinand) (1932) *Journey to the End of the Night* (translated by Marks, John). Chatto and Windus, London, 1934, 543 pp [p. 2].

Céline, Louis Ferdinand (Destouches, Louis Ferdinand) (1936) *Death on the Installment Plan* (translated by Manheim, Ralph). New Directions, New York, 1938, 592 pp.; pp. 15–17, 24–5, 32 [pp. 188–9, 221].

Chandler, Raymond (1943) *The Lady in the Lake*. Vintage Books, New York, 1976, 217 pp.; pp. 21–2, 129 [pp. 139, 201, 214, 226].

Chandler, Raymond (1953) *The Long Goodbye*. Pan, London, 1979, 285 pp.; pp. 85, 89, 98, 99–101, 131–5, 257 [pp. 25, 214].

Chase, James Hadley (Raymond, Rene Brabazon) (1959) Shock Treatment. In: *Three of Spades*. Robert Hale, London, 1974, 630 pp.; p. 2 [pp. 230–1].

Chaucer Geoffrey (*c.* 1390) The Canterbury Tales. In: Fisher, John H (ed.) *The Complete Poetry and Prose of Geoffrey Chaucer*. Holt, Rinehart and Winston, New York, 1977, 1032 pp.; pp. 17–18 [p. 104].

Cheever, Susan (1987) *Doctors and Women*. Methuen, London, 1988, 240 pp.; pp. 168–72, 197 [p. 146, 235–6].

Chekhov, Anton Pavlovich (1887) The Enemies (also titled Two Tragedies, also titled Antagonists). In: *Short Stories* (translated by Fen, Elisaveta). Folio Society, London, 1974, pp. 58–72 [pp. 141, 187–8].

Chekhov, Anton Pavlovich (1887–1889) Ivanov. In: *The Oxford Chekhov* (translated by Hingley, Ronald). *Volume 2*. Oxford University Press, London, 1967, pp. 163–227 [p. 5].

Chekhov, Anton Pavlovich (1888) An Awkward Business. In: *The Oxford Chekhov* (translated by Hingley, Ronald). *Volume 4*. Oxford University Press, London, 1980, pp. 99–115 [p. 5].

Chekhov, Anton Pavlovich (1892) The Butterfly. In: *The Oxford Chekhov* (translated by Hingley, Ronald). *Volume 6*. Oxford University Press, London, 1971, pp. 61–82 [pp. 18, 32, 143].

Chekhov, Anton Pavlovich (1892) My Wife. In: *The Oxford Chekhov* (translated by Hingley, Ronald). *Volume 6*. Oxford University Press, London, 1971, pp. 19–58 [p. 186].

Chekhov, Anton Pavlovich (1892) Ward Number Six. In: *The Oxford Chekhov* (translated by Hingley, Ronald). *Volume 6*. Oxford University Press, London, 1971, pp. 121–67, 129 [pp. 106–7, 185–6].

Chekhov, Anton Pavlovich (1896) The Seagull. In: *The Oxford Chekhov* (translated by Hingley, Ronald). *Volume 2*. Oxford University Press, London, 1967, pp. 239, 246, 252, 270, 231–81 [pp. 5–6, 186–7].

Chekhov, Anton Pavlovich (1897) Uncle Vanya. In: *The Oxford Chekhov* (translated by Hingley, Ronald). *Volume 3*. Oxford University Press, London, 1964, pp. 27, 38–40, 62, 66, 15–67 [pp. 5, 186].

Chekhov, Anton Pavlovich (1898) Doctor Startsev. In: *The Oxford Chekhov* (translated by Hingley, Ronald). *Volume 9*. Oxford University Press, London, 1975, pp. 51–66 [pp. 141–2].

Chekhov, Anton Pavlovich (1900–1901) Three Sisters. In: *The Oxford Chekhov* (translated by Hingley, Ronald). *Volume 3*. Oxford University Press, London, 1964, pp. 71–139, 74–7, 106, 113 [pp. 5, 142, 186].

Chellis, Mary Dwinnell (1870) *The Old Doctor's Son*. Henry A Young, Boston, MA, 354 pp.; pp. 14, 129, 175, 348–52 [pp. 17, 215].

Chevallier, Gabriel (1936) *Clochemerle* (translated by Godefroi, Jocelyn). Secker and Warburg, London, 1952, 317 pp.; pp. 58, 60–1, 182–3 [pp. 113–14, 142, 218–19].

Collier, John (1931) De Mortuis. In: *Fancies and Goodnights*. Time Life Books, Alexandria, VA, 1980, 328 pp.; pp. 11–19 [p. 20].

Collins, Wilkie (1868) *The Moonstone*. Perennial Classics, Harper and Row, New York, 1965, 462 pp.; pp. 222, 317–18, 361–71 [pp. 108, 206].

Cook, Robin (1977) *Coma*. Pan Books, London, 1978, 332 pp.; pp. 38–55 [p. 86].

Cook, Robin (1981) *Brain*. Pan Books, London, 235 pp.; pp. 42–53, 108–9, 119 [pp. 9, 86, 145, 178].

Cook, Robin (1993) *Fatal Cure*. Pan Books, London, 1995, 447 pp.; pp. 80, 112–13, 114–15 [pp. 9, 48–9, 177].

Coombs, Margaret (1990) *The Best Man for This Sort of Thing*. Black Swan, Sydney, 364 pp.; pp. 251–2 [p. 161].

Corris, Peter (1999) *The Other Side of Sorrow*. Bantam Books, Sydney, 216 pp.; pp. 107–23 [pp. 63–4].

Cozzens, James Gould (1933) *The Last Adam*. Harcourt Brace and Company, New York, 301 pp.; pp. 23, 31, 155–8, 161, 166, 173–4, 194, 203, 221–35, 250, 279, 301 [pp. 63, 77–8, 110, 224–5].

Crichton, Michael (Hudson, Jeffery*, pseudonym) (1968) *A Case of Need*. Signet, New York, 1969, 416 pp.; pp. 54, 60, 76–7, 124–5, 146, 210–12, 215–16, 308–11, 315–16, 379 [pp. 31, 46, 88, 94, 184].

Cronin, Archibald Joseph (1937) *The Citadel*. Gollancz, London, 446 pp.; pp. 77, 93, 156–9, 163–4, 173, 390–411, 426–46 [pp. 32, 70, 73–4, 123–4, 148, 181, 218, 220].

Cuthbert, Margaret (1998) *The Silent Cradle*. Simon and Schuster, London, 353 pp.; pp. 7, 140 [pp. 37, 116].

Danby, Frank (Frankau, Julia) (1887) *Dr Phillips: a Maida Vale Idyll*. Garland Publishing, New York, 1984, 342 pp.; pp. 27–30, 47, 52, 187, 250, 287, 316–21, 340–1, 335–40 [pp. 13, 106].

Daudet, Léon (Daudet, Alphonse Marie Léon) (1894) *Les Morticoles*. Fasquelle, Paris, 1956, 360 pp.; pp. 30–4, 42, 47, 144–6, 267–74 [pp. 75, 107, 126, 234–5].

Davies, Robertson (1985) *What's Bred in the Bone*. Penguin, Harmondsworth, 1988, 438 pp.; pp. 49–50 [p. 106].

Davies, Robertson (1994) *The Cunning Man*. Viking, New York, 1995, 469 pp.; pp. 26–7, pp. 48–9 [p. 219].

Dawson, William James (1900) *The Doctor Speaks*. Grant Richards, London, 334 pp.; pp. 20–8, 92–7, 169–204, 220 [pp. 62, 89, 128–9].

Dawson, William James (1900) A Surgical Operation. In: *The Doctor Speaks*. Grant Richards, London, 334 pp.; pp. 3–28 [p. 89].

Deeping, Warwick (1925) *Sorrell and Son*. Cassell, London, 1927, 394 pp.; pp. 252–3, 288–9, 297, 299–307, 312, 341–2, 350–5, 357, 361, 368 [pp. 19, 88, 206].

Dickens, Charles (1837) *The Pickwick Papers*. Signet Classics, New American Library, New York, 1964, 888 pp.; pp. 479–84, 583 [pp. 140–1, 143].

Dickens, Charles (1852–1853) *Bleak House*. Collins, London, 1953, 799 pp.; p. 796 [p. 39].

Diogenes Laertius (Third Century AD) Socrates. In: *The Lives of Eminent Philosophers*

---

* See footnote on p. xii.

(translated by Hicks, Robert Drew). *Volume 1*. Harvard University Press, Cambridge, MA, 1972, 549 pp.; p. 167 [p. 12].

Döblin, Alfred (1929) *Berlin Alexanderplatz* (translated by Jolas, Eugene). Continuum, New York, 2004, 635 pp.; pp. 593–4 [p. 79].

Doctor X (Nourse, Alan Edward) (1965) *Intern*. Harper and Row, New York, 404 pp.; pp. 87, 208, 216–21, 241, 247, 253–9 [pp. 9, 65, 79, 173, 234].

Dooling, Richard (1991) *Critical Care*. William Morrow, New York, 248 pp.; pp. 11–12, 17, 31, 93, 110–21, 126, 192–4 [pp. 16, 171–4, 179, 222–3].

Dostoyevsky, Fyodor (1880) *The Brothers Karamazov* (translated by Magarshack, David). Penguin, Harmondsworth, 1978, 913 pp.; *Volume 1*, pp. 211–12; *Volume 2*, pp. 789–95 [pp. 6, 64, 129].

Douglas, Lloyd Cassel (1935) *Green Light*. Angus and Robertson, Sydney, 1947, 329 pp.; pp. 21–4 [p. 86].

Douglas, Lloyd Cassel (1939) *Doctor Hudson's Secret Journal*. Grosset and Dunlap, New York, 295 pp.; p. 7, p. 32 [p. 171].

Doyle, Arthur Conan (1894) Behind the Times. In: *Round The Red Lamp*. John Murray, London, 1934, 328 pp.; pp. 1–8 [pp. 202, 227].

Doyle, Arthur Conan (1894) The Curse of Eve. In: *Round The Red Lamp*. John Murray, London, 1934, 328 pp.; pp. 89–108 [p. 91].

Doyle, Arthur Conan (1894) His First Operation. In: *Round the Red Lamp*. John Murray, London, 1934, 328 pp.; pp. 9–19 [p. 76].

Doyle, Arthur Conan (1894) A Physiologist's Wife. In: *Round the Red Lamp*. John Murray, London, 1934, 328 pp.; pp. 120–55 [p. 17].

Dreiser, Theodore (1919) The Country Doctor. In: *Twelve Men*. Constable, London, 1930, 320 pp.; pp. 102–22 [pp. 40, 202–3].

Dreiser, Theodore (1925) *An American Tragedy*. Signet Classics, New American Library, New York, 1964, 831 pp.; pp. 397–407 [pp. 124–5, 145].

Duhamel, Georges (1928) *Les Sept Dernières Plaies*. Mercure de France, Paris, 295 pp.; pp. 16–17, 52, 92, 105–17 [p. 210].

Eliot, George (Evans, Mary Ann) (1871–1872) *Middlemarch*. Penguin, Harmondsworth, 1988, 908 pp.; pp. 211, 212, 330, 335–6, 475, 497, 825, 850, 854, 858, 861, 893 [pp. 11–12, 33, 75, 105–6].

Eliot, Thomas Stearns (1939) Old Deuteronomy. In: *The Complete Poems and Plays of TS Eliot*. Faber and Faber, London, 1978, 608 pp.; p. 220 [p. 230].

Ellis, AE (Lindsay, Derek) (1958) *The Rack*. Penguin, Harmondsworth, 1988, 357 pp.; pp. 33, 64, 82–3, 97–8 [pp. 85, 204].

Ellison, Harlan (1957) Wanted in Surgery. In: *The Fantasies of Harlan Ellison*. Gregg Press, Boston, MA, 1979, 316 pp.; pp. 120–52 [p. 15].

El Saadawi, Nawal (1975) *Two Women in One* (translated by Nusairi, Osman and Gough, Jana). El Saqi Books, London, 1985, 124 pp.; pp. 23, 39, 60–4, 80 [pp. 147–8, 185].

Faulkner, William (1930) *As I Lay Dying*. Vintage Books, New York, 1985, 267 pp.; p. 89 [p. 63].

Faulkner, William (1933) Doctor Martino. In: *Doctor Martino and Other Stories*. Chatto and Windus, London, 1968, 320 pp.; pp. 163–83 [p. 7].

Faulkner, William (1939) *The Wild Palms*. Random House, New York, 339 pp.; pp. 4–16, 241–9, 274–306, 300 [pp. 26, 35–6, 169].

Fearing, Kenneth (1939) *The Hospital*. Ballantine Books, New York, 144 pp.; pp. 52–3, 55–8, 90–1 [pp. 146–7].

Fisher, Hazel (1982) *The Tender Heart*. Mills and Boon, London, 191 pp. [p. 16].

Fisher, Nancy (1994) *Side-Effects*. Hodder and Stoughton, London, 472 pp.; pp. 41–4 [p. 82].

Fitzgerald, Francis Scott (1932) Family in the Wind. In: *Taps at Reveille*. Charles Scribner's Sons, New York, 1935, 407 pp.; pp. 303–20 [pp. 219–20].

Fitzgerald, Francis Scott (1932) One Interne. In: *Taps at Reveille*. Charles Scribner's Sons, New York, 1935, 407 pp.; pp. 349–73 [pp. 174, 203].

Fitzgerald, Francis Scott (1934) *Tender is the Night*. Penguin, Harmondsworth, 1998, 358 pp.; pp. 129–30, 156, 169, 182, 182–8, 200, 206–11, 273–4, 303–6, 308, 323, 325, p. 338 [pp. 1, 4, 21–2, 152, 216–17].

Flaubert, Gustave (1857) *Madame Bovary* (translated by Steegmuller, Francis). Modern Library, New York, 1982, 396 pp.; pp. 7–9, 12, 13–23, 39–49, 68–9, 144–5, 204–5, 328, 360, 363, 364, 366, 394–6 [pp. 1, 10–11, 29, 32, 64, 66, 110–11, 140–1, 144, 180, 203].

Fontane, Theodor (1895) *Effi Briest* (translated by Parmée Douglas). Penguin, London, 1967, 267 pp; p. 250 [p. 82].

Frede, Richard (1960) *The Interns*. Corgi, London, 1965, 346 pp.; p. 23 [p. 86].

Frederic, Harold (1896) *The Damnation of Theron Ware*. Harvard University Press, Cambridge, MA, 1960, 355 pp.; pp. 69–78, 233 [p. 105].

Freedman, JF (1997) *Key Witness*. Dutton, New York, 532 pp.; p. 106 [p. 222].

Friel, Brian (1994) Molly Sweeney. In: *Plays. Volume 2*. Faber and Faber, London, 1999, pp. 455–509 [pp. 220–1].

Galgut, Damon (2003) *The Good Doctor*. Atlantic, London, 215 pp.; pp. 130, 139 [p. 9].

Garcia Marquez, Gabriel (1985) *Love in the Time of Cholera* (translated by Grossman, Edith). Jonathan Cape, London, 1988, 352 pp.; pp. 8–14, 15, 21, 24, 30, 32, 35, 40, 42, 47–8, 90, 109, 110–11, 112, 116–17, 126, 195, 196, 210–14, 225–6, 239–40, 253–4, 322–4, 349 [pp. 43–4, 80, 129–30, 159–60, 228, 233].

Gardner, John (1963) *Nickel Mountain*. Alfred A Knopf, New York, 1973, 312 pp.; p. 98 [pp. 66–7].

Gardner, John (1972) *The Sunlight Dialogues*. Ballantine Books, New York, 1973, 746 pp.; p. 665 [p. 35].

Gaskell, Elizabeth (1864–1866) *Wives and Daughters*. Oxford University Press, Oxford, 1987, 740 pp.; pp. 27, 32–8, 59, 98, 114, 125, 131, 147–8, 184–5, 337, 341, 398–405, 547, 683–4 [pp. 11, 62–3, 156, 226].

Gerritsen, Tess (1996) *Harvest*. Headline Publishing, London, 313 pp; pp. 10, 31–3, 45, 66–7, 124–34 [pp. 82, 109].

Glasgow, Ellen (1925) *Barren Ground*. Virago, London, 1986, 409 pp.; pp. 6, 64–71, 92, 128–31, 262, 360–2, 399 [pp. 119, 217–18, 232–3].

Glasser, Ronald J (1973) *Ward 402*. Garnstone Press, London, 1974, 240 pp.; pp. 55–6 [pp. 84–5].

Goethe, Johann Wolfgang von (1808) *Faust. Part I* (translated by Latham, Albert G). Dent, London, 1928, 464 pp.; pp. 30–1 [pp. 154, 190–1].

Goldsworthy, Peter (1988) The Nice Chinese Doctor. In: *Bleak Rooms*. Wakefield Press, Adelaide, 137 pp.; pp. 59–74 [pp. 74–5].

Goldsworthy, Peter (1992) *Honk If You Are Jesus*. Angus and Robertson, Sydney, 290 pp.; pp. 5, 17, 45–6, 48–9, 94–6, 289–90 [pp. 93, 111, 192].

Goldsworthy, Peter (2003) *Three Dog Night*. Penguin, Melbourne, 342 pp [p. 19 f.].

Gordon, Richard (Ostlere, Gordon Stanley) (1952) *Doctor in the House*. Michael Joseph, London, 1967, 190 pp.; pp. 69–71, 82 [p. 233].

Green, Gerald (1956) *The Last Angry Man*. Charles Scribner's Sons, New York, 494 pp.; pp. 2–9, 188, 217, 311, 324–33, 344, 356, 382, 420–4 [pp. 43, 63, 66, 79, 155, 159].

Green, Gerald (1979) *The Healers*. Melbourne House, London, 500 pp.; pp. 143, 178–9, 179–81, 221–2, 227, 236–7, 491–2 [pp. 26–7, 35, 116, 126, 182–3].

Greene, Graham (1940) *The Power and the Glory*. Heinemann, London, 1959, pp. 233–83 [p. 238].

Greene, Graham (1961) *A Burnt-Out Case*. The Bodley Head and William Heinemann, London, 1974, 236 pp.; pp. 15, 38–42, 68, 100–5, 143, 144–5, 159, 178–9 [p. 111].

Greene, Graham (1963) Dream of a Strange Land. In: *Collected Stories*. The Bodley Head and William Heinemann, London, 1972, 561 pp.; pp. 281–97 [p. 144].

Greene, Graham (1965) Doctor Crombie. In: *Collected Stories*. The Bodley Head and William Heinemann, London, 1972, 561 pp.; pp. 129–35 [p. 211].

Greene, Graham (1973) *The Honorary Consul*. Simon and Schuster, New York, 315 pp.; pp. 36, 255–67 [pp. 117–18].

Gregory of Tours (*c.* AD 580) The Miracles of the Bishop Saint Martin. In: *Saints and Their Miracles in Late Antique Gaul* (translated by Van Dam, Raymond). Princeton University Press, Princeton, NJ, 1993, 349 pp.; p. 238 [p. 104].

Grisham, John (1989) *A Time to Kill*. Island Books (Dell Publishing), New York, 1992, 515 pp.; p. 228 [p. 221].

Grisham, John (1995) *The Rainmaker*. Island Books (Dell Publishing), New York, 1996, 598 pp. [p. 8].

Guterson, David (1999) *East of the Mountains*. Bloomsbury, London, 279 pp.; pp. 3–11, 15–16, 47, 235–8, 256, 258–64, 274, 276–7 [pp. 43, 233–4].

Haggard, Henry Rider (1898) *Doctor Therne*. Hodder and Stoughton, London, 1923, 252 pp.; pp. 72, 86–8 [p. 76].

Hailey, Arthur (1959) *The Final Diagnosis*. Bantam Books, New York, 1967, 310 pp.; pp. 46–54, 141–7, 175, 195–9, 250–1, 302–5 [pp. 80, 228–9, 230].

Hailey, Arthur (1984) *Strong Medicine*. Dell, New York, 1986, 445 pp.; pp. 77–80, 82–3, 128–30, 137–41, 143, 210–17 [pp. 213–14, 221, 223–4].

Halle, John (1565) Preface to the Reader. In: Lanfranc of Milan (ed.) *The Herball*. John Daye, London, p. 5 [p. 204].

Hardy, Thomas (1886–1887) *The Woodlanders*. Oxford University Press, Oxford, 1988, 305 pp.; pp. 125–9, 274 [pp. 27, 107].

Haseltine, Florence (Yaw, Yvonne) (1976) *Woman Doctor*. Houghton Mifflin, Boston, MA, 336 pp.; p. 80 [p. 38].

Havard, Jonathan (1988) *Coming of Age*. Heinemann, London, 350 pp.; pp. 7–8, 21, 121–2, 154, 183–6, 220–4, 251–6 [pp. 88–9, 225].

Hawthorne, Nathaniel (1837) Dr Heidegger's Experiment. In: Pearson, Norman Holmes (ed.) *The Complete Novels and Selected Tales of Nathaniel Hawthorne*. Modern Library, New York, 1937, 1223 pp.; pp. 945–52 [p. 226].

Hawthorne, Nathaniel (1850) *The Scarlet Letter*. Ohio State University Press, Columbus, OH, 1971, 292 pp.; p. 119 [p. 105].

Hecht, Ben (1959) Miracle of the Fifteen Murderers. In: *A Treasury of Ben Hecht: collected stories and other writings*. Crown Publishers, New York, 397 pp.; p. 191 [p. 84].

Hejinian, John (1974) *Extreme Remedies*. St Martin's Press, New York, 342 pp.; pp. 221–5, 288–93 [p. 191].

Heller, Joseph (1955) *Catch 22*. Dell, New York, 1974, 463 pp.; pp. 32–3 [pp. 201–2].

Hellman, Lillian (1934) *The Children's Hour*. Dramatists Play Service, New York, 1981, 75 pp.; p. 63 [pp. 33–4].

Hemingway, Ernest (1925) The Doctor and the Doctor's Wife. In: *The Complete Short Stories of Ernest Hemingway*. Scribner Paperback Edition, Simon and Schuster, New York, 1998, 650 pp.; pp. 73–6 [p. 24].

Hemingway, Ernest (1929) *A Farewell to Arms*. Jonathan Cape, London, 349 pp.; p. 105 [p. 71].

Hemingway, Ernest (1933) God Rest You Merry, Gentlemen. In: *The Complete Short Stories of Ernest Hemingway*. Scribner Paperback Edition, Simon and Schuster, New York, 1998, 650 pp.; pp. 298–301 [pp. 149–50].

Herrick, Robert (1897) *The Man Who Wins*. Charles Scribner's Sons, New York, 125 pp.; pp. 98–109 [pp. 45–6].

Herrick, Robert (1900) *The Web of Life*. Macmillan, London, 356 pp. [p. 40].

Herrick, Robert (1908) *The Master of the Inn*. Charles Scribner's Sons, New York, 1913, 84 pp. [p. 181].

Herrick, Robert (1911) *The Healer*. Macmillan, New York, 455 pp.; pp. 50–51, 244–6, 426–7 [p. 181].

Hippocrates (fifth century BC) Aphorisms. In: *The Works of Hippocrates* (translated by Jones, WHS). *Volume 4*. Loeb's Classical Library, Heinemann, London, 1943, 521 pp.; p. 99 [p. 139].

Hippocrates (attrib.) (fifth century BC) The Physician. In: *The Works of Hippocrates* (translated by Jones, WHS). *Volume 2*. Loeb's Classical Library, Heinemann, London, 1923, 336 pp.; p. 311 [p. 204].

Hippocrates (attrib.) (fifth century BC) Precepts. In: *The Works of Hippocrates* (translated by Jones, WHS). *Volume 1*. Loeb's Classical Library, Heinemann, London, 1972, 392 pp.; p. 325 [p. 64].

Holmes, Oliver Wendell (1861) Elsie Venner. In: *The Works of Oliver Wendell Holmes*. *Volume 5*. Houghton Mifflin Company, Boston, MA, 1892, 487 pp.; pp. 210–11, 313–28 [pp. 122, 140].

Holmes, Oliver Wendell (1871) The Young Practitioner. In: *Medical Essays 1842–1882. The Works of Oliver Wendell Holmes. Volume 9*. Houghton Mifflin, Boston, MA, 1892, 445 pp.; p. 384 [pp. 139–40].

Hooker, Richard (Hornberger, Richard) (1968) *M.A.S.H.* William Morrow, New York, 219 pp.; pp. 19–27, 161–2 [pp. 63, 124].

Howard, Sidney (1932) The Late Christopher Bean. In: Warnock, Robert (ed.) *Representative Modern Plays*. Scott Foresman and Company, Chicago, 1952, 758 pp.; pp. 136–59 [p. 146].

Howells, William Dean (1881) *Dr Breen's Practice*. James Osgood, Boston, MA, 272 pp.; pp. 208–9 [p. 67].

Hulme, Kathryn (1956) *The Nun's Story*. Pan Books, London, 1959, 249 pp.; pp. 116–22 [p. 110].

Huyler, Frank (1999) Burn. In: *The Blood of Strangers*. University of California Press, Berkeley, CA, 154 pp.; pp. 93–8 [p. 154].

Huyler, Frank (1999) Faith. In: *The Blood of Strangers*. University of California Press, Berkeley, CA, 154 pp.; pp. 19–22. [p. 131].

Huyler, Frank (1999) The Prisoner. In: *The Blood of Strangers*. University of California Press, Berkeley, CA, 154 pp.; pp. 63–88 [p. 179].

Ibsen, Henrik (1884) The Wild Duck. In: *Three Plays* (translated by Ellis-Fermor, Una). Penguin, Harmondsworth, 1957, 368 pp.; pp. 189, 207, 223–4, 243–4, 253–60 [p. 217].

Irving, John (1981) *Hotel New Hampshire*. Corgi Books, London, 1984, 428 pp.; pp. 135–7 [p. 226].

Irving, John (1985) *Cider House Rules*. Bantam Books, New York, 1986, 587 pp.; pp. 59, 68 [pp. 7, 122].

Irving, John (2001) *The Fourth Hand*. Bloomsbury, London, 416 pp.; pp. 26–44, 149, 162–5, 170–1 [pp. 41, 84, 107–8].

Jackson, Shirley (1954) *The Bird's Nest*. Farrar, Straus and Young, New York, 276 pp.; pp. 32–5 [p. 78].

James, Henry (1881) *Washington Square*. Bantam Books, New York, 1959, 162 pp.; pp. 52–6, 127–32, 144, 150–2 [pp. 45, 232].

James, Henry (1884) Lady Barberina. In: *The New York Edition of Henry James. Volume 14.*

Augustus Kelley, Fairfield, NJ, 1976, 607 pp.; pp. 18, 23, 56–7, 79–81, 142 [pp. 12–13, 168–9].

James, Henry (1886) *The Bostonians*. Penguin, Harmondsworth, 1984, 438 pp.; pp. 58, 67–8, 73 [p. 120].

James, Henry (1893) *The Middle Years*. In: *The New York Edition of Henry James. Volume 16*. Charles Scribner's Sons, New York, 1937, 426 pp.; p. 87 [p. 142].

James, Montague Rhodes (1919) Two Doctors. In: Byatt, Antonia Susan (ed.) *The Oxford Book of English Short Stories*. Oxford University Press, Oxford, 1998, 439 pp.; pp. 97–104 [pp. 73, 103, 128].

James, PD (Phyllis Dorothy) (1971) *Shroud for a Nightingale*. Sphere Books, London, 1988, 300 pp.; pp. 178, 250–1, 275 [p. 26].

Jerome, Saint (Eusebius Sophronius Hieronymus) (AD 403) *Select Letters* (translated by Wright, Frederick Adam). Loeb's Classical Library, Harvard University Press, Cambridge, MA, 1980, 510 pp.; p. 363 [p. 209, footnote].

Jewett, Sarah Orne (1884) *A Country Doctor*. Houghton Mifflin Company, Boston, MA, 351 pp.; pp. 43, 56, 94, 105, 141 [pp. 7, 67, 68–9, 142–3, 167].

Kenealy, Arabella (1893) *Dr Janet of Harley Street*. Digby Long, London, 1894, 340 pp.; pp. 117–18 [p. 194].

Kingsley, Charles (1857) Two Years Ago. In: *The Works of Charles Kingsley. Volume 8*. Reprinted by Georg Olms, Hildesheim, Germany, 1969, 495 pp.; pp. 18–19, 26, 33–8, 36, 65, 71–2, 165, 303, 492–4 [pp. 111, 112, 117, 156, 180, 205, 215].

Kipling, Rudyard (1901) *Kim*. Pan Books, London, 1978, 322 pp.; p. 235 [p. 103].

Konner, Melvin (1987) *Becoming a Doctor*. Viking, New York, 390 pp.; pp. 2–4, p. 376 [p. 193].

Kornbluth, Cyril M (1950) The Little Black Bag. In: Conklin, Groff and Fabricant, Noah Daniel (eds) *Great Science Fiction About Doctors*. Collier Books, New York, 1963, 412 pp.; pp. 165–95 [p. 222].

Kundera, Milan (1976) *The Farewell Party* (translated by Kussi, Peter). Knopf, New York, 209 pp.; p. 36 [p. 184].

Kundera, Milan (1984) *The Unbearable Lightness of Being* (translated by Heim, Michael Henry). Faber and Faber, London, 1988, 314 pp.; pp. 10, 179–84, 230–2 [pp. 8, 83].

Leavitt, David (1989) *Equal Affections*. Penguin, Harmondsworth, 268 pp.; p. 175 [p. 5].

Lee, Harper (1960) *To Kill a Mockingbird*. Popular Library, New York, 1962, 284 pp.; pp. 108–9 [p. 160].

Le Sage, Alain-René (1715) *The Adventures of Gil Blas de Santillana* (translated by Smollett, Tobias George). *Volume 1*. Oxford University Press, London, 1907, 408 pp.; pp. 127–44 [pp. 28–9].

Levi, Primo (1975) *The Periodic Table*. Abacus, London, 1990, 233 pp.; pp. 13–15 [pp. 124–5].

Lewis, Sinclair (1920) *Main Street*. Harcourt Brace and Company, New York, 1948, 451 pp.; pp. 120, 175, 176–9, 302–3 [pp. 63, 73, 94, 148].

Lewis, Sinclair (1924) *Arrowsmith*. Signet Books, New York, 1961, 438 pp.; pp. 6–9, 16–17, 25–6, 82–5, 163–4, 167, 168–72, 193–7, 208–9, 211–12, 244–6, 262, 294, 309, 336, 351–2, 371, 374, 390–1, 395, 416, 426–7, 429, 430 [pp. 7, 8, 21, 42, 43, 67, 117, 123, 124, 144, 169, 181, 219].

Lightman, Alan (2000) *The Diagnosis*. Pantheon Books, New York, 369 pp.; pp. 267–8 [p. 170].

Lofting, Hugh (1923) *The Voyages of Doctor Dolittle*. Jonathan Cape, London, 223 pp [p. 190].

Maartens, Maarten (1906) *The Healers*. Constable, London, 379 pp.; p. 79 [p. 108].

McCarthy, Mary (1942) *The Company She Keeps*. Penguin, Harmondsworth, 1975, 224 pp.; pp. 185–6 [p. 155].

McCarthy, Mary (1954) *The Group*. Signet, New York, 1964, 397 pp.; pp. 311–22 [p. 33].

McCullers, Carson (Smith, Lula Carson) (1940) *The Heart is a Lonely Hunter*. Cresset Press, London, 1953, 350 pp.; pp. 77–8 [p. 29].

McEwan, Ian (2005). *Saturday*. Jonathan Cape, London, 279 pp. [pp. 45, 160, 167].

Malamud, Bernard (1973) In Retirement. In: *Rembrandt's Hat*. Farrar Straus Giroux, New York, 204 pp.; pp. 109–24 [p. 18].

Malègue, Joseph (1932) *Augustin, ou, Le maître est là. Volume 2*. Spes, Paris, 1935, 510 pp.; pp. 120, 277–83, 328, 415–16 [p. 151].

Mann, Thomas (1924) *The Magic Mountain* (translated by Lowe-Porter, Helen T). Penguin, Harmondsworth, 1960, 716 pp.; pp. 132–3 [pp. 203–4].

Mann, Thomas (1947) *Doctor Faustus* (translated by Lowe-Porter, Helen T). Secker and Warburg, London, 1949, 510 pp.; pp. 475–6 [p. 65].

Manzoni, Alessandro (1827) *The Betrothed* (translated by Penman, Bruce). Penguin, Harmondsworth, 1983, 719 pp.; pp. 566–76, 594, 603 [p. 118].

Marion, Robert (1989) *The Intern Blues*. William Morrow and Company, New York, 352 pp.; pp. 118–19 [pp. 178–9].

Marquis, Don (Marquis, Donald Robert Perry) (1939) Country Doctor. In: *The Best of Don Marquis*. Garden City Books, Garden City, NY, 670 pp.; pp. 444–63 [pp. 7, 231].

Martineau, Harriet (1839) *Deerbrook*. Virago Press, London, 1983, 523 pp.; pp. 39, 212, 472–509, 518 [pp. 15, 72–3, 117].

Martin du Gard, Roger (1922–1929) *The Thibaults* (translated by Gilbert, Stuart). John Lane, The Bodley Head, London, 1939, 889 pp.; pp. 532–40, 571–6, 870–89 [pp. 89, 119–20, 195].

Martin du Gard, Roger (1936–1940) *Summer 1914* (translated by Gilbert, Stuart). John Lane, The Bodley Head, London, 1940, 1078 pp.; pp. 814–24, 943–6, 976, 1021–6, 1057, 1071–5 [pp. 120, 202, 236–8].

Maugham, W Somerset (1909) Penelope. In: *The Collected Plays. Volume 1*. Heinemann, London, 1960, 110 pp.; p. 17 [p. 168].

Maugham, W Somerset (1915) *Of Human Bondage*. Signet Classics, New York, 1991, 680 pp.; pp. 346–51, 445–6, 476, 491, 512, 534–9, 645, 646–9, 652, 674–9 [pp. 7, 18–19, 76, 122, 142, 204].

Maugham, W Somerset (1920) Rain. In: *Collected Short Stories. Volume 1*. Pan Books, London, 1975, 476 pp.; pp. 9–48 [p. 115].

Maugham, W Somerset (1944) *The Razor's Edge*. Penguin, Harmondsworth, 1963, 314 pp.; pp. 94, 258–9 [pp. 124, 168].

Mauriac, François (1925) *The Desert of Love* (translated by Hopkins, Gerard). Eyre and Spottiswoode, London, 1949, 279 pp.; pp. 35–6, 55, 68, 82, 92, 151–8 [pp. 13, 27, 229, 230].

Mauriac, François (1927–1935) *Thérèse* (translated by Hopkins, Gerard). Penguin, Harmondsworth, 1959, 318 pp.; pp. 75, 119–38 [pp. 4, 24–5, 67–8].

Maurois, André (Herzog, Émile) (1921) *Colonel Bramble* (translated by Wake, Thurfrida). Jonathan Cape, London, 1937, 256 pp.; pp. 53–7, 88, 154, 180–81, 213, 215 [pp. 113, 158].

Maurois, André (Herzog, Émile) (1919–1950) *Les Silences du Colonel Bramble: les Discours et Nouveaux Discours du Dr O'Grady*. Grasset, Paris, 1950, 502 pp.; pp. 35, 244–57, 356–60, 378–86, 403, 483–7 [p. 158].

Melville, Hermann (*sic*)* (1847) *Omoo*. Dent, London, *c.* 1907, 328 pp.; pp. 9–10 [p. 152].

---

* In the Library of Congress Catalogue and Merriam Webster's Encyclopedia of Literature, Melville's first name is spelt Herman.

Melville, Herman (1850) *White Jacket*. LC Page, Boston, MA, 1892, 374 pp.; pp. 232–49 [p. 70].

Metalious, Grace (1956) *Peyton Place*. Dell, New York, 1958, 512 pp.; pp. 9, 33, 64 [pp. 7, 66, 110].

Miksanek, Tony (2004) An adverse reaction. *The Healing Muse*. 4: 65–70 [p. 176].

Miller, Andrew (1997) *Ingenious Pain*. Harcourt Brace, New York, 337 pp.; pp. 19, 31–3, 41, 138–40, 175, 177–9, 196–7, 287–9 [pp. 23, 107, 145, 211–12].

Miller, Arthur (1968) *The Price*. Secker and Warburg, London, 116 pp.; pp. 16–21, 53–4, 74, 82 [pp. 34, 220].

Mishnah (*c*. AD 180) (translated by Danby, Herbert). Oxford University Press, London, 1933, 844 pp.; p. 329 [pp. 103–4].

Mitchell, Margaret (1936) *Gone With the Wind*. Avon Books, New York, 1973, 1024 pp.; pp. 150, 184, 296, 807 [p. 42].

Mitchell, Paige (1965) *A Wilderness of Monkeys*. Arthur Barker, London, 379 pp.; pp. 13, 63, 78–81, 128, 158–63, 171–7, 185, 198–206, 247–8, 255, 275, 366–7 [pp. 36, 81, 87, 130].

Mitchell, Silas Weir (1885) *In War Time*. Century Company, New York, 1913, 423 pp.; pp. 3–7, 19–29, 45, 60–8, 103, 198, 208–15, 232–44, 293, 303, 323–7, 363, 375–90, 415–19, 422–3 [pp. 153, 171, 212–13].

Mitchell, Silas Weir (1900) *Dr North and His Friends*. Century Company, New York, 1900, 499 pp. [p. 154].

Mitchell, Silas Weir (1901) *Circumstance*. Century Company, New York, 1902, 495 pp.; pp. 31–52, 51–2, 53, 143, 146–7, 231–5, 276–7, 278–93, 331–42, 404, 444–52, 453 [pp. 18, 62, 78, 153, 157, 170, 175].

Molière, Jean Baptiste Poquelin (1665) Love's the Best Doctor. In: *The Plays of Molière* (translated by Waller, Alfred Rayney). *Volume 4*. John Grant, Edinburgh, 1926, 435 pp.; pp. 291–7 [p. 73].

Moore, Brian (1976) *The Doctor's Wife*. Jonathan Cape, London, 277 pp.; pp. 4–5, 80–2, 145–7, 207 [pp. 33, 148–9, 203].

Morgan, Joan (1956) *Doctor Jo*. Samuel French, London, 79 pp.; p. 45 [pp. 15–16].

Mortimer, John (1985) *Paradise Postponed*. Penguin, Harmondsworth, 1986, 447 pp.; pp. 57, 105 [pp. 122–3, 194].

Munthe, Axel (1929) *The Story of San Michele*. John Murray, London, 1950, 431 pp. [p. 160]

Nourse, Alan Edward (1978) *The Practice*. Futura Publications, London, 1979, 574 pp.; pp. 22–3, 27, 34, 36, 79–80, 108, 110–12, 124–6, 151, 157–8, 168, 298, 309–10, 423, 454, 573 [pp. 36–7, 72, 79, 83–4].

Oates, Joyce Carol (1969) How I Contemplated the World from the Detroit House of Correction and Began My Life Over Again. In: *The Wheel of Love and Other Stories*. Vanguard Press, New York, 1970, 440 pp.; pp. 170–89 [p. 46].

Oates, Joyce Carol (1971) *Wonderland*. Vanguard Press, New York, 512 pp.; pp. 50–71, 123–4, 138–44, 148, 162, 172, 185–97, 203–4, 246–50, 264–7, 297–300, 327–8, 371–9, 395, 430–4, 455, 485–6, 505–12 [pp. 46–7, 144–5].

O'Brian, Patrick (1992) *The Truelove*. WW Norton, New York, 256 pp.; pp. 14–17, 56, 67–73, 146–8, 200 [p. 159].

Odets, Clifford (1935) Awake and Sing. In: *Famous Plays of 1935–6*. Gollancz, London, 1936, 701 pp.; p. 545 [p. 226].

O'Hara, John (1962) The Properties of Love. In: *Forty-Nine Stories*. Modern Library, New York, 425 pp.; pp. 286–96 [pp. 232–3].

O'Neill, Eugene (1928) Strange Interlude. In: *The Plays of Eugene O'Neill. Volume 3*. Random House, New York, 1955, 633 pp.; p. 30 [p. 62].

Ozick, Cynthia (1971) The Doctor's Wife. In: *The Pagan Rabbi and Other Stories*. Penguin, New York, 1983, 270 pp.; pp. 181–90 [p. 183].

Palmer, Michael (1996) *Critical Judgment*. Bantam Books, New York, 386 pp.; pp. 7–14 [p. 82].

Palmer, Michael (1998) *Miracle Cure*. Arrow Books, London, 447 pp.; pp. 28–31, 51, 122–3, 144–5, 203, 220–2, 262–3 [pp. 65, 69, 214].

Pasternak, Boris (1957) *Doctor Zhivago* (translated by Hayward, Max and Harari, Manya). Pantheon, New York, 1958, 558 pp.; pp. 79, 404–21, 465, 523–58 [pp. 121, 153].

Percy, Edward (1940) *Doctor Brent's Household*. English Theatre Guild, London, 92 pp.; p. 24 [p. 92].

Percy, Walker (1977) *Lancelot*. Farrar Straus and Giroux, New York, 257 pp.; pp. 4–5 [p. 117].

Percy, Walker (1987) *The Thanatos Syndrome*. Ivy Books, New York, 1991, 404 pp.; pp. 13, 14–20, 27–9, 48, 104, 106, 125, 137, 384–6, 394–9 [pp. 127–8, 160, 218].

Perec, Georges (1978) *Life: a user's manual* (translated by Bellos, David). Collins Harvill, London, 1987, 581 pp.; pp. 47, 209, 474–80 [p. 182].

Plath, Sylvia (1963) *The Bell Jar*. Bantam Books, New York, 1972, 216 pp.; p. 106 [p. 38].

Plato (4th century BC) The Republic (translated by Jowett, Benjamin). In: Buchanan, Scott (ed.) *The Portable Plato*. Penguin, Harmondsworth, 1979, 696 pp.; pp. 283–5, 400 [pp. 202, 226].

Porter, Katherine Anne (1945–1962) *Ship of Fools*. Little Brown, Boston, MA, 1962, 497 pp.; pp. 16–17, 111–13, 113–15, 117–21, 196–205, 316, 346–50, 468–9, 492 [pp. 125, 203].

Pritchett, Victor Sawdon (1950) Passing the Ball. In: *The Complete Short Stories*. Chatto and Windus, London, 1990, 976 pp.; pp. 332–45 [p. 63].

Proust, Marcel (1913–1922) *Remembrance of Things Past* (translated by Moncrieff, CK Scott and Kilmartin, Terence). Penguin, Harmondsworth, 1985–7. Volume 1, 1197 pp.; pp. 102, 217–25, 233–4, 275–7, 467, 536. Volume 2, 1040 pp.; pp. 311–28, 354–5, p. 995 [pp. 24, 32, 78, 91, 140, 143–4, 149, 158, 160].

Pym, Barbara (1980) *A Few Green Leaves*. EP Dutton, New York, 250 pp.; pp. 2, 13, 18–19, 206–9, 242 [pp. 41, 116–17, 174–5].

Ravin, Neil (1981) *MD*. Delacorte Press/Seymour Lawrence, New York, 404 pp.; p. 70 [p. 95].

Ravin, Neil (1985) *Seven North*. EP Dutton/Seymour Lawrence, New York, 371 pp.; pp. 23, 66, 67–9, 145, 170 [pp. 172–3].

Ravin, Neil (1987) *Evidence*. Charles Scribner's Sons, New York, 292 pp.; pp. 23, 80, 132–51, 181–7, 229, 241–8, 291 [pp. 210–11].

Ravin, Neil (1989) *Mere Mortals*. Macdonald, London, 1990, 420 pp.; p. 204 [p. 69].

Reade, Charles (1863) *Hard Cash*. Chatto and Windus, London, 1894, 625 pp.; pp. 35, 180, 468. [pp. 39, 90].

Reed, Barry (1980) *The Verdict*. Simon and Schuster, New York, 282 pp.; pp. 31–3, 69 [pp. 87–8, 216].

Remarque, Erich Maria (1945) *Arch of Triumph* (translated by Sorell, Walter and Lindley, Denver). Appleton Century, New York, 455 pp.; pp. 38–48, 170, 178–84, 192, 252, 261–2 [pp. 6, 61–2, 115, 207–8].

Richardson, Henry Handel (Robertson, Ethel Florence Lindesay) (1917–1929) *The Fortunes of Richard Mahony*. Penguin, Harmondsworth, 1990, 841 pp.; pp. 30–1, 88, 120, 160–4, 164–8, 321–31, 369–70, 406–9, 453, 468, 488–97, 616, 676–703, 725, 788–92, 819–31, 838 (Afterword by Dorothy Green) [pp. 24, 63, 68, 73, 126–7, 152, 180–1, 209–10, 226–7].

Richardson, Samuel (1747–1748) The History of Clarissa Harlowe. In: Stephen, Leslie (ed.) *The Works of Samuel Richardson. Volume 8*. Henry Sotheran, London, 1883, 540 pp.; pp. 168, 341–2 [pp. 61, 70].

Rinehart, Mary Roberts (1935) *The Doctor*. Farrar and Rinehart, New York, 506 pp.; pp. 75,

91–5, 133–4, 136, 141, 161–6, 247–9, 277, 293, 308, 465, 495, 500–6 [pp. 9, 14, 23, 24, 27, 29, 62, 126, 131, 146, 171–2].

Roe, Francis (1989) *Doctors and Doctors' Wives*. Constable, London, 336 pp.; pp. 89–94, p. 241 [p. 178].

Rosenbaum, Edward E (1988) *The Doctor* (also titled *A Taste Of My Own Medicine*). Ivy Books, New York, 1991, 182 pp.; pp. 9–12, 40–2, 83–4, 130–43 [p. 236].

Ross, Lilian (1961) The Ordeal of Dr Blauberman. *The New Yorker*. 13 May, p. 13 [pp. 8, 151–2].

Roth, Philip (1969) *Portnoy's Complaint*. Random House, New York, 274 pp. [p. 194].

Russell, Robert (1985) *While You're Here, Doctor*. Souvenir Press, London, 254 pp.; pp. 177–84 [p. 41].

Salzman, Mark (2000) *Lying Awake*. Knopf, New York, 181 pp.; pp. 47, 121, 152, 159, 162 [p. 109].

Sams, Ferrol (1987) Big Star Woman. In: *The Widow's Mite and Other Stories*. Penguin, New York, 1989, 218 pp.; p. 161 [p. 2].

Sanders, Lawrence (1973) *The First Deadly Sin*. Berkley Books, New York, 1974, 576 pp.; p. 91 [p. 65].

Saramago, Jose (1995) *Blindness* (translated by Pontiero, Giovanni). Harvill Press, London, 1997, 309 pp.; pp. 15–21, 46, 21–30, 39, 169, 201–23, 224, 281, 309 [pp. 44, 154, 205].

Sava, George (1979) *No Man is Perfect*. Robert Hale, London, 256 pp. [p. 15].

Sayers, Dorothy (1923) *Whose Body*. Gollancz, London, 1971, 268 pp.; pp. 70–1 [p. 12].

Sayers, Dorothy (1928) The Vindictive Story of the Footsteps that Ran. In: *Lord Peter Views the Body*. Gollancz, London, 1979, 317 pp.; p. 167 [p. 82].

Schneiderman, Lawrence J (1972) *Sea Nymphs by the Hour*. Authors' Guild Backinprint.-Com, Lincoln, NE, 2000, 176 pp.; pp. 55–8 [pp. 85–6, 155–6].

Schnitzler, Arthur (1912) *Professor Bernhardi* (translated by Landstone, Hetty). Faber and Gwyer, London, 1927, 160 pp.; pp. 19, 23, 32–3, 59 [pp. 82, 118–19, 153].

Schnitzler, Arthur (1917) *Dr Graesler* (translated by Slade, EC). Thomas Seltzer, New York, 1923, 180 pp.; pp. 8, 11, 50, 53, 71–5, 94, 116–23, 148 [pp. 18, 183].

Scott, Walter (1831) The Surgeon's Daughter. In: *The Waverley Novels. Volume 25*. Adam and Charles Black, London, 1892, 424 pp.; pp. 3, 102, 147 [p. 168].

Segal, Erich (1988) *Doctors*. Bantam Books, New York, 1989, 678 pp.; p. 387 [p. 143].

Seifert, Elizabeth (1941) *Bright Scalpel*. Aeonian Press Inc., New York, 1973, 223 pp.; p. 27 [p. 68].

Seifert, Elizabeth (1969) *Bachelor Doctor*. Collins, London, 1971, 224 pp.; p. 17 [pp. 153–4].

Seifert, Elizabeth (1977) *Doctor Tuck*. Collins, London, 1979, 212 pp.; pp. 4–20, 81–2 [p. 16].

Selzer, Richard (1982) Imelda. In: *Letters to a Young Doctor*. Harcourt Brace, San Diego, CA, 1996, 205 pp.; pp. 21–36 [pp. 82, 191–2].

Shakespeare, William (1599–1600) *As You Like It*. Act II, Scene vii. Signet Classics, New York, 1963, p. 78 [p. 226].

Shaw, George Bernard (1906) The Doctor's Dilemma. In: *The Bodley Head Bernard Shaw: Collected Plays With Their Prefaces. Volume 3*. The Bodley Head, London, 1971, 914 pp.; pp. 338–45, 351, 423 [pp. 5, 64, 155, 201, 227].

Sheldon, Sidney (1994) *Nothing Lasts Forever*. Harper Collins, London, 293 pp.; pp. 102–5, 120–7, 293 [p. 223].

Shem, Samuel (Bergman, Steven) (1978) *The House of God*. Richard Marek, New York, 382 pp.; pp. 25, 29–30, 74–81, 91–8, 167–83, 209, 277, 354–9 [pp. 147, 193–4].

Shreve, Anita (1999) *Fortune's Rocks*. Abacus, London, 2000, 433 pp.; pp. 15–21, 42–56 [pp. 158–9].

Simenon, Georges (1941) The Country Doctor. In: *The White Horse Inn and Other Novels* (translated by Ellenbogen, Ellen). Hamish Hamilton, London, 1980, 330 pp.; pp. 203–27 [pp. 70–1].

Simenon, Georges (1963) *The Patient* (translated by Stewart, Jean). Hamish Hamilton, London, 1963, 236 pp.; pp. 45, 56, 78 [pp. 92–3, 151, 217].

Singer, Isaac Bashevis (1964) A Wedding in Brownsville (translated by Faerstein, C and Polley, E). In: *Short Friday and Other Stories*. Farrar Straus and Giroux, New York, 243 pp.; pp. 190–206 [p. 27].

Slaughter, Frank Gill (1942) *That None Should Die*. Jarrolds, London, 1958, 384 pp.; p. 7 [p. 160].

Slaughter, Frank Gill (1967) Doctors' Wives. In: *Four Complete Novels*. Avenel Books, New York, 1980, 804 pp.; p. 8 [p. 68].

Slaughter, Frank Gill (1969) Surgeon's Choice. In: *Four Complete Novels*. Avenel Books, New York, 1980, 804 pp.; pp. 241, 273 [pp. 30, 72].

Slaughter, Frank Gill (1972) *Convention MD*. Hutchinson, London, 1973, 351 pp.; pp. 32, 160, 191–4, 275, 292 [pp. 28, 30, 63, 87].

Slaughter, Frank Gill (1974) Women in White. In: *Four Complete Novels*. Avenel Books, New York, 1980, 804 pp.; pp. 438–46 [pp. 26, 30].

Slaughter, Frank Gill (1983) *Doctors at Risk*. Hutchinson, London, 274 pp.; pp. 37, 196–211 [pp. 31, 224].

Slaughter, Frank Gill (1985) *No Greater* Love. Hutchinson, London, 252 pp.; pp. 37–8, 43–4, 137–8 [p. 93].

Smollett, Tobias George (1748) *The Adventures of Roderick Random*. Dent, London, 1964, 479 pp.; pp. 33–7, 92–3, 424–8 [pp. 86, 124, 168].

Snow, Charles Percy (1958) The Conscience of the Rich. In: *Strangers and Brothers. Volume 1*. Charles Scribner's Sons, New York, 1972, 1071 pp.; pp. 702–4 [p. 182].

Sobel, Irwin Philip (1973) *The Hospital Makers*. Doubleday, Garden City, NY, 431 pp.; pp. 11–14, 63–71, 79, 349–58 [pp. 7, 69, 87, 91–2].

Söderberg, Hjalmar (1905) *Doctor Glas* (translated by Austin, Paul Britten). Chatto and Windus, London, 1963, 150 pp.; pp. 13–14, 17–19, 21, 23, 29–34, 40, 65–6, 95, 93–108 [pp. 5, 7, 114–15, 193, 208–9].

Solzhenitsyn, Aleksandr Isaevich (1968) *Cancer Ward* (translated by Bethell, Nicholas and Burg, David). Bodley Head, London, 1971, 619 pp.; pp. 55–7 [p. 122].

Soubiran, André (1947) *The Doctors* (translated by Coburn, Oliver). WH Allen, London, 1954, 288 pp.; pp. 133–41, 235–42 [p. 229].

Starkman, Elaine Marcus (1980) Anniversary. In: Mazow, Julia Wolf (ed.) *The Woman Who Lost Her Names*. Harper and Row, New York, 222 pp.; pp. 168–76 [p. 31].

Steinbeck, John (1936) *In Dubious Battle*. Heinemann, London, 1970, 290 pp.; p. 161 [pp. 120–1].

Stern, Richard Gustave (1980) Dr Cahn's Visit. In: *Noble Rot: Stories 1949–1988*. Grove Press, New York, 1989, 367 pp.; pp. 134–8 [p. 231].

Sterne, Lawrence (1759–1767) In: Work, James Aiken (ed.) *The Life and Opinions of Tristram Shandy, Gentleman*. Odyssey Press, New York, 1940, 647 pp.; pp. 106, 136 [pp. 104, 123].

Stevenson, Robert Louis (1883) *Treasure Island* (with *Kidnapped)*. Dent, London, 1925, 370 pp.; pp. 34, 149 [p. 180].

Stevenson, Robert Louis (1886) *The Strange Case of Dr Jekyll and Mr Hyde*. Heinemann, London, 1934, 216 pp. [p. 1].

Stoker, Bram (1897) *Dracula*. Penguin, Harmondsworth, 1993, 520 pp.; pp. 76, 147–59, 227–8, 353–7, 428 [pp. 8, 89, 156–7].

Straub, Peter (1988) *Koko*. Penguin, Harmondsworth, 1989, 634 pp.; pp. 90–5, 299 [pp. 27–8, 83, 181].

Strindberg, Johan August (1887) The Father. In: *Twelve Plays* (translated by Sprigge, Elizabeth). Constable, London, 1962, 689 pp.; p. 47 [p. 107].

Swift, Jonathan (1726) *Gulliver's Travels*. Asimov, Isaac (ed.). Clarkson Potter, New York, 1980, 298 pp.; pp. 4–6, 210–11, 285 [p. 190].

Tennyson, Alfred Lord (1880) In the Children's Hospital. In: Ricks, Christopher (ed.) *The Poems of Tennyson*. Longmans, London, 1969, 1835 pp.; pp. 1261–3 [p. 110].

Thackeray, William Makepeace (1848–1850) *The History of Pendennis: his fortunes and misfortunes, his friends and his greatest enemy. Volume 1*. Smith Elder, London, 1879, p. 11 [p. 168].

Theroux, Paul (1989) *My Secret History*. Penguin, Harmondsworth, 1990, 544 pp.; pp. 164–86 [p. 221].

Thomas, Donald M (1993) *Pictures at an Exhibition*. Bloomsbury, London, 278 pp.; pp. 28–9, 79–84, 110–11, 121–3, 165, 181, 195–7, 219 [pp. 27, 37].

Thompson, Morton (1951) *The Cry and the Covenant*. Pan Books, London, 1969, 474 pp.; pp. 462–9 [pp. 81, 231].

Thompson, Morton (1955) *Not as a Stranger*. Michael Joseph, London, 702 pp.; pp. 141–2, 189–92, 237–9, 429, 509–10, 648–57, 693–4 [pp. 15, 81, 147, 223, 230].

Tucker, Augusta (1939) *Miss Susan Slagle's*. Heinemann, London, 1940, 328 pp. [pp. 21–2 f., 24].

Updike, John (1961) The Doctor's Wife. In: *Pigeon Feathers and Other Stories*. Andre Deutsch, London, 1963, 278 pp.; pp. 197–210 [p. 33].

Updike, John (1963) The Persistence of Desire. In: *Pigeon Feathers and Other Stories*. Andre Deutsch, London, 278 pp.; pp. 12–26 [p. 146].

Van Der Meersch, Maxence (1943) *Bodies and Souls* (translated by Wilkins, Eithne). William Kimber, London, 1953, 463 pp.; pp. 62–3, 120, 232–5, 231–43, 309, 396–401 [pp. 71, 79, 139, 230].

Van Gogh, Vincent (1873–1890) *Complete Letters* (translated by Van Gogh-Bonger, Johanna Gesina and de Dood, C). *Volume 3*. Thames and Hudson, London, 1958, Letter 637, p. 271 and Letter 648, p. 294 [pp. vi, 204].

Waltari, Mika (1945) *The Egyptian* (translated by Walford, Naomi). Panther Books, London, 1960, 352 pp.; p. 5, 31–3, 51–2, 151, 167, 240, 255, 298, 340–7, 348–50 [pp. 121, 189–90].

Warren, Robert Penn (1946) *All the King's Men*. Modern Library, New York, 1953, 464 pp. [p. 7].

Watson, Robert (1977) Tale of a Physician. In: *Lily Lang*. St Martin's Press, New York, 212 pp.; pp. 161–72 [pp. 22–3].

Weldon, Fay (Birkinshaw, Franklin) (1976) *Remember Me*. Coronet, London, 1983, 223 pp.; pp. 98, 118, 177 [pp. 25–6].

Wells, HG (Herbert George) (1894–1895) The Time Machine. In: *Selected Short Stories*. Penguin, Harmondsworth, 1958, 352 pp.; pp. 7–83 [p. 158].

Wells, HG (Herbert George) (1909) Tono Bungay. In: *The Essex Edition of the Works of HG Wells. Volume 7*. Ernest Benn, London, 1926, 445 pp.; p. 414 [p. 143].

Wharton, William (1981) *Dad*. Alfred A Knopf, New York, 449 pp.; pp. 130, 159–62 [pp. 89, 170].

Wilder, Thornton (1938) *Our Town*. Longmans, London, 1965, 128 pp.; pp. 8, 26, 40–1, 59, 97 [pp. 41, 176].

Williams, Tennessee (1948) Summer and Smoke. In: *The Theatre of Tennessee Williams. Volume 2*. New Directions, New York, 1971, 591 pp.; pp. 130, 132–4, 154, 211, 218–19, 221, 227, 248–50 [pp. 20–1, 111–12].

Williams, William Carlos (1928) *Voyage to Pagany*. New Directions, New York, 1970, 270 pp.; p. 148 [p. 75].

Williams, William Carlos (1932) Mind and Body. In: *The Doctor Stories*. New Directions, New York, 1984, 142 pp.; pp. 6–7 [p. 160].

Williams, William Carlos (1932) Old Doc Rivers. In: *The Doctor Stories*. New Directions, New York, 1984, 142 pp.; pp. 13–41, 16–17 [pp. 10, 216, 218].

Williams, William Carlos (1934) Jean Beicke. In: *The Doctor Stories*. New Directions, New York, 1984, 142 pp.; pp. 69–77 [p. 82].

Williams, William Carlos (1948) A Dream of Love. In: *Many Loves and Other Plays. The Collected Plays of William Carlos Williams*. New Directions, Norfolk, VA, 1961, 437 pp.; p. 156 [p. 10].

Williams, William Carlos (1952) *The Build-Up*. Random House, New York, 335 pp.; pp. 77–81 [p. 5].

Wilner, Herbert (1966) *All the Little Heroes*. Bobbs-Merrill, Indianapolis, IN, 487 pp.; pp. 42–50, 130, 145, 200–10, 251, 258, 273, 305, 311, 482 [pp. 8, 192–3].

Wolfe, Thomas (1929) *Look Homeward Angel*. Charles Scribner's Sons, New York, 1936, 626 pp.; pp. 170–80, 353 [pp. 108–9, 150, 218].

Wolfe, Thomas (1939) *The Web and the Rock*. Heinemann, London, 1969, 642 pp.; p. 627 [p. 38].

Woolf, Virginia (1925) *Mrs Dalloway*. Zodiac Press, London, 1947, 213 pp.; pp. 106, 108, 110–12 [pp. 24, 64, 65, 144].

Wouk, Herman (1951) *The Caine Mutiny*. Cape, London, 1954, 479 pp.; pp. 61, 63 [pp. 131, 182].

Yonge, Charlotte Mary (1856) *The Daisy Chain*. Virago, London, 1988, 673 pp. [p. 39].

Young, Francis Brett (1919) *The Young Physician*. Heinemann, London, 1934, 470 pp.; pp. 184–6, 466–7 [pp. 6, 19–20, 232].

Young, Francis Brett (1928) *My Brother Jonathan*. Heinemann, London, 595 pp.; pp. 83, 127, 202–11, 228–9, 287, 309, 341, 431–6, 553, 568, 575–95 [pp. 6, 19 f., 20, 72, 169, 215–16].

Young, Francis Brett (1938) *Dr Bradley Remembers*. Heinemann, London, 745 pp.; pp. 32–5, 631, 670, 744 [pp. 46, 227].

Zola, Émile (Zola, Émile Édouard Charles Antoine) (1892) *The Downfall* (translated by Vizetelly, Ernest Alfred). Chatto and Windus, London, 534 pp. [pp. 160–1].

Zola, Émile (Zola, Émile Édouard Charles Antoine) (1893) *Doctor Pascal* (translated by Kean, Vladimir). Elek Books, London, 1957, 292 pp.; pp. 30–1, 102, 144, 198, 257 [pp. 152–3].

Zola, Émile (Zola, Émile Édouard Charles Antoine) (1894) *Lourdes* (translated by Vizetelly, Ernest Alfred). Chatto and Windus, London, 1896, 491 pp.; pp. 142–3, 450 [p. 116].

Selected secondary sources

Aach RD, Girard DE, Humphrey H *et al.* (1992) Alcohol and other substance abuse and impairment among physicians in residency training. *Ann Intern Med.*. **116**: 245–54.

American Medical Association Council on Mental Health (1973) The sick physician: impairment by psychiatric disorders including alcoholism and drug dependency. *JAMA*. **223**: 684–7.

Ballantyne J (ed.) (1995) *Bedside Manners*. Virgin, London, 266 pp.

Bamforth I (ed.) (2003) *The Body in the Library*. Verso, London, 418 pp.

Bennet G (1998) Coping with loss: the doctor's losses: ideals versus realities. *BMJ*. **316**: 1238–40.

Book of Common Prayer According to the Use of the Church of England. Cambridge University Press, Cambridge, 1968, p. 42.

Bosch X (1999) Too many physicians in Spain. *JAMA.* **282:** 1025–6.

Bosk CL (1980) Occupational rituals in patient management. *NEJM.* **303:** 71–6.

Ceccio J (ed.) (1978) *Medicine in Literature.* Longmans, New York, 324 pp.

Charon R, Banks JT, Connelly JE *et al.* (1995) Literature and medicine: contributions to clinical practice. *Ann Intern Med.* **122:** 599–606.

Choudhry NK, Fletcher RH and Soumerai SB (2005) Systematic review: the relationship between clinical experience and quality of health care. *Ann Intern Med.* **142:** 260–73.

Cole H (ed.) (1963) *Under the Doctor.* Heinemann, London, 301 pp.

Coulehan J (1998) Chekhov's doctors. 18. The Zemstvo Doctor. *JAMA.* **279:** 270.

Cousins N (ed.) (1982) *The Physician in Literature.* Saunders, Philadelphia, PA, 477 pp.

Curran WS (1961) Arthur Lee and the secret diplomacy of the American Revolution. *NEJM.* **264:** 240–42.

Donzelot J (1977) *The Policing of Families* (translated by Hurley R). Hutchinson, London, 1980, 243 pp.; p. 172.

Franks P, Clancy CM and Nutting PA (1992) Gatekeeping revisited: protecting patients from overtreatment. *NEJM.* **327:** 424–9.

Frenk J, Alagon J, Nigenda G *et al.* (1991) Patterns of medical employment: a survey of imbalances in urban Mexico. *Am J Public Health.* **81:** 23–9.

Gordon R (Ostlere GS) (ed.) (1993) *The Literary Companion to Medicine.* St Martin's Press, New York, 1996, 431 pp.

Grecco S (1980) A physician healing himself: Chekhov's treatment of doctors in the major plays. In: Peschel ER (ed.) *Medicine and Literature.* Neale Watson Academic Publications, New York, 204 pp.; pp. 3–10.

Green JP (1993) Physicians practicing other occupations, especially literature. *Mt Sinai J Med.* **60:** 132–55.

Grim JA (1983) *The Shaman.* University of Oklahoma Press, Norman, OK, 258 pp.

Groves JE (1978) Taking care of the hateful patient. *NEJM.* **298:** 883–7.

Gutheil TG and Gabbard GO (1993) The concept of boundaries in clinical practice: theoretical and risk management dimensions. *Am J Psychiatry.* **150:** 188–96.

Harper GP (1969) Ernesto (Che) Guevara: physician – revolutionary physician – revolutionary. *NEJM.* **281:** 1285–91.

Hughes PH, Brandenburg N, Baldwin DC *et al.* (1992) Prevalence of substance use among US physicians. *JAMA.* **267:** 2333–9.

Hunter KM (1991) *Doctors' Stories: the narrative structure of medical knowledge.* Princeton University Press, Princeton, NJ, 205 pp.

Hyppola H, Kumpusalo E, Neittaanmaki L *et al.* (1998) Becoming a doctor: was it the wrong career choice? *Soc Sci Med.* **47:** 1383–7.

Jones AH (1997) Literature and medicine: Garcia Marquez' *Love in the Time of Cholera.* *Lancet.* **350:** 1169–72.

Kassirer JP (1998) Doctor discontent. *NEJM.* **339:** 1543–5.

Kolin PC (1975) The Elizabethan stage doctor as a dramatic convention. In: Hogg J (ed.) *Elizabethan and Renaissance Studies.* Institut für Englische Sprache und Literatur, Universität Salzburg, Salzburg, Austria, 212 pp.

Lindgren KM (1966) Doctor Thornton and his Capitol. *NEJM.* **274:** 790–1.

Little M (2001) Does reading poetry make you a better clinician? *Int Med J.* **31:** 60–1.

Manian FA (1998) Should we accept mediocrity? *NEJM.* **338:** 1067–9.

Meier DE, Emmons CA, Wallenstein S, Quill T, Morrison RS and Cassel CK (1998) A national survey of physician-assisted suicide and euthanasia in the United States. *NEJM.* **338:** 1193–202.

Mitchell SW (1888) *Doctor and Patient.* Arno Press, New York, 1972, 177 pp.; pp. 58, 99.

Moynihan BGA (Lord Moynihan) (1936) *Truants: the story of those who deserted medicine, yet triumphed*. Cambridge University Press, Cambridge, 109 pp.; pp. 32–7.

Mukand J (ed.) (1990) *Vital Lines*. St Martin's Press, New York, 426 pp.

Nitzberg EM (1991) *Hippocrates' Handmaidens: women married to physicians*. Haworth Press, New York, 401 pp.; pp. 62–8, 72–3, 177–83, 194–8.

Norris CB (1969) *The Image of the Physician in Modern American Literature*. PhD Dissertation, University of Maryland, Baltimore, MD, 434 pp.; pp. 37–43, 93, 155.

Osler W (1903) The master-word in medicine. In: *Aequanimitas*. HK Lewis, London, 1920, 474 pp.; pp. 365–88.

Osler W (1906) Unity, peace and concord. In: *Aequanimitas*. HK Lewis, London, 1920, 474 pp.; pp. 447–65.

Paré A (1564) *Ten Books of Surgery* (translated by Linker RW and Womack N). University of Georgia Press, Athens, GA, 1969, 264 pp.; p. 153.

Pedrotti L (1981) Chekhov's major plays: a doctor in the house. In: Barricelli JP (ed.) *Chekhov's Great Plays*. New York University Press, New York, 268 pp.; pp. 233–50.

Petro JA (1992) Collegiality in history. *Bull N Y Acad Med*. **68**: 286–91.

Posen S (2005) *The Doctor in Literature. Volume 1. Satisfaction or resentment?* Radcliffe Publishing, Oxford, 298 pp.; pp. 3–7, 72–8, 195–6.

Reynolds R and Stone J (eds) (1991) *On Doctoring: stories, poems, essays*. Simon and Schuster, New York, 428 pp.

Rollman BL, Mead LA, Wang NY and Klag MJ (1997) Medical specialty and the incidence of divorce. *NEJM*. **336**: 800–3.

Rothfield L (1992) *Vital Signs: medical realism in nineteenth-century fiction*. Princeton University Press, Princeton, NJ, 235 pp.; pp. 46, 114.

Rushmore S (1934) The care of the patient as the religion of the physician. *NEJM*. **211**: 1081–7.

Saltzman C (1999) *Portrait of Dr Gachet*. Penguin, New York, 409 pp.; p. 32.

Schneck SA (1998) 'Doctoring' doctors and their families. *JAMA*. **280**: 2039–42.

Shanafelt TD, Bradley KA, Wipf JE and Back AL (2002) Burnout and self-reported patient care in an internal medicine residency program. *Ann Intern Med*. **136**: 384–93.

Simon SR, Pan RJD, Sullivan AM *et al*. (1999) Views of managed care: a survey of students, residents, faculty and deans at medical schools in the United States. *NEJM*. **340**: 928–36.

Smithers DW (1989) *This Idle Trade*. Dragonfly Press, Tunbridge Wells, 272 pp.

Snow CP (1973) Human care. *JAMA*. **225**: 617–21.

Talbott GD, Gallegos KV, Wilson PO and Porter TL (1987) The Medical Association of Georgia's impaired physicians program. Review of the first 1000 physicians: analysis of specialty. *JAMA*. **257**: 2927–30.

Toyry S, Rasanen K, Kujala S *et al*. (2000) Self-reported health, illness and self-care among Finnish physicians. *Arch Fam Med*. **9**: 1079–85.

Trautmann J and Pollard C (1982) *Literature and Medicine: an annotated bibliography*. University of Pittsburgh Press, Pittsburgh, PA, 228 pp.

Winick C (1963) The psychiatrist in fiction. *J Nerv Ment Dis*. **136**: 43–57.

Name index

Titles of works of fiction cited in this book. Also listed are some non-fictional works, place names and fictional characters. The title 'Dr' is awarded to professional healers even if they are called 'Mr' or 'Monsieur' by their patients. The numbers indicate the pages in this book where the relevant doctors, patients, place names or literary works are mentioned. Dr and Doctor are alphabetised separately.

Subject index